Complexities of Spiritual Care in Plural Societies

Studies in Spiritual Care

Edited by
Simon Peng-Keller, Eckhard Frick,
Christina Puchalski, and John Swinton

Volume 8

Complexities of Spiritual Care in Plural Societies

Education, Praxis and Concepts

Edited by
Anne Hege Grung

DE GRUYTER

ISBN 978-3-11-071723-5
e-ISBN (PDF) 978-3-11-071736-5
e-ISBN (EPUB) 978-3-11-071738-9
ISSN 2511-8838
DOI https://doi.org/10.1515/9783110717365

Library of Congress Control Number: 2022944032

Bibliographic information published by the Deutsche Nationalbibliothek
The Deutsche Nationalbibliothek lists this publication in the Deutsche Nationalbibliografie; detailed bibliographic data are available on the internet at http://dnb.dnb.de.

Printing and Binding: LSC Communications, United States

www.degruyter.com

Table of Contents

Anne Hege Grung

Complexities of spiritual care in plural societies: An introduction

Spiritual care could be approached as one of the most meaningful activities of re-humanization and meaning-making in challenging human situations. A spiritual caregiver may in certain situations of human trauma be as pivotal as a medical practitioner. The aim of spiritual care, in whatever way one understands the concept, is to enhance people's lives, to foster resilient communities, to allow people to flourish, and to build human hope. People receiving spiritual care do not belong to any specific human category – everyone is potentially needy and a possible receiver of such care under circumstances marked by crisis and loss.

Investigating the conceptual meaning of spiritual care reflects that the broad understanding of the term in a hospital context is connected to specific care seeking to address and encounter existential and spiritual needs, and challenges connected to illness and crisis (Hvidt et al 2020, 2). In hospitals, research show that spiritual care increases the quality of life for the spiritual care receivers, and that failure to provide such care may have negative consequences for the patients' health and well-being (Hvidt et al 2020, 2).

Spiritual care is of interest beyond health institutions and hospitals, and the practice has an everyday perspective: Social communities such as family and friends share necessary meaning-making, counselling and mutual care. This everyday perspective is hidden within most scholarly or political discourses of spiritual care, and the perspective of the everyday is not our main focus in this volume. To keep this perspective in sight, however, is necessary as a reminder of the deeply human and common practice of seeking hope in community with others and mutual meaning-making as a life-giving, crucial activity. Most of the actually performed spiritual care is thus not limited to specific realms of life or to specific people, and its everyday performance is not under the control of experts, or professionals as such.

What spiritual care means in practice within plural societies would differ, and this is one of the starting points for the contributors in this book. In an encounter of spiritual care, there is a need to establish communication and trust. The question is not only if you as a receiver of spiritual care could communicate with and trust someone having a different cultural and religious background than yourself. The question is also if such an encounter provides meaning-mak-

 https://doi.org/10.1515/9783110717365-001

ing and hope enhancing elements that would make deep sense to you in a situation where you seek spiritual care.

This volume addresses professional aspects of spiritual care in plural societies. This kind of care is integrated in public institutions of care and caretaking, such as hospitals, nursing homes, hospices, and correctional facilities/prisons in most of Europe and North America. Spiritual care through chaplaincy is also present in the armed forces, in institutions of higher education, and elsewhere. Leaders and staff in faith communities provide spiritual care in local communities. The challenges connected to pluralization of spiritual and existential care to encounter a pluralized population are conceptual, educational, institutional and political. Novel languages and scholarly discourses have to emerge in order to encounter both the current plurality and the complexity of the field. This volume aims to bring a substantial contribution to this field in the making.

The contributions focus on three areas: 1) The professional language and discourses of spiritual care, 2) Religious as well as existential concepts connected to spiritual care and 3) The education of spiritual caregivers. While *plural* and *plurality* is relating to actual, acknowledged, and sometimes embraced, human differences, *complexity* as a concept relates to the relations between these. There are two overarching complexities intersecting with the three areas listed above: The complexity of organizing spiritual care in specific plural contexts, and the complexity of the spiritual care's actual content in such contexts.

In practices and education related to plural spiritual and existential care in Europe and North America, religious and worldview differences are displayed and structured in various ways. Both from the inside – the actual praxis of spiritual and existential care and its content – and from the outside – including structure, education, and policy making – the structuring of the field could be based on a plural or a complex understanding, or on a combination of these. In the plural understanding, spiritual care relates to different practices and understandings according to various religious and worldview traditions. This perspective may emphasize the differences between the various ways to understand and practice spiritual care while seeking to keep the integrity of the various traditions, and establish education and chaplaincy parallel for each of them. With a complex perspective, however, spiritual care is regarded more generically across religious and worldview divides. This leads to concepts such as "interfaith spiritual care" and "interfaith chaplains", indicating a non-confessional service of spiritual care. In the Netherlands and Norway, these concepts also include the Secular Humanist worldview, one (but not the only) reason why "existential" pairs up with "spiritual" in the description of such care. Viewed through complexity as a lens, the focus is less on content and resources located within each religious and worldview tradition and their communities, and more on spiritual and existential care and chaplaincy as a possibly hybrid practice regarding religions and worldviews. The content as well as the practice would be more connected to the specific contexts and more specialized, for instance within health care or correctional facilities/prisons.

Complexity as a term can also refer to established relations between the involved partners in spiritual and existential care, crisscrossing religious and worldview boundaries, such as a religiously and worldview diverse team of chaplains in an institution. Using complexity as the main lens when describing the field, the religious and worldview traditions may become less significant as identity markers understood as respectively confined structures of meaning-making. One of the challenges of engaging with complexity in this way is that it may entail confirming religious and cultural hegemonies within the respective contexts because of this downplaying of religion and worldview as identity markers, with the possible result of overlooking or neglecting needs of religious and worldview minorities in specific contexts. Critical research on the inclusion of immigrants within Nordic welfare states suggests that the term "subordinated inclusion" reflects how these are included only on the premises of the majority, establishing "welfare state nationalism" (Keskinen, Tuori, Irni and Mullinari 2009, 5). Professional spiritual care as parts of the welfare structure should certainly be investigated through this critical lens.

Kwok Pui-Lan and others have insisted on introducing a post-colonial critical lens when exploring religious ministry in Christian churches (Pui-Lan and Burns 2016)). A postcolonial critical lens is also useful when exploring spiritual care and chaplaincy as a field. The plural societies figuring in the book: Canada, Germany, Denmark, Sweden, the Netherlands, the US and Norway are all societies deeply shaped by Christian traditions. Gé Speelman's chapter in the book reflects over the practice of pastoral and spiritual care in the Netherlands from the 1830's until today. She shows how pastoral care started as a disciplining practice from the Church's side to ensure that the churchgoers were in a proper spiritual state before receiving the holy communion, and to prepare the sick and dying to face the divine judgement. The most significant shift Speelman identifies between the 1830's and the contemporary Dutch context is the shift from focus on the collective to focus on the individual in spiritual care. This shift corresponds with the societies' transformation from traditional to post-traditional – as a general trend – in the Netherlands as well as in Europe and North America. In a post-traditional society, the individual has rights, duties and possibilities to make significant life choices on an individual basis. This does not entail that traditions, for instance based on culture or religion, have vanished or become irrelevant, but that the increased emphasis on the individual shapes how these traditions are conveyed and positioned. This unfolds differently within various contexts, and within cultural and religious groups in these contexts.

As the general populations in North America and Europe are becoming more plural and more post-traditional, the adequate way to assess these areas is to shift the perspective from spiritual care as a mono-religious (Christian) activity to a multi-religious, an inter- or trans-religious activity. In a reflection over pluralization of theologies at European universities, these three modes of scholarly interaction in a pluralized academia is suggested (Leirvik 2020, 26–27). Speelman, in her contribution argues that spiritual caregivers need to recognize difference among the care-receivers on an individual basis in order to recognize the human dignity of the other. Most of the contributors in this book address one or several of the focused areas within the frames of different religious backgrounds such as Muslim, Buddhist, Hindu and Christian, within an inter- or trans-religious frame. The discussion is unpacked in various ways throughout the chapters: Is spiritual care to be understood as a religious (or worldview) based service, or as a general service of improving spiritual or existential health? Is professional spiritual care to be regarded as a generic activity, where the competence of the spiritual caregiver should be disentangled from religious and worldview traditions, or is it a specific, confessional activity, where the spiritual caregiver needs skills and background from a particular religious or worldview tradition in order to enter into the caregiving space? Different contexts answer these questions disparately. It seems that the overarching understanding and policies of governing religious and worldview plurality in a specific society plays a role in how these questions are answered, and in how professional spiritual care is organized in relation to this plurality.

One of the main discussions connected to spiritual and existential care in plural societies is thus whether one should follow a "plural" or a "complex" model regarding both organization and content. In addition, there are questions about whether personnel performing this care should be specialists, that is, people trained and educated in the field, or ordinary health workers such as nurses and doctors in hospitals. Anke Liefbroer, a contributor to one of the chapters in this book, has contributed to an article exploring various modes for integrating spiritual care into healthcare. Combining the questions "who should provide spiritual care", and "what is the role of the caregiver's spirituality when providing spiritual care", the article suggests a matrix where "generalists" and "specialists" ("generalists" refer to all health personnel, "specialists" to educated spiritual caregivers) on the two ends of one continuum, and "particularists" and "universalists"are establishing the two ends of another. "Particularists" refers to generalists or specialists who provides spiritual care to patients of the same religion or worldview, and "universalists" to providers who offer this care to all (Liefbroer, Ganzevoort, Olsman 2019, 249). The latter continuum refers to a plural vs. complex model of spiritual care regarding organization related to religious affiliations and worldviews, but the first continuum referring to generalists vs. specialists includes a pluralization related to various professions involved in spiritual care. We could therefore speak about the presence of a double pluralism of structuring spiritual care in healthcare, both referring to religion/worldview and referring to professions.

The professional aspect: Transforming the professional paradigm of the spiritual caregiver in plural contexts

When investigating the professional paradigm of spiritual and existential caregivers, we ask not only about the professional vetting of the work, but about the quest for integrity and the skills of the caregivers themselves. In religiously plural contexts several parties have interests in the matter: The institutions providing the care, faith and worldview communities, as well as the caregivers themselves. The chapter by Liefbroer, Lauwers, Coppens and Lalbahadoersing describes how Buddhist, Muslim and Hindu spiritual care in the Netherlands is framed and performed in the Dutch context, and how chaplains carrying out this care has a double affiliation: to the institution where they are employed and to their faith community.

Chaplaincy and spiritual care have been formatted by the Catholic and the Protestant churches in Europe and North America. This entails that developing spiritual care practices from other traditions need to negotiate and evaluate their own stances, teachings and practices related to the Christian heritage concerning education, the professional language and discourses of spiritual care as well as religious concepts embedded in the practice. I addition, many of the contexts appearing in this volume's contributions are secular societies – formatted by particular Christian confessions. For some contexts, such as Sweden, Norway and the Netherlands, this has established a situation where the religious (Christian) element in spiritual care in public institutions has been significantly downplayed, and spiritual caregivers who are educated as Christian theologians highlight their ability and will to serve all, regardless of their religious affiliation or lack thereof (Ruyter 2014). But when spiritual caregivers from new religious and worldview backgrounds enter the field, the discussion returns about the religious or worldview identity of the service. This may lead to contestations over the content of spiritual care, and discussions around the professional paradigm.

In the Norwegian context, there has been a discussion over whether spiritual caregivers in hospitals as employed chaplains are to be legally regarded as health workers. Health workers have full access to the medical history of patients, and they regularly share information in working teams around the patients. The Norwegian ministry of health has decided that hospital chaplains are not to be included in the category of health workers, and among the chaplains, there has been diverging views of this ruling.[1] This is a question related to the professional paradigm: A health worker is anticipated to be serving all on equal footing, and not to be affiliated in her work with faith communities. The wish among many Norwegian hospital chaplains ordained to service by the Church of Norway to be regarded as health workers may therefore indicate that they regard their work to be religiously neutral or "secular". This could further lead to a position where employing people of other faiths and worldviews as spiritual caregivers seem to be unnecessary, or even unwanted if they represent a re-introduction of religion and worldview as a marker of spiritual care. Other hospital chaplains are content with the decision of the ministry of health, because they claim this protects the chaplains' confidentiality regime and uphold spiritual care as a protected area, outside of the curative and sometimes instrumental perspective of the health institutions[2]. Confidentiality is regarded as a crucial part of the confessional paradigm but the interpretation of what it means, may differ.

In discussing transformation of the professional paradigm for spiritual and existential caregivers, the actual needs and wishes among the receivers and potential receivers of the care needs to be heard. The challenge is that there has been little research mapping this across North America and Europe. There are exceptions, such as Abu Ras and Laird (Abu Ras and Laird 2011), Liefbroer and Nagel (Liefbroer and Nagel 2021), and the chaplaincy research conducted by European Research Institute for Chaplains in Healthcare (ERICH), which mostly conducts large surveys[3]. The general lack of research may be surprising, but given the vulnerable position of patients, inmates and other receiving groups of this kind of care in institutions, it is ethically challenging to execute such re-

1 https://www.helsedirektoratet.no/rundskriv/helsepersonelloven-med-kommentarer/lovens-formal-virkeomrade-og-definisjoner/-3.definisjoner (accessed December 21, 2021); see also https://www.regjeringen.no/contentassets/3810c6a1d2eb412485319c1dfbef00e4/333-uio-tilleggsnotat-prestetjenesten.pdf?uid=Oslo_universitetssykehus_HF_-_tilleggsmerknad_prestetjenesten (accessed December 21, 2021).

2 https://www.ahus.no/avdelinger/medisinsk-divisjon/prestetjenesten#samtaler-og-sjelesorg (accessed December 21, 2021).

3 https://www.pastoralezorg.be/page/erich/ (accessed December 10, 2021).

search. This means that we need a sharp empirical turn in the study of spiritual care in order to get research based knowledge about the needs and how to meet this in an adequate way. The current professional paradigm puts the receiver of professional spiritual care as the decisive part: The needs of the patient, the student, the prison inmate should be in focus. At the same time, a pluralized population in the institutions – not only regarding religious/non-religious and cultural background, but also regarding the care receivers' mother tongue, gender, social belonging, makes it difficult to establish a perfect match between the caregiver and the care receiver. Some research show that such match is not required for experiencing high quality spiritual care for the involved parties (Liefbroer and Nagel 2021). However, there would be particular cultural and religious resources that would be unavailable for the care receivers if the caregiver does not have knowledge and skills about specific narratives or rituals outside of her realm. Whether these narratives and rituals are parts of the patients', students' or inmates' need would have to be further explored before deciding on whether a cultural/religious match – at least to a certain degree – is important. Then there is a question about whether the care receivers and potential care receivers are in a position to articulate their needs, or if they restrict themselves to ask for what they consider possible to obtain (Abu Ras and Lance 2011). This is where we indeed need empirical research in order to map the field.

The professional paradigm for spiritual caregivers may change if results of such research is consulted. There is however, a transformation which is clearly required in order to tune in to more pluralized populations: To include a more religiously and culturally plural group of spiritual caregivers to reflect the population more adequately. In some contexts such as the Netherlands, the US and Canada spiritual caregiver and chaplaincy teams have undergone such transformations. In Germany, Denmark, Norway and Sweden this is implemented to a much lesser degree.

An important matter connected to the discourse on professional paradigms is the question of authority, addressed in Beret Bråten's contribution in this volume. Drawing on fieldwork in Norwegian hospitals, Bråten claims that hospital chaplains affiliated to the Church of Norway – the country's by far largest religious organization and community – tend to downplay their traditional authority as religious leaders and signify their legal authority as well educated and qualified hospital employees. For Muslim chaplains in a Norwegian context, Bråten finds that they generally lack the same level of education as their Church of Norway colleagues, and that most of them lack a formal position as employed by the hospitals – they are engaged as volunteers ("lay chaplains") or part-time employees. Their access to authority in their role is primarily connected to traditional religious leadership within their communities. Bråten's findings show how the structuring and organization of chaplaincy may generate differences in anchoring the professional authority for spiritual caregivers for the majority versus minorities, in this case the Muslim minority. This influences the position (or lack of position) of Muslim chaplains in Norwegian hospitals, but also the professional interaction between chaplains with different affiliations and legal status, which in its turn may lead to a less coherent understanding of the professional paradigm and the conduct of spiritual care.

The professional language and discourses of spiritual care: Plural, complex

Scholarly as well as political discourses on spiritual care are often connected to discourses on chaplaincy and religious leadership. Chaplaincy and religious leadership as positions executing spiritual care are seen as "spiritual care experts", and several of the contributions will include reflections over chaplaincy work, and indirectly also religious leadership.

The scholarly discourses on spiritual care in Europe and North America includes broad disciplines such as psychology and theology. These two disciplines are in themselves constructed very differently and have different methods and aims. Psychology is using qualitative and quantitative methods and is mostly concerned with descriptive and therapeutic perspectives. Theologies in all its shapes increasingly engages with various methods, and are concerned with meaning-making and the use of religious resources such as scriptures, rituals and specific perspectives on human life. But psychology is also engaging with existential questions and health beyond the therapeutic, such as the contribution by Cecilia Melder in this volume shows. Melder explores the existential dimension of health through studies conducted by the World's Health Organization (WHO) and suggests how to relate developed methods and interventions from these studies into plural and interfaith spiritual care contexts. Taking on a public health perspective, Melder suggests that extended collaborations between interfaith actors and faith communities on the one hand, and health institutions on the other establishes resilient and effective care structures within societies.

Within discourses of Practical Theology, the traditional academic locus for spiritual care, Christian theology is still the main hermeneutical framework although a more plural shaping of Practical Theology is emerging in some institutions. If we extend the field of Practical Theology to discourses of chaplaincy, there is, particularly in the UK, North America and the Netherlands a substantial and vivid discourse connected to this.

It seems obvious that a pluralization of spiritual care requires a pluralization of theologies, in the sense that other religious traditions than the Christian are included at the table as well as in the institutional corridors. Philosophy has emerged as a small, but significant contributor to the field through the concept Philosophical Practice. For some Secular Humanists, this provides a framework for their spiritual and existential care (Schuhmann 2015). One of the most significant tasks yet to be accomplished could be to integrate the Secular Humanists' take on philosophical practice and philosophy in the broader religiously marked discourse on spiritual care. Within Islamic, Buddhist, Hindu, Jewish, and other traditions people are equipping themselves theoretically and practically to meet requirements and standards for spiritual caregivers in Europe and North America. For some of these traditions, considerable translation and hermeneutical work is needed to adapt these religious resources to a Northern American and European context of spiritual care. Several of the contributions to this book reflect such work: Schröer, Roloff, Baig, Isgandarova as well as the chapter by Liefbroer Lauwers, Coppens and Lalbahadoersing.

How to include the work done within Islamic, Buddhist, Hindu, Jewish, and other traditions as full partners within discourses of spiritual care in Europe and North America is a salient question reflecting a comprehensive task. We can find resources to address this within interreligious hermeneutics and interreligious studies, where the relational aspects of religious pluralism is explored, and theorized (Leirvik 2014). This includes critical reflection over power relations and postcolonial perspectives (Grung 2020). There has also been some work on inter-rituality, exploring what inter- and trans-religious encounters through rituals may entail (Moyaert 2019). This is relevant also in the discourse of plural spiritual care. Performing religious rituals is sometimes expected from spiritual caregivers, sometimes outside religious and worldview concordance. Moyaert describes inter-ritual spaces as "(...) far messier, the identities of the parties involved are multilayered and complex, and their intentions ambivalent" (Moyaert 2019, 6). She claims that in contexts of inter-rituality, the involved parties have to make strategic decisions about how they want to relate ritually to other traditions.

The praxis of Spiritual Care is not necessarily reflected well in the scholarly discourse. In praxis, spiritual caregivers as well as the receivers of such care and the institutions with the overarching responsibility have to find pragmatic solutions in urgent situations. Spiritual Care as a field is by some claimed to only slowly recognize a necessary main focus on praxis (Grung, Danbolt, and Stifoss-Hanssen 2016).

Religious and existential concepts of spiritual care

To establish a more relevant cluster of resources regarding spiritual and existential care in religiously and worldview diverse societies, there is not only a need to reflect over the plurality or complexity in itself, but also to obtain knowledge about how other religious and worldview communities than the Christian articulate and approach their interpretation of this care. In this volume, we have in particular focused on Buddhist, Christian and Islamic traditions and included both empirical and philosophical/religious/theological research on these. The chapter by Gé Speelman reflects changes within the Churches' conceptualization of spiritual care in the Netherlands over the last two decades. Carola Roloff's chapter discusses the emerging concept of Buddhist chaplaincy, shows how Buddhist care practices connect to Buddhist teachings, and how these practices can work in secular institutions. She also discusses the intra-religious plurality within Buddhism and how Buddhist care practices offer resources for interreligious spiritual care.

The chapters by Naveed Baig, Jussra Schröer and Nazila Isgandarova all discuss concepts and practices of Islamic spiritual care, but relate to different contexts and highlight various aspects. Baig discusses Islamic spiritual care in relation to core concepts he identifies in Islamic theology to make a strong connection between theology and care practices. He also reflects over Islamic chaplaincy in the West. Schröer relates to the German context and includes an empirical study on Islamic spiritual care in Germany. She also gives an overview of the German state of the art, including the current pressing challenges related to education, available positions and integration of Islamic spiritual care in the German society. Isgandarova focuses on women's voices in Islamic spiritual care. Throughout her contribution she reflects critically over the power relations connected to the gendered understanding of spiritual care as well as religious leadership within Islamic traditions. Isgandarova identifies issues Muslim women spiritual caregivers may face and provides resources to encounter these and transform Islamic care practices to fully include women.

Education of spiritual caregivers

Spiritual care as an organized, institutional activity has been affiliated to Christian religious communities and churches in North America and Europe, and categorized as pastoral care, connected to the role of the clergy (Sullivan

2014). This entails that this kind of care has been integrated in the Churches' mission, but is also deeply rooted in their identity. The practice of spiritual care (pastoral care) has been reflected on within Christian theological discourses such as Practical Theology, and necessary skills conveyed within Christian theological education. Due to the increasing pluralization, other traditions than the Christian have engaged in discourses of spiritual care. Some Buddhist, Islamic, and Secular humanist scholars and practitioners have taken up a comprehensive task of developing necessary tools, concepts and language from their traditions' resources to provide an adequate framework and an understanding of what Buddhist, Islamic and Secular Humanist spiritual care could be in the context of plural contexts shaped by Christian and/or secular majority populations. This is to some extent – and increasingly – reflected in a pluralization of the education of spiritual caregivers. A growing number of institutions of higher education are offering programs for the training of spiritual caregivers from various religious and worldview traditions in Europe and North America. Most of the institutions offering this are traditionally educators of Christian clergy. Jennifer Peace claims that in order for these institutions to make an integrated plural turn, there needs to be a focus on co-formation, not only formation. Co-formation entails that students do not learn about people from other religious and worldview affiliations, but learn from them and with them (Peace 2020).

Su-Yon Pak and Gregory Snyder's contribution to this volume reflects over challenges and possibilities in a Buddhist chaplaincy education at a Protestant Seminary in New York. The education highlights formative aspects of the education, including theological reflection and self-inquiry, and their question is how to create a pedagogy "that allows meaningful religious difference to endure while cultivating the possibility for connections to be realized across that difference" (Pak and Snyder, 263). An inter- or transreligious mode of chaplaincy education requires, according to Pak and Snyder, that all involved parties engage with "practical vulnerability" – including not only teachers and students, but the institution itself. They claim that normativity is a necessary frame to establish interreligious wisdom, but this normativity should be open enough for all engaged to be able to find and express themselves within it.

Acknowledgements

This volume aims to provide valuable resources for scholars and practitioners in the field of spiritual care in plural societies. The contributors represent a plural group of scholars regarding religious affiliation, scholarly discipline, gender, age and cultural backgrounds. All contributors met physically in two workshops conducted by the Faculty of Theology, University of Oslo, in June 2018 and June 2019. Thanks to the Faculty of Theology, UiO for providing the resources to hold these workshops, and for providing funds to publish the volume as Open Access. The contributors have shown engagement and patience throughout the pandemic times that delayed all of us – thank you to each one. A particular thank go to PhD Helena Strandli Schmidt, who contributed to the editing and offered valuable comments.

Ataullah Siddiqui, who was supposed to be one of the contributors, stated in one of the workshops we had to share our work on spiritual care proceeding this publication, that the best qualification for a religious leader was to undergo training in spiritual care and chaplaincy work. Ataullah Siddiqui passed away in November 2020. This volume is dedicated to him. Not only was he a significant pioneer and entrepreneur of Muslim chaplaincy and spiritual care in the UK as well as to the education of Muslim spiritual caregivers, he also contributed substantially to the development of Islamic spiritual care in other contexts such as the Danish and the Norwegian.

References

Abu Ras, Wahiba, and Laird Lance. 2011. "How Muslim and Non-Muslim Chaplains Serve Muslim Patients: Does the Interfaith Chaplaincy Model have Room for Muslims' experiences?" *Journal of Religious Health* 50: 46 – 61. DOI: https://doi.org/10.1007/s10943-010-9357-4

Grung, Anne Hege, Lars Johan Danbolt, and Hans Stifoss-Hanssen. 2016. "Sjelesorg på plass. På sporet av dagens sjelesorgpraksis i Den norske kirke." *Tidsskrift for praktisk teologi* 1: 28 – 43.

Grung, Anne Hege. 2020. "Interreligious or Transreligious?" In: Hans Gustafson (ed.) *Interreligious Studies: Dispatches from an Emerging Field.* Wako: Baylor University Press. 58 – 65.

Hvidt, Niels Christian, Kristina Tomra Nielsen, Alex K. Kørup, et al. 2020. "What is spiritual care? Professional perspectives on the concept of spiritual care identified through group concept mapping." *BMJ Open*; 10:e042142. DOI: 10.1136/bmjopen-2020 – 042142

Keskinen, Suvi, Salla Tuori, Sari Irni, and Diana Mulinari (eds.). 2009. *Complying with Colonialism: Gender, Race and Ethnicity in the Nordic Region.* Farnham, Burlington: Ashgate.

Leirvik, Oddbjørn. 2020. "Pluralisation of Theologies at Universities. Approaches and Concepts." In: Wolfram Weisse, Julia Ipgrave, Oddbjørn Leirvik, and Muna Tatari (eds.) *Pluralisation of Theologies at European Universities.* Münster, New York: Waxmann. 25 – 34.

Leirvik, Oddbjørn. 2014. *Interreligious Studies: A Relational Approach to Religious Activism and the Study of Religion.* London, New York: Bloomsbury Academic.

Liefbroer, Anke, Ruard R. Ganzevoort and Erik Olsman. 2019. "Addressing the spiritual domain in a plural society: what is the best mode of integrating spiritual care into healthcare?" *Mental Health, Religion & Culture* 22/3: 244–260. DOI: 10.1080/13674676.2019.1590806

Liefbroer, Anke, and Ineke Nagel. 2021. "Does Faith Concordance Matter? A Comparison of Clients' Perceptions in Same Versus Interfaith Spiritual Care Encounters with Chaplains in Hospitals." *Pastoral Psychology* 70: 349–377. DOI: 10.1007/s11089-021-00947-4.

Moyaert, Marianne. 2019. "Broadening the Scope of Interreligious Studies: Interrituality." In: Marianne Moyaert (ed.) *Interreligious Relations and the Negotiation of Ritual Boundaries: Exploration of Interrituality.* Cham: Palgrave Macmillan. 1–34.

Peace, Jennifer. 2020. "Religious Self, Religious Other: Coformation as a Model for Interreligious Education." In Najeeba Syeed and Heidi Hadsell (eds.) *Critical Perspectives on Interreligious Education: Experiments of Empathy.* Leiden: Brill Rodopi. 201–219.

Pui-Lan, Kwok, and Stephen Burns (eds). 2016. *Postcolonial Practice of Ministry: Leadership, Liturgy and Interfaith Engagement.* Lanham, Boulder, New York, London: Lexington Books.

Ruyter, Knut. 2014. "Space for Religion in Public Hospitals." In: Rosemarie van den Breemer, José Casanova, and Trygve Wyller (eds.) *Secular and Sacred? The Scandinavian Case of Religion in Human Rights, Law and Public Space.* Göttingen: Vandenhoek & Ruprecht. 197–220.

Schuhmann, Carmen. 2015. "Counselling and the Humanist Worldview." In: Andrew Copson and A.C. Greyling (eds.) *The Wiley-Blackwell Handbook of Humanism.* Hoboken: Wiley-Blackwell. 173–193.

Sullivan, Winnifred Fallers. 2014. *A Ministry of Presence: Chaplaincy, Spiritual Care, and the Law.* Chicago, London: University of Chicago Press.

Gé Speelman

Shifting concepts of pastoral care in the Christian tradition: from the past to the present to the future

Abstract: This contribution deals with the historical development of different views of pastoral care in the Western-European Protestant Christian tradition. Four dimensions of pastoral care can be distinguished: healing, sustaining, guidance and reconciliation. Each requires specific roles of pastoral care givers. In the modern context important shifts have been made in these different dimensions of pastoral care. This is due to an increasing diversity, individualization and loss of authority of the tradition. The four dimensions take shape in one-to-one meetings, where the life stories of care-receivers are connected to the large Christian narratives. In the postmodern, intercultural approach, the diversity of master narratives requires a modest, hospitable and open attitude from the care-giver. All dimensions need to be addressed in new dynamic ways that takes otherness and difference seriously.

A pastoral visit in 1830: the shift towards the individual

In 1830, the Dutch minister Cornelis Eliza van Koetsveld, a young graduate from Leiden University, took his first post as a minister in the village of Westmaas. More than ten years later, he published a humoristic book about his experiences under the title 'Sketches from Mastland Parsonage' (van Koetsveld 1978 (1848)). In the book, he gives a vivid description of a pastoral visit in his first year as a minister. In the Dutch Reformed church at that time, the Eucharist was celebrated only once a year, at Easter. Together with a presbyter, van Koetsveld reserves one fine spring day for a visit to all the households in the village to invite everybody personally to this important event. The young minister describes his own fear and tribulation as he is making his rounds through the village. In each house, they are received by the whole household, everybody from the grandmother to the scullery maid gathered together in the visitors room in total silence. The minister begins the conversation by informing who lives in the household, noting down the names in a pocket book that he has brought along. Then he continues with the almost ritual formula: "You all know the reason for my coming; in a few days, it is Eucharist, and you all know the importance of this event, etc." The hosts answer in a tone that has the same ritual quality:

The householder said in a solemn tone of voice: "I thank the reverend minister", and continued: "The reverend does not have the best kind of weather on his rounds". The housewife looked up again, resumed her work on a half-peeled potato; the maid and the farm-

 https://doi.org/10.1515/9783110717365-002

> hand skulked away without anything else, and then this house had received a pastoral visit. (van Koetsveld 1978 (1848), 123)

Pastoral care in this period was seen in the light of the need for the church to discipline the believers in a right frame of mind for the Eucharist. In the period van Koetsveld describes, there was a strong tendency among more orthodox believers, in the book called 'Folks for the Good' (van Koetsveld 1978 (1848), 186), who were critical of the moderate, liberal tone of their ministers. They avoided attendance of the Eucharist out of fear to jeopardize their eternal souls and 'meat and drink damnation unto themselves'.[1] In his visits to their households, van Koetsveld would engage in discussions, trying to correct their – in his eyes- too rigid views (van Koetsveld 1978 (1848) 129 – 145). House visits were in this period seen as essential for the maintenance of the Christian community, as the population, although in name all members of the Reformed Church, were not always enthusiastic church goers. So, the pastoral visit to the household denoted a struggle between pastor and parishioners about the meaning of Eucharist, sin and forgiveness. These issues were not often discussed at length during the visits however, they were the implicit background. House visits are a ritualistic and collective affair.

The only other recognized form of pastoral care at the time was the visit to the sick. This type of visit was not only aimed at providing comfort and a listening ear. For the young minister, most of the sick people he visited were in fact on the point of dying, and the subject of the conversation was the preparedness of the patient to face the end of her/his life and his need to confess his or her sins. The conversation would turn to the issue of guilt, sin and forgiveness, and sometimes the pastor was able to bring some relief to the sufferer by preaching the message of God's reconciliation with the sinner (van Koetsveld 1978 (1848), 187). The opportunities of speaking with the patient in private were limited, as family members and neighbors were customarily assembled around the sickbed. Again, there is a strong frame of expectation among the parishioners about the shape and contents of such a visit, although there are possibilities of improvisation for the minister.

From the way he describes these practices at the onset of his career, the reader can infer already that van Koetsveld is not satisfied with his prescribed role as a pastor. In his student days, as an avid reader of Friedrich Schleiermacher, he became aware that something was lacking in the Calvinistic ritual of the pastoral

1 1 Corinthians 11: 29, King James Version: http://www.gutenberg.org/ebooks/10, accessed March 10, 2021.

visit in his day and age. The very publicness of the event, he comments, prevents people from baring their souls to the minister. In the course of his ministry, he develops the practice to visit some of the households again on his own, to find an opportunity to speak to individual members of the household in private. The practice of pastorate as individual conversation that van Koetsveld is developing in 1830, becomes later on part of a budding new branch of theology. Thirty years after the events described in the *Sketches*, the first professor in the Netherlands in the field of 'Practical Theology', professor Muurling, made a distinction between *cura specialis* (individual spiritual care) and *cura generalis* (collective spiritual care with an eye to discipline).[2] Pastoral care after that becomes more and more focused on the care for the individual, besides the still important aspect of care in a more communal and ritualistic setting.

Christian tradition as a chain of memory

All religious traditions engage in practices in the field of spiritual care. In the context of this article, I see 'spiritual care' as a response from representatives of a religious tradition to individuals or groups in need, in order to help them in their search for meaning and making sense of life.

I take 'tradition' here as a cumulative set of discourses and practices with roots in the past, institutionalized forms in the present and strategies for the future. As Talal Asad writes:

> A tradition consists essentially of discourses that seek to instruct practitioners regarding the correct form and purpose of a given practice that, precisely because it is established, has a history. These discourses relate conceptually to a *past* (when the practice was instituted, and from which the knowledge of its point and proper performance has been transmitted) and a *future* (how the point of that practice can best be secured in the short or long term, or why it should be modified or abandoned), through a *present* (how it is linked to other practices, institutions, and social conditions). (Asad 1986, 14)

Asad remarks that, contrary to certain conceptions of 'tradition', religious traditions are never homogeneous, but always subject to contestation from within and from the outside (hence his addition of the term 'discursive' to the conception of Islam as a tradition). Nevertheless, actors who want to take part in a tradition strive for internal coherence (Asad 1986, 7).

---

2 Quoted in Gerben Heitink, *Biografie van de dominee.* Baarn 2001: ten Have, 122.

In a similar line of reasoning, Danielle Hervieu-Léger (2000) argues that *religion* needs to be distinguished from *the sacred* in modern societies precisely because what is commonly known as *a religion* is a social system embedded in its particular tradition. She introduces the concept *chain of memory* as a paraphrase for tradition. In many ways, individuals in modern societies are preoccupied with spiritual growth and rituals embodying *the sacred* in their lives. Yet, these practices do not form *a religion*, and the practitioners would not view themselves as *religious* people. Religion is not just a set of emotional experiences or beliefs about the meaning of life, but is rooted in a tradition that is seen as authoritative. According to Hervieu-Léger: "There is no religion without the authority of a tradition being invoked (whether explicitly, half-explicitly or implicitly) in support of the act of believing" (2000, 76).

The content of the beliefs of people who are conscious members of a religious community is authorized by the larger tradition of which they are a part. This community then becomes a form of social identification, through incorporation and differentiation from others, who belong to other 'chains of memory' (Hervieu-Léger 2000, 81). Practices and narratives of belief are forming a coherent, albeit constantly shifting and adapting whole. Tradition is for Hervieu-Léger as much a dynamic concept as it is for Asad. It involves those parts of the past that must be accepted in the present as normative, but these elements are susceptible to re-interpretations and innovative inventions (ibid.).

Hervieu-Léger points out that all religious traditions (as well as other e.g. legal, artistic, political traditions) are undergoing strong erosion in modern, de-traditionalizing societies. Not only are religious communities losing members, but also the members that remain inside the community no longer interpret their tradition as authoritative for their daily lives.

> How can religious institutions, with their prime purpose of preserving and transmitting a tradition, reform their own system of authority- essential for the continuity of a line of belief- when the tradition, even by the believers, not as a sacred trust, but as an ethical-cultural heritage, a fund of memory and a reservoir of signs at the disposal of individuals? (Hervieu-Léger 2000, 168)

This article does not deal with religious institutions and the possible reformation of their structures of authority. Rather, it addresses the shifts in the field of Christian pastoral care in the late Twentieth Century in order to understand the setting of practices of present-day spiritual care in Western Europe. If we want to understand the future of spiritual care, we need to look at both the present and the past.

In the fast developing field of interreligious spiritual care, attention needs to be paid to the origins of, and the developments within particular religious traditions in order to see the genealogy of certain taken-for-granted assumptions about the concept of 'spiritual care'. These shifts took place within different churches and locations in different ways. To describe them all at great length would be impossible. Also, this type of question cannot be answered from a neutral perspective. In the introduction to this article, the starting point was a particular historical, local and cultural context, i. e. that of the Netherlands in the Nineteenth Century, even more specifically that of the Protestant (Calvinistic) variety of the Christian tradition. In what follows, I want to take a step back and try to catch the larger picture of the Western Christian tradition, before focusing again on the context of which I am a part: that of the present-day Protestant Church in the Netherlands. In doing so, I am aware of the fact that the Dutch Protestant tradition in pastoral care owes much to earlier and more widely disseminated Christian traditions, while at the same time it is formed in interaction with the specific context it operates in.

The traditions of Christian pastoral care and their dimensions

In the Christian tradition in the sense Hervieu-Léger gives to the concept, the term most used for spiritual care is *pastoral care*. This refers back to the biblical image of the religious leader as a shepherd (pastor) who is leading his flock, by caring for their needs. Even the terminology used by Christians for the practice of spiritual care is loaded with concepts derived from their specific tradition. What are the classical dimensions of the Christian tradition of pastoral care, and how have these elements reacted to the shift towards modernity?

In the broader Christian tradition, pastoral care has many dimensions. Stephen Pattison mentions four interrelated aspects: healing, sustaining, reconciling and guiding. In different periods in time, different aspects took the foreground.(Pattison 2000, 7). I will expand very briefly on these aspects in what follows.

Healing is already an important aspect of the pastoral work of Jesus and the first apostles described in the New Testament. In an important essay, Eric Cassell (1976) defines disease as biochemical or structural abnormality and illness as the set of altered feelings the sick person experiences. Disease is something an organ has while illness is something a person has.(Cassell 1976, 27–37)

It is clear from the stories in the early Christian tradition, that illness is not conceptualized as either illness of the body or of the mind, but as a combination of both. Also, illness is seen in biblical narratives as something that isolates the sufferer from the community. In order to heal the illness, all these aspects have to be addressed. Some of the rituals addressing the bodily or spiritual ills of the person in need are prayer and the laying of hands, or anointing. In some cases, diseases are conceptualized as caused by evil spirits, that could be exorcised by the pastor. Collective prayer and the laying of hands are in many present-day Christian communities employed in healing rituals.

Sustaining, or supporting the person in need may mean either comforting people or affirming them in their identity as they struggle with life-decisions. Here again, next to words, rituals can be important. An example are rituals around death and mourning.

When we think of *reconciliation*, then the work of Christian pastors knows two orientation points: reconciliation between one person and the other, and reconciliation between humans and God. The first aspect asks of the pastor the qualities of a good mediator, connecting the interests of the different parties in a conflict, either groups or individuals. This involves listening to the stories of the conflict and putting them in the perspective of the tradition, drawing from biblical narratives, lives of the saints or moral preaching. The conflict between individual humans and God is often cast in terms of sin and human failure. The pastor can become the recipient of the confessions of sin from the person in need, on behalf of God. In the medieval period, this led to a detailed practice of confession, in which the pastor (if he were an ordained priest) would have the ritual authority to convey God's forgiveness of the sins that were confessed.

In the field of *guidance*, the importance of discipline has always been very important. The work of the pastor involves from this perspective not only ritual knowledge or diplomatic skills, but also the didactic ability to support a training of the virtues. In the past, as we saw from the example of van Koetsveld, the visits of clergy to family homes was often cast in the mold of moral exhortation. People would react as if the pastor was inspecting the quality of their religious life. Pattison calls the pastor in the past "[...] a mix of schoolmaster, saint and policeman" (2000, 13). The disciplinary character of pastoral care is emphasized when churches see themselves more as countercultural gatherings of faithful disciples, who distinguish themselves from the outside world by their moral excellence. (Pattison 2000, 66) One particular aspect of the pastoral guidance of believers is the incitement to have a disciplined life of prayer and spiritual sources. The monastery is one of the leading institutions in this respect, and for many lay Christians, the life of monks and nuns has been an inspiration for their own prayer life. (Pattison 2000, 70)

The four different dimensions are interrelated and the boundaries between them are permeable. Healing can be thought of as a form of inner reconciliation to suffering, or as a reconciliatory restoration between the patient and his social environment. There is a strong link between guidance and reconciliation, and between guiding and sustaining.

In various historical periods and locations, different dimensions are most prominent. In the context of van Koetsveld for instance, moral exhortation and therefore guidance seemed to be the most important part of pastoral care, with sustaining and reconciliation as secondary dimensions, whereas healing was seen as pertaining to the domain of professional medical specialists.

Another thing to be noted is the intertwining of knowledge, faith and practices in each of the dimensions. Healing is a combination of convictions and knowledge coming from narratives at the center of the Christian tradition, and it is acted out in practices like prayer, and rituals like the lighting of candles and exorcisms. Reconciliation can be a social interaction guided by knowledge of the meaning of it in the Christian tradition, performed in rituals like the confessional or other ritual forms. Moral discipline may be embodied in regular participation in ritual activities.

In what ways do the four dimensions of pastoral care function in a present-day setting in the Protestant Church in the Netherlands? And in what way are they different from the dimensions in the time of van Koetsveld?

The present praxis in parish pastoral care: personal experiences

My experiences as a pastor in a village in the Netherlands, where I worked from 2001–2006 show the shift in pastoral care, if I compare them to the past as described by van Koetsveld. In the village, there is a lively tradition of visits from the church- regular one-monthly visits to the elderly and people in need of a listening ear. One of the most striking differences is in the actors who perform a pastoral role. Although the professional pastor is called in in a crisis, as the specialist for 'difficult cases', that is for people with special needs, for most parishioners pastoral care was seen as a task for the whole of the religious community. Although the pastor functions as *primus inter pares*, [3]as she was trained in hermeneutical and ritual skills, nevertheless the equality of all believers was translated into a sharing out of tasks. There is a declining stress on the religious authority of the professional pastor. This has its roots in the Calvinistic tradition, where from the 16th Century onwards, the authority of the minister was always shared with the members of the church council, and it has been strengthened

3 First among equals.

in a more egalitarian society. We organized groups of lay pastoral visitors, sharing the work of visiting everyone who wanted to receive visits from the church.

Another shift is that from ceremonial household visits to individual visits. This stress on the individual, which started in early modernity, was not confined to the Reformers. The spiritual exercises of Loyola as well as the modern Devotion movement of Thomas à Kempis addressed the individual soul in its search for spiritual fulfillment (Gerkin 1997, 43). Pastoral care was increasingly taking place in a face-to-face meeting of pastor and care-receiver. The shift from the community as recipient to the individual was a therefore a development with roots in early modernity, but it was still far from finished in the time of van Koetsveld.

Nevertheless, there are also traces of the type of collective visit that van Koetsveld described in my present-day village. Parishioners would once a year meet in gatherings called 'greater house visits'. These visits would usually be led by a prominent member of the parish. The people invited were church members living in the same neighborhood, and about 10–20 people would attend. For the whole parish five or six such sessions would be planned. The meetings took place in the private home of a parishioner. The topics discussed during the meeting were chosen and prepared by the ministers, the church council and volunteers who facilitated a visit. Typical topics would be: "What is the meaning of 'faith' for you?", or "How can we pray?" The participants were invited to share stories and experiences with each other. Although the greater house visits gave an opportunity to share spiritual questions and experiences with each other, they were typically not framed as forms of spiritual care, but rather as an educational activity.

A third shift is one in focus. In some instances, the image of the pastor as a moral disciplinarian still lingered. People might assume that their pastoral visitors would disapprove of them, because of their divorce or their sexual orientation. But on the whole, the topic of the typical pastoral conversation would not be guilt, but meaning: "Why is this happening to me?", "What is the meaning of my illness?" The visits would be understood both by the pastoral care-giver and the receiver of pastoral care to address the existential questions of people in need. There was no expectation that the pastor would be able to cure physical or psychological diseases. Rather, healing was seen more as "learning to live in a positive way with my disease". Sometimes, there was an expectation that a pastor would be able to guide into the reconciliation with quarreling family members. The pastor would also address the topic of reconciliation with God. But the meaning of 'reconciliation' had shifted slightly. Again, not "sin" but "meaning" was the main focus of many care-receivers. They wanted to understand how some good might come out of their suffering, and how God could have a hand in that good. They also needed guidance about the opening up of more disciplined spiritual practices that would help them in their daily lives. Meditation, regular prayer practices and celebrations in small groups would answer to their need to find meaning.

Pastoral caregiving as I experienced it, is taking its shape in a context where the professional care-giver is not automatically a person with authority, where the receiver of care is approached as an individual, and where the aim of receiving and giving pastoral care is in the field of existential meaning-giving. In spite of the differences, there are also similarities between my present-day village and the *Mastland* of van Koetsveld. The parish religious tradition and the religious community as a whole are in both contexts the assumed frames for pastoral care. The term *pastoral* connects with a situation where the pastor and the parishioner are sharing the same religious frame of reference. This is still largely the case in my work in my parish. Usually, our conversation ends in Bible reading and prayer.

Yet, the diversity in orientation is considerable. The pastor needs hermeneutical skills to reframe her common ground with care-receiver who may combine his or her Bible reading with the books of Deepak Chopra, Thich Nhat Hanh or Rumi. Some church members go to Catholic monasteries to 'load up their batteries', others visit Zen-Do's.

When the Christian religious tradition is still important to both pastor and care- receiver, but the authority of the institution and of the pastor as a representative of that institution is weakened, how is the connection between tradition and individuals maintained? And what is the role of the pastor? I turn to American practical theologian and Methodist clergy Charles Gerkin for possible answers.

The shifting role of pastors: interpreters, healers, counselors and friends

Charles Gerkin sees Christian pastoral care in the classical period as a process that takes place in the interaction between four poles: the Christian tradition, as shaped by narratives and practices that are rooted in the past (1), the society in which the Christian community functions (2), Christian individuals and families (3), and the Christian community (4). In modernity and postmodernity, tradition and the community have almost completely fallen out of the square. Even when people regard themselves as active members of the church, they do not take on the whole tradition that it represents. Research has shown that in many respects, the attitude towards the Christian tradition of church members is not radically different from that of people outside the church. Rather, there is a gradual difference as to the degree of authority the tradition carries for them. Within the church, many people are combining Christian traditions, convictions and rituals with those of other faiths (Berndts, Berghuis, 63–83).

The appropriation of elements of the tradition in a more individual, bricolage-like manner means that the representatives of that tradition, the professional pastors, are losing their grip on the faithful. What remains are individuals, who take an autonomous stance vis-a vis the tradition and the community on the one hand, and society, seen as the total anonymous carrier of the larger culture on the other hand. Mediating communities between the individual and society have lost their meaning. Nevertheless, when individuals are seeking for ways to restore a certain connection between themselves and the Christian traditions, they tend to focus on the role of the pastor. The pastor has traditionally always functioned as mediator, giver of moral and spiritual guidance, and as the handler of the sacraments, a ritual leader (Gerkin 1997, 81). Therefore, in the line of reasoning of Gerkin, the pastor is in the one-to-one meeting with Christian individuals as it were the sole representative of that tradition, the mediator between individual, tradition and the Christian community, echoes of which are still remaining somewhere at the background. That community is the guardian of the typical "grammar" of Christian faith, the repository where the narratives from that faith tradition are being kept.

Gerkin sees pastoral care as a meeting point where the pastor connects the narratives of the lives of individuals in his or her care with the larger narrative of the Christian community.

The pastor functions primarily as the interpreter of the stories both of the people s/he meets and the collection of narratives that gives shape to the collective authoritative Christian tradition. These authoritative narratives are the starting point for the individual Christian. They are the idiom of her first language, the language she grew up with as a child and which gave her the words to retell her own life- story. Later in life, she may learn to use other idioms and speak other languages as well. , She may find other traditions and narratives outside the Christian community which may be illuminating and helpful. Yet, there are times when one returns to the original language and structure of thought/worldview (Gerkin 1997, 148).

Gerkin's hermeneutical approach to pastoral care evolving around life-stories has found many followers. In the Dutch context, an influential textbook on pastoral care that is used by many theological training centers has as its title: *Care for the Story* (Ganzevoort and Visser 2018). In this book, pastoral care is characterized as taking care of the life-narratives of people. By *taking care* the authors intend helping people to discover the deeper meaning of their life- stories, guiding them in making sense of these stories, learning to *read* them as meaning-making narratives. The handbook sees the role of the pastor as that of a listener and of an interpreter, who is *translating* the stories in terms that make them fit in with the other existing Christian narratives, and handing back metaphors and elements of these Christian stories to the story-tellers, enabling them to make more sense of their life-narratives. The different roles pastors assume in this hermeneutical process can be ordered in a fourfold typology.

Model 1 is that of *kerygmatic pastoral care (Ganzevoort and Visser 2018).*[4] 'Witness' is the keyword here. The care-giver here stands for the Christian tradition and the community, he or she is an office holder on behalf of the community. S/he is out there by divine command, an officer of the great King. The care-giver takes on the role of witness to the kingdom of God. Our human stories falter and fail, and the care-giver needs to proclaim the great story that gives meaning to it all, to set the person opposite him/her really free. This can take the form where the pastor looks for the work of the healing Spirit of God, where s/he gives spiritual guidance so that the other may discover this liberating message. A pitfall for this type of pastorate is that the care-giver may be so busy proclaiming that s/he forgets to listen.

Model 2 will be found mainly among Christian care-givers active in specialized care, i.e. in hospitals, in the army or prison. The nucleus here is 'outreach'. The care-giver can see her/himself as a professional, specialized therapist, hence the name *therapeutical pastoral care (Ganzevoort and Visser 2018).* Theologians have studied, and they are among other things also religious and ritual experts. The story of the person opposite gives clues to the problems s/he is wrestling with in their lives. The role of the care-giver is to give names to these problems and helps the client to find solutions. Christ, the great healer, never feared to name the problems of the people he met, and give them concrete clues how to live a better life. A criticism here may be that by concentrating on individual problems, the sick-making context in which they arose is ignored. There is a variety called systemic pastorate, where the context, the systems in which the client is functioning, is part of the diagnosis.

Model 3 is called *inter-human pastoral care (Ganzevoort and Visser 2018).* Here, the care-giver is like a friend, a companion. The authenticity and charisma of the care-giver are very important in this model. The authority of the care-giver is not based on his/her official function, nor on specialist knowledge, but on his/her qualities as a human being and abilities to maintain a meaningful relation.

---

4 Kerygmatic means oriented towards Christian witness.

The care-giver can never be the specialist in the field of the life-story of this particular person: the specialist is always the one who is telling the story. The care-giver does not try to manipulate, has faith in the work of the Spirit and creates the space to listen. A risk here is that the boundaries between care-giver and the care-receiver are blurring to such an extent that a false intimacy comes into existence. The care-giver should always also guard boundaries. In urban mission, there is a variety of inter-human care called pastoral care of presence. In this variety, the pitfall of the pastor may be that s/he desires to become a counselor or mediator, trying to solve the problems of the care-receiver. The role of the care-giver as one who is present as a witness to the life of the care-receiver requires that s/he refrains from interventions.

Model 4 is aware that good pastoral care always has elements of witness, outreach *and* presence (Ganzevoort and Visser 2018). So, the typologies must never become static. They must all play a role in the unfolding of the life-stories of the person with whom one is meeting. This can be done by concentrating on the stories themselves. By seeing the person in care as a living human document. Listening, 'reading' the stories told, the care-giver and the care-receiver may come to new points of understanding the world they live in. A new understanding of this person and of the world as a whole sends us back to the tradition, the Scriptures that we learn to read with new eyes. A model is the narrative of the two who were going to Emmaus. The companion is going part of the way, asks about their experience and explains Scripture in a novel way. The ritual of breaking bread discloses a new way of seeing the world. The care-giver in this model becomes an *interpreter*, both of the human and the Divine stories.

There is much to be valued in this hermeneutical, narrative approach of care. It gives place to the different roles of pastors that are connected to the four dimensions of pastoral care: healing, sustaining, reconciliation and guidance. In kerygmatic pastoral care, guidance and reconciliation are the key terms. The pastor, in interpreting the life-story of the care-receiver, ties it up to the grand Christian narrative of forgiveness, and guides the care-receiver into a more meaningful life. The pastor who sees her or himself as a spiritual therapeutic helper will combine the roles of healer and guide. A role concept of the pastor as a friend gives space to a more sustaining and comforting role. Whatever the role the pastor takes on, there is always the need to function as a hermeneutical bridge between the Christian tradition and the care-receiver.

Neither the Christian tradition nor the individual life- narratives are static wholes however. They are diverse and shifting. Church, cultural background, class and gender have an influence on the ways these stories are told. Missiologist Mechteld Jansen problematizes the narrative approach in multicultural Christian pastoral care. There are master-plots, serving as a framework for the individual life-story, which differ between cultures. Life-stories combine biography (based on an account of the things that happened) with a stock of inherited master-narratives in a certain cultural setting, that supply frames from culturally available sets. These frames shift over time.

For my grandmother, the first question she asked about persons she met for the first time was: "Who is her family, what region does she come from?" For a later generation, the achievements of the person they met were more important: 'What did he study, what kind of carrier does he have?', whereas for the post-modern generations these questions are less prominent. This has an influence on the way people present themselves to others in their life-narrative. The life-story is nowadays individualized, more 'the things I did' than 'where I come from and who my people are'.

For Christians, grand narratives from the Christian tradition help people to get a grip on their life- stories. But again, the Christian tradition provides a different sets of frames that can be employed. For some, the core of that tradition is a triumphant story of sin overcome and sickness healed, whereas for others it is the story of human frailty and the inability to do good (Jansen 2011, 44).

If the pastor and the care-receiver come from different backgrounds, the care for the story requires that the pastor is aware of these differences and has the ability to deal with them in a thoughtful and democratic way.

Diversity in spiritual care: dialogue and the model of hospitality

Pastoral care in a Church setting has undergone changes. It is now seen as a hermeneutical process in which both the care-giver and the care-receiver are engaged in a conversation where they try to make sense of and give meaning to the life-stories of the care-receiver in the light of the Christian tradition.

Yet another shift occurs when Christian pastors function outside of the Church in government funded institutions, to give spiritual care to patients, prison inmates or military personnel of diverse religious and life-stance backgrounds. In institutionalized spiritual care in the Netherlands, most spiritual accompaniment is given by professionally trained care-givers who are from a secular humanist or a Christian background.

Most care-givers have an institutional tie with a religious institution like a church, a humanist organization or a mosque organization, although there have been debates in the professional Organization for Spiritual Care, the VGVZ, on the desirability of such a tie. Some VGVZ members opted in 2007 for the possibility to become an 'unattached' spiritual care-giver, arguing that they would be more acceptable to the larger part of the population that does not have any ties with a religious or life-stance community.[5] They saw both the care-giver and the care-receiver as individuals who have developed their own spiritual identity without having recourse to a particular religious tradition (Schilderman 2010). Of the 1000 members of the Dutch professional organisation for spiritual care-givers, the VGVZ, 300 have a Roman Catholic background [6], 420 are Protestants[7], 120 are secular humanists[8] and 120 are non-aligned[9]. The conclusion must be that the numbers of Jewish, Hindu, Buddhist and Muslim care-givers are small.[10]

In spite of the fact that the large majority of the GVGZ members derive their authority from a *sending agency*, that is that they have a formal tie with a particular religious tradition, the expectation is that as spiritual care givers in secular institutions, they are able to function in a neutral secularized context. They receive a professional training with among others the aim to develop the hermeneutical skills that enable them to guide and accompany people of different cultures and religious and life-stance backgrounds. How can they be sensitive to these differences?

In his book on the multicultural setting in Christian pastoral care, Emmanuel Lartey distinguishes four types of approach towards cultural difference:

1. The monoculturalist or universalistic approach. Here cultural differences in the telling of the stories are approached in a colorblind manner. The care-giver assumes that 'we are really all the same', and universalizes particular sets of norms and values, cultural beliefs and practices that are actually only his/her own norms and values (Lartey 2003, 164).The cross-culturalist approach. Here, there is an openness to cultural differences. Differences are acknowledged, but perceived of as static wholes instead of continually evolving living traditions (Lartey 2003, 166).
2. The multi-culturalist approach. Care-givers working with this model try to seek as much information about the other as possible, but at the cost of not seeing the individuality of the other.

---

5 https://vgvz.nl/wp-content/uploads/2016/06/VGVZ-Cahier4-AmbtelijkeBinding_eindversie_totaal.pdf (accessed July 9, 2021).
6 https://vgvz.nl/sectoren/katholiek/ (accessed March 19, 2020).
7 https://vgvz.nl/sectoren/protestant/ (accessed March 19, 2020).
8 https://vgvz.nl/sectoren/humanistisch/ (accessed March 19, 2020).
9 https://vgvz.nl/sectoren/sing-institutioneel-niet-gezonden/ (accessed March 19, 2020).
10 https://vgvz.nl/sectoren/ (accessed March 19, 2020).

3. Intercultural care and counseling. This is for Lartey the preferred model. It departs from the assumption that every human person is in certain respects at the same time like all others (1), like some others (2), and like no other (3) (Lartey 2003, 171).

Although Lartey writes from a Christian context, his distinctions are relevant as well for the practice of interreligious spiritual care that has developed in the Dutch context.

In the Netherlands, policy makers and managers of care need to take diversity into account in three different contexts. These are the broader field of multicultural care-giving, moral deliberation and spiritual care as accompaniment (Walton 2017, 107–120).

In the context of care-giving, diversity is the point of departure and practices are culturally aware in order to optimize the care praxis. Institutions, be they prisons, hospitals or homes for the aged, try to attract personnel of different cultural backgrounds in order to optimize their communications with clients. A recruitment policy that is culturally aware is the hallmark of a modern, open institution. It makes a difference if the nurse or doctor can communicate more easily with patients who share the same religious background. Here, diversity is an asset.

In moral deliberation, cultural and religious/life-stance diversity is seen as potentially problematic. Diversity and lack of consensus about the good life and the morally good is often the starting point to have moral deliberation in the first place. In the exploratory stage of a process of moral deliberation, diversity can be seen as enriching- and yet, the often implicit aim is to reach moral consensus in the light of ethical rationality. This directs the participants of the deliberation toward a general shared viewpoint.

In spiritual care, there is a paradoxical situation. On the one hand, institutions strive for a religiously/life stance-wise diverse team of care-givers, on the other hand, the professional ability of each team member requires that s/he is available for each client or patient. That implies that the role perception of Protestant spiritual care-givers, for instance, makes another shift again. Whereas in the modern approach of the pastor as a hermeneutical mediator between the care-receiver and the Christian tradition, be it as a comforter, a counselor, a healer or a reconciler, here the Pastor turns into a spiritual care-giver that caters to care-receivers of any kind of religious background. How can this role be combined with a continuous connection with the Protestant Church (in the case of the protestant spiritual care-giver the 'sending organization')?

In practice, the universalistic approach that Lartey mentions is a course that is often pursued. The care-giver sees him or herself as a generalist, who is an expert in listening and interpreting the life-narrative of the care-receiver. The study of Cadge and Sigalow of spiritual care given in an American hospital shows that such a color-blind approach is often followed. They call this approach 'neutralizing'. The patient needs someone who really listens, and the hermeneutical interpretation of the life-narrative by the care-giver is not problematic, as 'everybody has a spirituality'. Another type of strategy is called 'code-switching'. It relates to the use of the religious language, symbols and even rituals of the other. A pastor can say a prayer, read a text or tell a story derived from the religious tradition of the care-receiver, thus appropriating another tradition than his or her own. This can extend to the use of rituals from the other tradition, such as anointing or blessing. One respondent in the research of Cadge and Sigalow called this use of ritual 'mimicking'. In Code-switching, the multi-cultural approach mentioned by Lartey is followed: the spiritual care-giver takes the religious and cultural tradition of the other seriously by making use of elements from it, but what remains problematic is that it is the care-giver who decides what elements can be used in which way. A third strategy that occurred occasionally is called 'referral'. The care-giver can ask a colleague who shares the religious tradition of the patient to step in for the performing of a ritual. Here, one sees the cross-cultural approach mentioned by Laherty.

These three strategies can be commented on as follows:

- They do not address difference, but ignore it/approach it passively
- They do not take into account individuality of the patient
- The pastor acts from a 'knowing' position, as the expert who 'knows' that fundamentally she believes the same, or that she has the better insight into the tradition of the other
- This puts the care-giver in a position of power and has a blind spot for their own religious/life stance position (Walton 2017, 111).

A better strategy would recognize difference, 'touch' difference, have respect for individuality, make the care-giver vulnerable as one who does not know, give openness to deal with uncertainty, correction and control and would be open to discuss the position of the pastor herself.

In the approach of Lartey, every human person is in certain respects like all others, like some others, like no other. This calls for three tasks: recognition for the human dignity of the other as a creature of God, recognition of difference in culture, context and power and seeing the other as an individual.

Conclusion

The traditions of Christian pastoral care are never static. They undergo changes, are under debate and scrutiny and take different shapes in different contexts. At the same time, they are rooted in an ongoing practice that is not always explicitly addressed. Much of what happens is implicit, invisible.

The *Sketches from Mastland Parsonage* give an insight into a situation where pastoral care was given and received from an assumed shared religious common ground, rooted in the Protestant Christian tradition of the Netherlands. The book also shows that there were dissidents in the village. The minister had sometimes difficulty to establish his authority when it was challenged by the more orthodox villagers.

In the present-day context in B, diversity was present and acknowledged. Parishioners were playing an active part in pastoral care in its many shapes and practices. Yet, the minister was a reference figure for them. She was to many villagers the representative of the local church community. For people who were less active in the church, the minister could be the only link between them and the Christian tradition. In the model of Gerkin as well as that of Ganzevoort, this role is emphasized. Here, the pastor becomes the interpreter of the Christian master narratives, bringing them into conversation with the life-stories of care-receivers. S/he, and much less the Christian community, becomes the bridge between Christian tradition and the everyday life and search for meaning of ordinary people.

The life-story approach may work well in a mono-cultural setting, although even there, there is the risk of misunderstanding. It becomes more problematic when there is a considerable cultural and religious difference between the care-giver and the care-receiver. Then the authority of the Christian master narratives is less obvious, although it functions as the background narrative for care-givers who have been raised in the Christian tradition. They may assume that they operate from a neutral position as skilled interpreters and listeners, and even stress their ability to employ and appropriate elements of other religious and life-stance traditions, without confronting possible differences between them and their clients.

In a multicultural and multi-religious setting, there is a need to devise strategies to bring the difference in traditions into the conversation, because if they remain implicit, then the dominant tradition tends to become normative. This is especially a risk if the care-giver belongs to the dominant tradition in society.

References

Asad, Talal. 1986. "The Idea of an anthropology of Islam" *Occasional Paper Series.* Georgetown University, Washington.

Berndts, Ton, and Joantine Berghuis. 2016. *God in Nederland 1966–2015.* Utrecht: Ten Have.

Cadge, Wendy, and Emily Sigalow. 2013. "Negotiating Religious Differences: Strategies of Interfaith Chaplains in Healthcare." *Journal for the Scientific Study of Religion* 52/1: 146–158.

Cassell, Eric J. 1976. "Illness and Disease: Treating Patients for Both is the Healer's Art." *Hastings Centre Report* 6/2.

Ganzevoort, Ruard, and Jan Visser. 2018. *Zorg voor het verhaal.* Zoetermeer: Boekencentrum.

Gerkin, Charles. 1997. *An Introduction to Pastoral Care.* Nashville: Abingdon Press.

Heitink, Gerben. 2001. *Biografie van de dominee.* Baarn: ten Have.

Hervieu-Léger, Danielle. 2000. *Religion as a Chain of Memory.* Cambridge: Polity Press.

Jansen, Mechteld. 2011. *Interrelated Stories: Intercultural Pastoral Theology.* Muenster: LIT.

Lartey, Emmanuel. 2003. *In Living Color: An intercultural Approach to Pastoral Care and Counselling.* London, Philadelphia: Jessica Kingsley Publishers.

Pattison, Stephen. 2000. *A Critique of Pastoral Care.* London: SCM Press.

Schilderman, Hans. 2010. "De identiteit en positie van geestelijke verzorgers in de zorg." *VGVZ Cahiers* 4.

van Koetsveld, Eliza. 1978. *Schetsen uit de pastorij te Mastland: Ernst en luim uit het leven van de Nederlandse Dorpsleraar.* Wageningen : L.J.Veen. https://www.dbnl.nl/tekst/koet003sche01_01/

Walton, Martin. 2017. "Wat maakt het verschil? Levensbeschouwelijke diversiteit in zorginstellingen." *Religie en Samenleving* 2: 107–120.

Beret Bråten

The authority of Norwegian hospital chaplains

Abstract: The questions handled in this chapter concern 1) how Norwegian hospital chaplains reflect on their authority while relating to staff and patients in a multi-faith setting, and 2) whether there are differences in how chaplains from the Church of Norway (CofN) compared to Muslim chaplains, relate to authority. These questions are discussed based on Max Weber' theory of authority and an empirical material comprising qualitative interviews with 22 hospital chaplains. Results show that hospital chaplains rely on legal and traditional as well as charismatic authority. This goes for Muslim as well as CofN chaplains. There are however differences. Muslim chaplains do not have the same chances to capitalize on legal authority, a fact making traditional authority more important to them.

Introduction

> I try, but this is a rather hazardous project ... I think, however, that it is important, although it is laborious, to make sure that in the wards where I am responsible [for chaplaincy] at this hospital, the staff are going to know who I am. They are not supposed to call for a chaplain, they are supposed to call for a chaplain named [mentioning his own first name]. That is me, who they have experienced and who they can recommend to the patient. They are supposed to be sure and feel secure: If we ask him to come, we'll get something that is watertight. The problem is that the staff in the wards are replaced all the time. (Hospital chaplain *C2*[1], *CofN)*

This quote from an interview with a hospital chaplain from the Church of Norway (CofN) illustrates how a Norwegian hospital chaplain works to establish his position as part of hospital services. Three or four decades ago, hospital chaplains like this one walked the wards and offered their services to patients who they met on their way. They were present and visible. Back then, being a hospital patient meant being exposed to religious staff on a par with medical staff. Religious leaders, more precisely chaplains ordained as priests in the Lutheran Church of Norway, the (former) state church, were self-evident parts of the institutions of the welfare state, such as hospitals. This has changed and

1 The interviewees are anonymized and given an alias based on a randomly chosen letter of the alphabet and a number.

 https://doi.org/10.1515/9783110717365-003

so has the position and work of chaplains. Norwegian hospital chaplains no longer walk the wards offering their services to patients they meet on their way. They need to be sent for by a patient and/or by doctors and nurses. Meaning that it is no longer self-evident meeting a chaplain as part of services offered at a hospital, and that the position of the chaplain in terms of visibility and authority has become more blurred.

These changes in the position of chaplains as part of Norwegian hospitals is due to changes in how religion and faith is present in society at large; how it is part of institutions, communities, relations and individual ponderings over existential questions. The UK sociologist Grace Davie ([2007] 2013) underlines how the postmodern turn in cultural life in the 1980s and 1990s challenged all kinds of certainties. The whole idea of grand narratives, scientific as well as political and religious, became suspect, turning religion away from something that is imposed or inherited into a matter of personal inclination (Davie [2007] 2013, 95–97). These changes as well as immigration to Norway from every part of the world, have caused increasing plurality in beliefs and belief practices among citizens. Religious pluralization challenges the hegemony of the Lutheran Church in the Northern part of Europe (Schmidt 2010). State-church systems are suspended in Norway as well as Sweden (although not in Denmark), and there are ongoing changes in the management of religion in public institutions (Kühle, Schmidt, Jacobsen and Petterson 2018). Concentrating on the Norwegian case, religion is still present in public institutions such as hospitals, but in an increasingly plural way: Chapels are accompanied by prayer rooms, multi-faith rooms and quiet rooms. Facilities and procedures have been put in place to facilitate Muslim rituals after a patient has died. Special diets offering halal as well as vegetarian meals have been developed. Staff uniforms include hijabs and sometimes long-sleeved coats. And interfaith chaplaincy is put on the agenda.[2] Chaplains from the CofN are, however, still dominant as hospital specialists in spiritual and existential care. They have a mandate to serve all patients, regardless of belief, unless the patient asks for someone else (NOU 2013:1). A development towards interfaith chaplaincy has been initiated at just a few hospitals – but has nevertheless begun (Bråten 2019). Equally important, the practices of hospital chaplains have gradually changed from a "religious service" model to an "existential care" model, emphasizing dialogue and professionalism. A practice affected by the increasingly multi-religious and secular profile of the population (Stifoss-Hanssen, Danbolt and Frøkedal 2019, 60).

2 Information from a survey conducted in hospitals in 2017 by the Ministry of Health on behalf of the Ministry of Culture (and Church). I had permission to access the data material.

Hospital chaplains as of today serve in a shifting context when it comes to religious leadership (Henriksen 2012), influencing how chaplains shape their authority as professionals in secular institutions. Max Weber elaborates on legal authority in a text which is among the sociological classics (Weber [1947] 1959). Here, authority is defined as "power with a reason" – something that makes power legitimate (ibid., 218). This is an approach to power well suited an ambition to explore and discuss the position of chaplains in Norwegian hospitals. Power, when related to hospital chaplains, is not in the form of domination, but more subtly in the form of influence, knowledge and organizing, enabling professionals who are listened to and who matter as part of hospital care. Richard Coble (2018) writes, from a US-perspective, on how a chaplain functions "[...] through innumerable connections and vast networks", how they are connected to a department, to patients, to hospital staff and to hospital administration (Coble 2018, 4). Why is the authority of chaplains at all important? The study of religion in public institutions is, Sophie Gilliat-Ray argues: "[...] an ideal context for mapping the evolution of new religious discourses because of the way in which it is possible to see far larger issues in microcosm [...]" (Gilliat-Ray 2018, 193). Hospital chaplains are placed at the very epicentre of changes in how faith is made or not made part of public institutions in societies marked by individualization, secularization and religious plurality. Therefore, it is an important question how they engage with authority as part of hospital staff, as hospital professionals.

The questions asked and explored in the following are: 1) How do Norwegian hospital chaplains reflect on their authority in relating to staff and patients in a multi-faith setting? 2) Are there differences in how CofN chaplains (who constitute a majority among hospital chaplains) compared to Muslim chaplains (who constitute a minority among hospital chaplains) relate to authority?

The data material I analyse are qualitative interviews made with 17 hospital chaplains from the CofN and five hospital chaplains/volunteers from Muslim communities (a total of 22 interviews). I start by introducing hospital chaplaincy in a Norwegian context before I present the interview material, analytical strategies and theoretical perspectives. I use theory, mainly on different kinds of authority and different kinds of spiritual counselling, to structure the analysis on how chaplains talk about authority when they reflect on their role and practices in the hospital. Results are presented based on the three types of authority coined by Weber ([1947]1995). Finally, I discuss results and compare chaplains from different denominations.

The Norwegian context

Social change due to welfare, individualism and immigration reshape and reinvent religion and belief in different ways (Davie ([2007] 2013; Thorbjørnsrud/Døving [2012] 2017, 11–12). Swedish scholar Magdalena Nordin describes these changes as shaping a "blurred religious situation": There is increased religious plurality, a decline in religious belonging and in religious practices, but openness to spiritual beliefs and no decrease in belief in God (Nordin 2018, 162). The current situation when it comes to individual belief is, however, difficult to "measure". One way of doing so is to count members in faith communities: The share of the population that is part of the protestant, former state church, the Church of Norway (CofN), is declining steadily, but 64,9 per cent still count as members.[3] At the same time, the number of members of religious and faith communities outside the CofN has been on the increase and counts for 13 per cent of the population. The majority are Christians (most of them Catholics) and member of Islamic communities.[4] Counting members might, however, paint a somewhat inaccurate or incomplete picture. In the Norwegian survey on quality of life (2017), one question is whether the respondents consider themselves as part of a religion or belief: Only 47 per cent concur,[5] implying that individuals might be religiously affiliated without identifying closely with their community – a tendency which might be described as "belonging without believing" (Davie 2015). At the same time there might be individuals who do believe, but who lack a religious affiliation. They are "believing without belonging" (ibid. 2015). In a macro perspective, this is the plural group of people whom chaplains meet in a Norwegian hospital.

Chaplains provide religious and spiritual care within a secular institutional setting, such as a hospital, nursing home, prison, university, part of military forces or an airport (Gilliat-Ray et al. 2013, Sullivan 2014). The role has evolved from within Christian churches, but the term chaplain is, in an English-speaking context, used across different religious confessions, including humanist life stances. Interfaith hospital chaplaincy units are customary in countries such as the UK, Netherlands, the United States and Canada (Liefbroer 2020; Gillat-Ray et al. 2013; Cadge 2012; Isgandarova 2012) but are, so far, scarce in the Nordic region (Kühle et al. 2018).

3 Religion (ssb.no) (read 25.05.2022).

4 Religious communities and life stance communities (ssb.no) (read 25.05.2022).

5 Sekularisering i Norge (ssb.no) (read 25.05.2022).

In Norwegian and other Scandinavian languages, we also lack terms equivalent to chaplaincy and the related term, pastoral care. The term used in Norway to capture how priests and deacons ordained in the CofN talk about faith and existential questions with individuals who need it, is "sjelesorg", or spiritual and existential care. The term "sjelesorg" is borrowed from the German term "seelensorge", meaning "care for the soul" (Okkenhaug 2002, 7). Care for the soul is part of the practical theological work clergy and deacons in the CofN do, as well as part of public institutional caring practices: Norwegian hospital chaplains are employed and funded by the twenty public health trusts and by the relatively few private (often diaconal) hospitals. All public health trusts have what is known as a pastoral service, but a health trust usually consists of several hospitals, and not all hospitals have their own chaplain. When necessary, hospitals without a chaplain on staff use staff from the local community of the CofN and sometimes other denominations (Bråten 2019). Although they are employed at the hospital, hospital chaplains are supposed to have an authorization from their faith community – and the local CofN bishops are supposed to monitor the pastoral service at hospital units, although from a distance. The Lutheran dominance is inherited from the relationship between church and state. Kühle and Christensen (2019) refer to the political scientist Tim Knudsen and his argument that "the Nordic welfare states owes to the post-Reformation state appropriation of the church, which transformed local pastors into state officials" (Kühle/Christensen 2019, 187). Pastors were made into important local actors as part of "a religious infrastructure" in education and social services as well as health care (ibid. 187). While there is no longer a state church, CofN representatives are still very much present as part of Norwegian welfare services.

There are but four Norwegian hospital trusts with heterogeneous chaplaincy departments. The Pastoral and Counselling Department at St. Olav in Trondheim has, since 2010, engaged what is called a cultural consultant in a 30 % position working as a chaplain alongside colleges from the CofN. From the start different employees in the position as cultural consultant has been a Muslim, but since none of them have had the title imam they have been presented as *the hospital Muslim*. In the period 2015–2018 this department also had a hospital Humanist in a full-time position, replacing a CofN chaplain on a leave of absence. The second heterogeneous pastoral department is at the health trust in Bergen (Helse Bergen), where they have hired a hospital imam in a 20 % position. Additionally, Helse Bergen has a cultural adviser in a part-time position who is a Buddhist and does spiritual and existential care when needed (Bråten 2019). Recently the hospital trust in Tromsø has hired a hospital humanist. This is done in cooperation with the Humanist organization in Norway. Finally, there is at the Oslo University Hospital (OUS) established a temporary part time position (30 %) as a Muslim conversation partner. This is a temporary arrangement financed through the Norwegian Ministry of Children and Family, which at the time, where responsible for religious matters. The initiative came from Oslo University Hospital in cooperation with the nursing homes in Oslo. OUS established, back in 2012, a team of voluntary conversation partners recruited from different local belief communities. The team got a specially designed training program at the Faculty of Theology at the University of Oslo. From 2019 the Pastoral Department at OUS has had the responsibility of administrating this team of volunteers. Patients who ask for a chaplain who is not from the CofN might be visited by one of the volunteers, who receive a fee for each visit. If the patient defines herself as a Muslim, one of the Muslim conversation partners is asked. If the patient defines himself as a Humanist, one of the Humanist conversation partners are asked. The volunteers at OUS and employed chaplains from other denominations in part-time positions, differ from those who have a full-time position. The former primarily visit patients who share their belief, while the fully employed chaplains have a mandate to visit all patients regardless of beliefs (Bråten 2019; Grung/Bråten 2019).

There is no standardized level or content of specialist skills required of those who are hospital chaplains (Stifoss-Hansen, Danbolt and Frøkedal 2019, 66). A kind of specialist competence known as Clinical Pastoral Education (CPE) is, however, recommended (Okkenhaug 2002, 20–21). CPE was started in Norway during the 1970s, inspired by similar training facilities in the United States, and focuses on psychological and communicative skills as well as theory (Stifoss-Hansen, Danbolt and Frøkedal 2019, 66). Until now CPE, has been reserved for those who are clergy or deacons in the CofN. It is considered as further training to clergy/deacons and access requires a master's degree. Qualification requirements are, however, slowly changing. An important change occurred in 2019 with a new master programme on Interreligious Chaplaincy and Leadership at the Faculty of Theology, University of Oslo (Grung/Bråten 2019).

Hospital chaplains have a mandate to provide counselling, support patients and their next of kin during crises and grief, perform rituals and act as a resource for the rest of the hospital staff regarding ethical and spiritual issues (Kühle, Schmidt, Jacobsen and Petterson 2018, 109). They relate to patients and their next of kin – but also to health professionals and the hospital as an institution. A Danish study among hospital, prison and military chaplains revealed that the top three tasks among hospital chaplains were: 1) Pastoral care/conversation 2) Religious services and devotionals and 3) Religious ceremonies (baptisms, weddings) (Kühle/Christensen 2019, 190). There is no similar survey made in a Norwegian context, but my interviews show a similar pattern. Attention is directed towards an authoritative ambition in health care policy to provide holistic care. Palliative care is, for example, explicitly targeted at providing physical, psychological, as well as social and spiritual/existential care (Meld. St. 24 2019 – 2020). Nurses and physicians are expected to take care of spiritual and existential care as generalists, while chaplains are the specialists on these matters (e. g. Liefbroer et al. 2019). Chaplains are, however, a kind of deviant specialist among hospital staff. While the medical discourse is based on natural science, existential questions – the expertise of chaplains – follow a broader and more hermeneutic logic, actualizing core questions on coherence and meaning. Joy and hope and love are essential matters. Chaplains engage in how these notions are expressed in relations, towards our self, our nearest and dearest. Society, nature as well as spiritual figures and beliefs are at the core of chaplaincy services (Boelsbjerg 2013; Walderhaug 2018).

Authority

Norwegian professor in Interreligious Studies, Oddbjørn Leirvik, differs between two kinds of religious leadership: Spiritual leadership (conducted in formal or informal positions) and organizational leadership (Leirvik [2012] 2017). While Henriksen ([2012]2017) writing about power and powerlessness among leaders in the CofN differs between what he conceptualizes as the power to lead the CofN, versus religious authority as having an impact on how people ponder over faith. The latter is, he argues, a kind of power that is more ambiguous and less transparent (ibid. 201). Henriksen regards ordained priests in the CofN in the first row among leaders in the church (ibid. 202). Hospital chaplains are, I would argue, conducting a kind of spiritual leadership. This is due to their position as legalized and certified specialists on handling spiritual and existential questions in relation to patients – but also in relation to the rest of the group of health professionals. They do not have a local church or community to lead organizationally, but they are authorized by their faith community (CofN). When the group of professional hospital chaplains also include chaplains from outside the majority Church, these chaplains sometimes also have commitments outside the hospital setting linked to their faith community – making them into both spiritual and organizational leaders. Gilliat-Ray et.al (2013) conducting research among Muslim hospital and prison chaplains in a UK context, simply consider them a kind of Islamic religious leaders.

But how to approach authority when it comes to hospital chaplains? According to Max Weber, authority is – as underlined in the introduction – power with a reason. These are reasons making power legitimate and justified. Weber conceptualizes three pure types of *legitimate* authority: Authority based on 1) legal/normative grounds, 2) traditional grounds and 3) charismatic grounds (Weber [1947]

1995, 218). *Legal grounds* rest on patterns of normative rules and the right of those who have authority under such rules to issue command. *Traditional grounds* rest on an established belief (among people) in immemorial traditions and the status of those exercising authority under them, while *charismatic grounds* rest on devotion to the specific sanctity, heroism or exemplary character of an individual person and of the normative patterns or order revealed or ordered by him (ibid.).

The three kinds of authority differ in the way they capitalize on factors inside or outside the person in a leading position. Legal authority is a kind of impersonal order. It can be exercised by all who inherit the position with a legal mandate to lead. Traditional authority is gained by those – the individual persons – who inherit the sanctioned position as leaders, and rests on traditions at hand (for example disqualifying women from inheriting leadership in some religious communities). Charismatic authority is dependent on the person and might be conceptualized as "the gift of grace" (Weber [1947]1995). It is, as Weber describes it, accessible to those who are "obeyed by virtue of personal trust in him and his revelation" (ibid.) Charismatic authority is, however, not everlasting. It has to be proved and renewed: "the charismatic ruler has to show that he is a ruler by the 'grace of God'" (Weber [1922]1990, 100, my translation).

These grounds of authority are applicable to chaplaincy framed as a kind of spiritual leadership. The Norwegian theologian and teacher in "care for the soul", Berit Okkenhaug (2002), differs between three approaches to or kinds of care for the soul (see also Grevbo 2006). One type is based on "kerygma", which means message or news. Then, the task of the spiritual caring person is to take a lead in the conversation and pass on or explain the word of God, based on normative theology. An alternative type is based on the other in the conversation, in Norwegian referred to as "konfidenten". The spiritual caring person is brought into the conversation by the other. The task is to create an atmosphere that is safe and non-judgemental in a way that allows the other to dare to talk about difficult feelings and themes. While the *kerygma* approach is based on a theological platform, the *konfident* approach relies on a therapeutic psychological platform, paving the way for a third alternative – a kind of golden mean: A *Church-based belief and life help*, an approach that takes into consideration that listening to and understanding the other is not enough, the spiritual caring person also needs to point in the direction of God (Okkenhaug 2002, 15–17).

In my interpretation, Okkenhaug's first two alternative approaches resemble the distinction between a directive and a non-directive approach in pastoral counselling (see for example Rassool 2016, 16–17). A directive approach means that the counsellor takes the lead and acts as an adviser or teacher, while a non-directive approach is client or person-centred: The counsellor is supposed to be non-judgemental, genuine, and more concerned about the client's perception of the problem than of the problem per se. These concepts explicitly attach theology to both alternatives. A chaplain might use his or her knowledge about religion and belief in a directive or not-so-directive way. While the chaplain in the directive kind of relation has a message based on an evangelist intention, the chaplain in a non-directive relation pays full attention to the needs of the other as they evolve in the conversation. However, the last one might also turn to religion and belief – turning toward Okkenhaug's (2002) third alternative, belief- and life help.

If we, again, turn to Max Weber's different forms of legal authority, a directive approach in chaplaincy practice might be said to rest on tradition: The CofN-chaplain has a historical position interpreting the gospel. But the authority of chaplains might rest on law as well, at least in a hospital setting making formal competence claims to chaplains employed as part of hospital staff. Finally, authority might rest on charisma inherited by individual chaplains – on the trust he or she manage to create in relationships with patients and the rest of the staff. Given what we know about the resonance for people of belief and their eagerness to make choices for themselves, traditional authority might be the least familiar and the least useful in relating to patients in hospitals of today. Before we turn to how hospital chaplains as of today talk about authority and whether these approaches can be categorized as legal or traditional or charismatic – or perhaps all three, I will present the data material.

Interview data and analysis

The empirical analysis is based on qualitative interviews made with hospital chaplains from the CofN (17) and Muslim chaplains (5). All the CofN chaplains are employed at Norwegian hospital trusts, while the Muslim chaplains are partly employees, partly volunteers. The 22 chaplains "belong" to seven different hospitals located all over the country, six public and one private. Among the interviewed CofN chaplains there are nine women and eight men, while among the Muslim chaplains there are four men and one woman. While some of the CofN chaplains have worked in hospitals for several decades (some since the early 1980s), others have just a few years of chaplaincy experience. Compared to the CofN chaplains, the Muslim chaplains have less experience in their role.

The interviews were conducted as part of my post-doc project on palliative care in a multicultural society (2017–2020) located at the Health Services Research Unit at Akershus University Hospital and financed by the Research Council of Norway.[6] The research project's main ambition was to reveal potential challenges in palliative care relating to a social and cultural plural group of patients and their next of kin. I soon realized that spiritual and existential care as part of palliative care was one such potential challenge. Palliative care is supposed to meet physical, psychological, social, as well as spiritual and existential needs. And with a religious plural group of patients it seemed like a paradox that hospital chaplains turned out to be mainly from the CofN. Simultaneously, I noticed that there were discussions and changes going on. The Norwegian hospital context provided access to interfaith chaplaincy in the making.

The research project was presented to the Norwegian Regional Committee for Medical Research Ethics. The Research Ethics Committee deemed the study to fall outside their remit as specified by the Norwegian Health Research Act.[7] The study was approved by the Privacy Ombudsman at Akershus University Hospital.[8] All the interviewees signed a consent form.

The interviews with hospital chaplains follow a prepared protocol of questions, but I have tried to be open to unexpected turns – to depart from the plan for a while and "go with the flow" (Johnson 2001). The interview guide starts out by asking the chaplain at hand who they are, about education and job experience, as well as why they wanted to become chaplains. Then we talked about what they do and how they do it when they are asked to visit a patient and/or their next of kin: How they are asked to come? Who asks for them? How do they prepare? How do they relate to the patient when they enter the room and in the conversation? What are they asked to do? What are the conversations about? How is religion and belief part or not part of it? We also talked about what they do when the patient in the encounter does not share their belief, about their experiences with a religiously plural patient group. My main interest has been to get access to their practices, or more precisely – since I have not observed what they do – the way they talk about and interpret their practices.

All the interviews were taped, except for two where detailed notes were made. Afterwards I transcribed the taped interviews. Then I read through the transcripts and, partly inspired by what the chaplains said, partly by theory and former research, I have defined themes and identified patterns in the interview material. The analysis is inspired by the thematic analytical method of Braun and Clark (2013). Thematic analysis can, as they describe it, be descriptive. Descriptive analysis tries to capture what is said and how the interviewees

6 ref: 256431.
7 ref: 2017/553 – 1.
8 ref: 17_101.

understand practices, situations and themes. Thematic analysis can also be theoretical, using theory to interpret and discuss what is said (ibid. 2013). The analysis presented in the following started out identifying how chaplains talked about their role and position in the hospital. Since authority was mostly talked about implicitly as part of their role, I asked reading the interview transcripts how chaplains define their role as chaplain – towards the hospital, the belief community they are part of (including how they relate to belief/God) and in relation to the patient. The next step was to use theory, mainly on different kinds of authority and different kinds of spiritual counselling, to structure what is said about roles and positions, and to interpret and discuss what is said. Results are presented based on the three types of authority coined by Weber ([1947]1995).

Legal authority: Insiders as well as outsiders in the hospital institution

Some of the Muslim hospital chaplains and all from the CofN are, as described earlier, employed at the regional hospital trusts, while the rest of the Muslim chaplains are volunteers. They are, however, a special kind of volunteer since they have agreed to be trained and join a particular group of lay chaplains. The job or appointment at the hospital and the knowledge requirements they are supposed to fulfil, give employed chaplains legal authority as professionals in their field. Employed chaplains also have a legal position as part of the hospital staff. This is providing authority they can rest on in relations to the rest of the hospital professionals and to patients. Their institutional belonging is, however, seldom made into a theme in the interviews.

Some CofN chaplains mention, though, the fact that chaplains who are not ordained as clergy or deacons in the CofN do not have the same educational background they as CofN chaplains have. As mentioned earlier, Clinical Pastoral Education (CPE) has not been accessible to those who are not part of the CofN. The alternative training chaplains from other denominations have had is insufficient, some CofN chaplains argue. In that way they establish a distinction between themselves and chaplains from other denominations, a distinction that indirectly downplays the professional authority of these "other" chaplains.

Additionally, the group of lay chaplains is not part of the hospital as an institution in the same way as employees are. They are asked for when needed in patient relations only. They are not asked to educate and supervise hospital staff or take part in ethical guidance at the hospital – something those who are employed do. In that way their legal authority is limited toward staff and the hospital as an institution. The position the group of lay chaplains inherit, may all the same give them authority in relations with patients, who are not that familiar with the distinction between employees and volunteers. One Muslim chaplain explains, for example, how people he meets and who are immigrants, tend to think of him as a kind of governmental representative since he has a position at the hospital. That gives authority, but also obligations since some perceive him as someone who can sort out almost everything relating to public authorities in general and particularly in relation to health authorities.

Hospital affiliation gives legal authority through professional positions and by regulatory means. But as an institution, a hospital is also comprised of normative and cultural elements (Scott 2008, 48). In a hospital there are specific ways of relating to problems and humans who carry these problems along, this is a medical discourse focused on fixing problems (Bondevik, Madsen and Solbrække 2017). The discourse on curing and healing – and in that way solving the problems of the patient, is strong. This establishes a certain frame for how professionals relate to patients and how patients are supposed to respond, an approach easily making the way professionals relate towards patients, pretty directive. Increasing individualization and reflexivity, as described by Davie ([2007] 2013) referred to in the introduction, have shifted the medical discourse somewhat in favour of the patient as a competent agent and towards shared decision-making. There is however still a tendency to see patient choices not consistent with medical advice as illogical or deviant (cf. Blaxter [2004] 2010, 83–84). Contrary to this pretty directive approach, there is a tendency among the chaplains to explicitly define their role – in relation to the patients and their next of kin – in a non-directive way: Chaplains tend to define themselves as helpers, but helpers that are present not to heal or cure. The helper they speak of themselves as has an ambition to make it easier for patients/families to deal with difficult life experiences, but not to fix any problem. One CofN chaplain defines himself as a "pilot boat": There are difficult weather conditions for a while, and a need for some assistance, but these are temporary conditions patient manage to handle themselves – with a little help. Others talk of being someone who walks with the patient for a while.

As an underlying consequence, patients are constructed not as helpless and in need of rescue and fixing, but as capable of figuring things out themselves – with some assistance from a fellow who is trained in facing existential difficulties, a professional who does not evade hard questions and themes. Some of the chaplains explicitly talk of this as a contradictory way of relating to patients, when compared to a traditional medical approach towards patients. They talk about themselves and their practices as contrary to what they interpret as a dominant medical discourse. This is underlined when some chaplains refer to the hospital as an institution relating to humans as if they were constructed in fragments, and to treat them as cars, where different parts are possible to fix or replace. In that way they point towards a tendency in medicine to deny a genuinely holistic approach towards humans, to overemphasize medical possibilities and make it difficult to accept death as part of life. These are approaches chaplains tend to emphasize that they do not share, underlined by one CofN chaplain who says ironically: "Hospitals do not prevent death, they postpone it."

Chaplains stress that to grieve, for example, is part of life, and is not a diagnosis. To grieve, to encounter death and experience crisis are part of normality; something that is difficult, but possible to deal with. And it is their mission, as chaplains, to assist others in facing reality. Some explicitly emphasise that they take this approach, representing a kind of complementary or even counter cultural competence inside hospitals. This counterculture is, for example, brought to the fore when patients are facing death. Here are two chaplains:

> [...] We all have an inherent capability to be born. We know how to do it. We do. In the same way all humans have an inherent capability to die. So, it is all about having people trust their capabilities: I have all that I need to manage to face this. Bottom line, I have (*Hospital chaplain B1, CofN).*

> You need to accept that you are going to die. However, ... the doctor says that I am going to die, but no one really knows ... God decides. That gives him (the patient) a glimpse of hope, at the same time we have to prepare him. He has to accept that he is going to die. That is the way life is. And if he has something to sort out in his life, I can help him; if he has children and is concerned about the inheritance, if he has a family. Some want to be sent off to their country of origin when they die. Others don't, they let me know (*Hospital chaplain K1, Muslim).*

These two quotes by a CofN and a Muslim chaplain, respectively, treat death and dying as realities to be faced and handled. The two chaplains have their attention fixed on the capabilities of the dying, on their resources and ability to accept and handle. Their role, as chaplains, is to be by their side as "pilot boats" and guides, not as healers.

Another difference the chaplains are proud to represent inside the hospital, is their special code of confidentiality. Chaplains do not need to tell the rest of the staff what has been going on in the conversation with a patient; the content of the conversation does not become part of the medical records. They are supposed to follow their own duty of confidentiality, not sharing knowledge about the patient unless it is necessary due to life and death. In this way, some chaplains argue, they have an ability to perceive the other as a human, not as a patient – and to create a "space" inside the hospital where the patient can be who they are beyond the patient role.

Hospital chaplains are part of the hospital institution and they extract legal authority from their professional position. At the same time, chaplains position themselves as a contrary culture to a medicalized hospital discourse focused on fixing humans who have a defect. They tend to define a counterculture based on a genuinely holistic stance towards people. In that way they construct an alternative to the medical hospital discourse, and a fundament for their own professional authority.

Traditional authority: Belief managers

Traditional authority rests, according to Weber, on an established belief in immemorial traditions and the status of those exercising authority under them. Traditional authority is, historically, a way to inherit authority easily applicable to understand the role and position of clergy and others who inherit spiritual leading positions as part of faith communities.

Inside the hospital, chaplains across denominations, share having a belief, or as some of the interviewed chaplains from the CofN state: "We are the ones who carry hope with us". Hope is, used like this, a rather ambiguous concept, but it is as I interpret it, linked to God or faith or – something that might work as resources to patients finding themselves in distressful situations. Implicitly, they carry God/the gospel with them – something that might be comforting and/or useful tools in relations to patients in need of support in dealing with severe problems.

This is, however, contradictory – especially in the way CofN chaplains tend to talk about it. Most of them stress that they first and foremost are professionals who carry their unique competence inherited through Clinical Pastoral Education (CPE) and through experience. They are qualified, as they talk of it, to meet all kinds of people, something that is described like this by one chaplain:

> Competence is an absolute demand. We are hired on competence, not on our belief. We have an education on world views and health, and we are supposed to take care of this for all patients. Our education is supposed to make us capable to see, understand and meet (clients) [...] (*Hospital chaplain F, CofN).*

Chaplains are, as spelled out here by a CofN chaplain, hired on competence, on their dialogical capability to address difficult existential matters meeting patients, regardless of who the patient is and what she believes in. CofN chaplain F tends to position belief contradictory to competence, an approach underlined by the words: "hired on competence, not on our belief". Others are more ambivalent or nuanced, as one CofN chaplain puts it: "I believe. I am a clergy after all". Approached like this, belief is underlined as an important asset in the professional job they do as hospital chaplains. It is linked to their position as believers and to their position as ordained by or representatives of their religious community. This is, however, an asset talked about as important to handle wisely as part of their professional work. Something that is expressed in different ways in the interviews, sometimes while underlining that they do not preach; they are not directive in that way. Here are two chaplains:

> [...] I can't have salvation from evil for people facing death as my main motivation. That would have made me crazy (laughs) if I considered that as my responsibility. There are, however, Christian gospels/beliefs resonating like that, holding it as the most important. And it might be important to me, as well, beneath a lot of layers, but not in the professional job I do. [...] (*Hospital chaplain W2, CofN)*

> [...] you know, I believe in a great God who is tolerant. We are allowed respecting the beliefs of each other. But if you had asked me, as a Christian, I would have wished that the whole world was becoming Christians. Because I have a comforting belief and feel that Jesus is my best friend. But as a hospital chaplain, I think that what is most important is to take care of and meet the needs they (patients and their next of kin) have. And I am willing to go an extra mile when it comes to that, because that is – if you ask me – what is most important. [...] (*Hospital chaplain D2, CofN)*

These two chaplains reflect on how a task of proselytizing in one way is built into who they are as Christians and as clergy. They experience their own belief as a benefit, as something they find support and comfort in – and something they love to share with others. But, as both these CofN chaplains underline in their interpretations of their mandates, this is not the main part of the professional job they are supposed to do as hospital chaplains. This is explicitly underlined in the last quote, where the chaplain pinpoints that their mandate is to meet the patient and to figure out what the patient needs; a practice focusing the other, in a non-directive way. Meetings with patients and their next of kin are underlined by all the interviewees as vitally important, some even described them as almost sacred meetings.

Hospital chaplains and patients ideally relate to each other in an open and mutual way. If such a meeting is not possible to create, it might be that no relationship is established. This might be due to lack of personal chemistry (I will get back to that). But first and foremost, it depends, chaplains argue, on the chaplain's ability as a professional, on their ability to be open, respectful, humble and inquisitive in order to reveal the needs of the other person. Sometimes patients are not fully aware of their needs and the meeting is a golden opportunity to search for it. Sometimes the conversations do not encompass God, belief or religion in any way; sometimes it is "only" a patient who wants to tell the story of his life, to reflect on difficult close relationships, or to talk about existential questions not involving religion. But sometimes the conversation comprises God, belief, or religion. This might be because the patient explicitly highlights these subjects. Some chaplains emphasise that they do not bring belief into the conversation unless the patient does. But it might also be the chaplain who brings religion into the conversation without a "signal" from the patient. Here is one chaplain reflecting:

> [...] To intercede for someone (gå i forbønn), it is quite surprisingly many who either signal or who agree when I find it natural to bring it up. They want me to do so, even if they do not define themselves as Christians or religious. They are more kind of Christians because of the crisis. Or they agree to light a candle. But I am a bit careful to suggest it. I need to be confident that the patient finds it all right. (*Hospital chaplain Y2, CofN)*

The quote illustrates situations where chaplains are the ones who put God on the agenda. This is, however, addressed as something that needs to be done very carefully, without being insistent or intrusive. Some CofN-chaplains describe how they might say something like: "You know I am a clergy, is there anything you want me to do?" The reasons for bringing this into the conversation are several. One is a perceived lack of spiritual language among people, a kind of embarrassment concerning God and religion. The patient may not know whether they need or want to talk about belief or do symbolic things like lighting a candle. Or it might be that God is needed because a crisis has occurred. But a tendency to hint at belief and/or symbolic practices also concerns who the chaplains perceive themselves to be in the relationship and the tools they keep in reserve: They are the ones who carry hope, who carry God and belief with them. Although it is underlined in the interviews that it is often difficult to tell how they, as hospital chaplains, are interpreted by others, they tend to think that patients are well aware of their role as members of the clergy. One CofN-chaplain talks about how some patients, for example, mention angels in the conversation in a way they perhaps would not have brought up while relating to any other kind of professional:

> [...] I think that, even if I do not believe in angels – at least not very much – I think that this is part of the symbolic universe of a Christian culture and a Muslim culture as well, this is part of their tradition. A lot of people believe in angels and relate to angels. Angels might mean a lot of things. Many carry this picture of an angel watching you, like the picture you used to have beside your bed as a child. Angels are related to safety, and I think it is part of the symbolic universe I as a clergyman carry with me, even if I do not mention it at all. But because I am a clergyman, it is with me [...]. *(Hospital chaplain H1, CofN)*

Even if this hospital chaplain does not mention God and religion and angels, this is something he expects people to think is possible to bring into a conversation with him. The chaplain expects people to expect that these themes are part of his mandate, something he can handle based on the toolbox in a chaplain's disposition. Chaplains tend to think that these are expectations making it natural to bring religious matters into the conversation for patients, and from such a viewpoint it is also plausible for chaplains to bring religion into the agenda.

CofN-chaplains report a tendency among patients who have asked for or agreed to meet the chaplain to underline that they are not very religious. Patients tend to refer to their belief from childhood (in Norwegian: *barnetro*), they talk about how they are baptized and have married in church, how they used to pray in the evenings, but still – that they perceive themselves as not that religious, or only a little religious. Chaplains interpret this way of talking as a kind of religious embarrassment and as a need for religious privacy considered common among Norwegian Lutherans. I will argue that an additional interpretation is possible: That this is a way to ask the chaplain whether they qualify as Christians, whether their belief is sustainable and good enough. CofN chaplains are, in my interpretation, read as religious authorities by the patient, as someone who is in a position not just to carry God with them, but to know how God resonates. The tendency among the interviewed chaplains is not to step back and refuse to be an authority on such matters. They tend to meet these questions with reassurances that all kinds of belief are good enough. Indirectly, they accept their position as religious authorities, although these incidents are not talked about as situations where they exercise or display authority. When they explicitly talk about being religious authorities, it is usually as part of narratives involving sacraments.

Sometimes chaplains are asked for advice. This might – as we have seen earlier – be practical advice, but it might also be ethical questions: What is right and wrong? How ought a person to live the rest of their life? Chaplains talk about how they respond by giving practical advice, but also by attempting to activate belief as a mastering tool. The patient's image of/relation to God is brought to the fore. Sometimes this is a relation that is experienced as good by the patient, sometimes it is experienced as bad. If it is bad, then it is necessary to change or reform or adjust it. Some chaplains tell how they reflect together with the patient on how it is possible to use belief as an asset, how it is possible to activate resources the patient inherits. This might include praying for, or together with, the patient, blessings, confessions and on some occasions (for chaplains from the CofN) Communion. These are talked about as powerful "tools" brought into the meeting by the patient or by the chaplain. However, they usually ask patients or their next of kin for permission:

> [...] Sometimes, a few times, I am allowed to be clergy and confessor. It is seldom, but it happens. [...] (*Hospital chaplain D2, CofN)*

Are there differences when it comes to being religious authorities, comparing CofN and Muslim chaplains? Are Muslims chaplains more directive based on religious tradition, more eager to give concrete advice? When it comes to focusing on law and legal interpretation of the Qur'an I find a tendency in my interviews with Muslim chaplains to emphasize this. For example, one voluntary Muslim conversation partner underlines how on several occasions he has been asked (by hospital staff) to come to wards to clarify in disagreements between patient and health professionals:

> [...] A classic is Ramadan and medicalization. The patient needs to get his medicine at the exact time, and then the patient wishes to fast at the same time. And then a dilemma occurs ... and then I have been asked to come to talk to the patient and the next of kin and tell them that it is ok, you can do it (to fast) when you are getting better, now it is your health and getting well that have to be first priority. (*Hospital chaplain, E2, Muslim)*

The Muslim chaplain is asked to come to talk to the patient. The mission, the reason why health professionals ask him to come, is the need to sort out a difficult situation at the hospital ward. Hospital staff find that they lack authority on a religious matter. Consequently, they need to get someone the patient and the patient's family will listen to. This concrete hospital had no Muslim chaplain among their employees and the voluntary Muslim chaplain was asked to come. Entering the disagreement, it turns out that this chaplain inherits the kind of authority required. How this is achieved in relation to the patient, on what grounds, is not elaborated on when he talks about such occurrences. However, the chaplain reports that when he arrives as a Muslim chaplain, patients often tend to think that he is an imam. At least he thinks that they think he is an imam. And although he is not, he usually does not tell them. Anyway, he has the authority – and I interpret it as traditional, in addition to the legal authority he inherits from being paged by hospital staff as a Muslim chaplain. The paging is important, because an important reason for Muslim chaplains to be preoccupied with giving legal advice based on their religious expertise is that this is asked for by hospital staff. They are explicitly asked to be traditional religious experts because that is what the hospital needs in some patient encounters. Sometimes, when there are critical situations and no Muslim chaplain is available, hospital staff ask a CofN chaplain to come and solve the problem via law and a legal interpretation of the Qur'an. That might work as well, but then the CofN chaplain acts based on knowledge about Muslim belief (a kind of professional and legal authority) not on their own belief or authority inherited through tradition. These situations differ from those where they face patients who want a Christian chaplain's opinion on their status as believers.

Charismatic authority: Partly personality, partly expertise

Finally, we turn to charismatic authority. This is the most mysterious kind of authority the way Weber describes it. It rests on the individual person and the person's sanctity, heroism (something done/achieved) and character. Weber refers to it as a gift of grace. As a gift of grace, it can be considered as granted to some, but not to others. At the same time, Weber underlines, that this is dependent on trust – a kind of personal trust individuals must struggle to inherit. In that way it is not given, it needs to be activated or constructed. When I ask about their chaplaincy practices, there is a tendency among the interviewees to state that they "use" themselves. To use oneself differs from using legal position, pastoral care techniques or traditional religious authority. What is it that they use when they use themselves? In the following quote from an interview, the interviewer (me) and a CofN chaplain elaborate on this:

> CofN chaplain, I1: [...] You need to be present as a person, in the situation. [...] I often think, what is my competence? Well, I am a theologian and therefor I have conducted an extensive program of professional study. I have studied other subjects as well and I have worked as a clergywoman in a congregation and now ... here. But then I think ... that it (the things she does) is not in a way possible to ... it can't be formalized, it's just there. I tend to think that I do not know very much, but then I get these responses; it was good, it was really important that you asked those questions, it was just so good that you were present with those people, or they managed to calm down when you had visited and talked with them. So, I think ... I do not know what it is that I am good at, but I am.
>
> Interviewer: A bit like riding a bicycle?
>
> CofN chaplain, I1: Yes, a bit like that ... and when you ask, what do you say to them? Well, what *am I* saying? When I have greeted people and looked them straight into their eyes, then it just goes on ... in a way. It starts where it starts. I do not know what I am saying ... actually.
>
> Interviewer: And at the same time, you know, because as you have told me: You need to be really present, something can't just slip out.
>
> CofN chaplain, I1: No, it can't for sure. And I am pretty conscious asking open questions, giving people a possibility to "go and get" some of the things they are struggling with and thinking about, if they want to share it. [...]

In the conversation we – the chaplain and the interviewer – try to capture what it is that makes this chaplain good, what it is that makes patients and hospital staff telling her that her presence is important. This is talked about like trying to capture and name something that can't be captured. It can't be "formalized", she says – "it's just there". Chaplain I1 talks about a capacity that is present and real, in a rather general and abstract way. But many interviewees, Muslim and CofN chaplains alike, use examples when they talk about their practices, sometimes to illustrate typical or difficult situations and questions, but also to present a kind of best practice. I do not interpret this as bragging or something they do to "sell in" chaplaincy in hospitals, I rather interpret it as a technique to explain to me something that is difficult to put into concrete words. An example is a Muslim chaplain who tells about a patient who reassured him, when he entered the patient room, that she "knew everything about Islam" and "that she had told the nurses that she did not need anyone to talk to". But, the patient added, "since this was what the Muslim chaplain did for a living, he was welcome to sit down and talk to her". A rather unwelcoming start, but after five minutes, the chaplain explains: "She told me the story of her life". When I ask him to elaborate, he explains:

> [...] She did not know who I was. It's not enough to tell them that you are a conversation partner and that's it. It is no use thinking; that is what it takes to create safety necessary to talk to me about almost everything. That is not the way it works, unfortunately. We humans, we are all different and we need time. But the minute she understood that this is someone who is completely independent, he does not care about who I am and what I do and ... he is present only in order to listen to me. He is here to me ... then she started to tell. (*Hospital chaplain B2, Muslim)*

Based on the story of the patient who did not need to talk to anyone, but who ended up telling the Muslim chaplain the story of her life, the more abstract considerations of chaplain I1 and the quote in the introduction, it is possible to trace a couple of marks distinctive to these chaplains and their practices. The CofN chaplain quoted in the introduction talks about being not any chaplain, but the chaplain *he is* – the watertight one. All three touch trust and safety as notions in need of construction, not present when they enter the room, but possible to construct in the relation. They "use" themselves and who they are, their personality as well as a trained intuition. This is perhaps why Weber writes about charisma as a gift of grace in need of activating. But there is more to it, they activate distinctive techniques using time and patience to signal an ambition to be present and to listen, having no other agenda. To be able to communicate this, can be interpreted as a kind of expertise, possible to learn and cultivate. It is about a genuine interest in the other person, about asking open questions (and not fearing any reply or follow-up questions), about strength and inner security – an ability to be beside other people when life is at its most difficult. Interpreted like that, the x-factor of charismatic authority is also a technique. Something it is possible to learn and train to be proficient in.

Concluding discussion

The questions posed in the introduction concerned how Norwegian hospital chaplains reflect on their authority in relating to staff and patients in a multi-faith setting. Secondly, whether there are differences in how CofN chaplains (in majority) compared to Muslim chaplains (in minority) relate to authority.

Norwegian hospital chaplains shape their work relating to staff and patients in a religiously plural setting. They need to be recommended (by staff) and asked for (by patients). This is an institutional fact placing them in a position where they need to build authority in one way or another. An important question is how they legitimize a role as an expert in a context and a time when people's belief is chosen, not inherited. Hospital chaplains not necessarily inherit authority as automatically attached to their position.

In the introductory quote, a CofN chaplain is concerned about the personal factor: He wants staff to know him and to perceive him as good with the patients. The reference to the personal factor points to charisma as an important asset, a kind of grace or intuition or x-factor, but at the same time – as we have seen – techniques and part of training, an expertise. To be watertight is also to be a convincing professional, someone who identifies what is needed and who is capable of handling it. Chaplaincy work is, however, professional work without an accurate manual. The personal factor is assets chaplains carry with them in their professional work, their way of relating to people of faith and those who do not know what to believe in.

Traditional authority is easily applicable when the leaders at hand are spiritual, being part of a tradition of spiritual leadership. This might be the way the spiritual part of religious leadership and authority is historically portrayed. Those who are clergy in the CofN also have legal authority as employees in the hospital institution; they are part of Norwegian hospital history, of a tradition where first Roman Catholic and then Protestant clergymen were important cornerstones in the first caring hospitals, forerunners to the curing hospitals. When the very first curing hospital with a national mandate (Rikshospitalet) where established in the Norwegian capital almost two hundred years ago, the group of employees included two professors in medicine, two physicians, four candidates (physicians to be) and an hospital chaplain (additionally, administrative personal and those who should look after the patients during the day) (Evensen 2017). When curing hospitals were established, medical and theological professions where both present. Hospital chaplains from the CofN have been present since. But the hospital environment and the role of religion as part of it, has changed tremendously – making traditional authority less important. Hospital CofN chaplains as of today are required to have theological academic education (as they always have had) but they are also required to have additional training and professional expertise in spiritual and existential care, *and* they are ordained as clergy by the Church. As a vicar/pastor in a protestant Church, they are preachers, managers of sacraments and rituals and spiritual advisers.[9] They are religious leaders by law. The interviewed CofN chaplains tend to downplay their traditional authority compared to their legal – and especially the professional part of their legal authority. This may be interpreted as caused by the environment they work in, health workers are professional workers, building their authority on their professional expertise. CofN-chaplains underline that so are they. Additionally, focusing professional capacity is focusing on the entrance requirement (cf. Leseth & Solbrække 2011) to the chaplain profession. That said, CofN-chaplains are also aware that they are framed and approached as clergy by patients, positioning them as someone possible to talk to on spiritual and existential questions. They tend to underline how they differ from other health professionals, having a guiding and supporting role as complementary or counter to the curing role.

Traditional authority, as Weber ([1947]1995) coined the term, is plausible to interpret as working through a directive approach to patients. However, as we have seen, it does not need to be so in a plural and individualized setting. When chaplains from the CofN meet with patients who underline that they are not very religious, and in that way indirectly ask the chaplain to evaluate their belief, chaplains take on the role as evaluators. But they do this in a rather non-directive way, by reassuring people that there are no definite standards attached to belief. They act, in such relations, as religious authorities, an authority not easy to frame as based on their clinical pastoral care education. Their practice as trusted evaluators are more likely to rely on their traditional authority as clergy.

Muslim chaplains who are imams or have other positions/roles in Muslim communities and mosques, lack a formal legal confirmation as religious leaders in a Norwegian context. Although some of them have had some official training in spiritual and existential care, they have not had permission to Clinical Pastor-

9 https://snl.no/prest (read 15.11.20).

al Education (CPE). Compared to their Lutheran colleagues, Muslim chaplains in a Norwegian context are more dependent on traditions when it comes to authority construction. Most of them lack a formal position as hospital staff and the professional requirements attached to it, both important assets to legal authority. They are however, by patients who are not that into formal legal requirements, often interpreted as part of the hospital institution – since they are send for by hospital staff and have a kind of position in the institution. Still, when Muslim chaplains are trusted on their legal advice, it seem to be part of the traditional authority patients, their families and staff ascribe to them as religious leaders. This is an authority not caused by formalized education or their capacity as hospital employee – they might lack both – but in their position as part of a Muslim tradition, as an imam (some are), as part of a specific mosque or religious community.

Gilliat-Ray et al. (2013) have done empirical research on Muslim chaplaincy in institutions in the UK and state that "there is no formal institutional tradition of pastoral care in Islam" (ibid, 2), a point of departure making it important how the interviewed Muslim chaplains understand what they do in their capacity as chaplains. Gilliat-Ray et al. (2013) find that Christian and Muslims chaplaincy practices are very much alike – in a UK context. They are both influenced by an assumption that public spaces and institutions "will not be used to evangelize or coerce captive or needy people into particular belief systems" (ibid. 169). The focus of their work "lies with supporting people as they cope with the realities of institutional life, and the challenges of illness, death, imprisonment or other transitions" (ibid. 173). This is pretty much in line with what I find in the Norwegian hospital context – comparing Christian protestant and Muslim chaplains. However, Gilliat-Ray et al. (2013) argue that there are also differences when Muslim and Christian practices and understandings are compared: one being that Muslim chaplains more often need to facilitate a range of Islamic practices, another that Muslim chaplains more often have to explain their role to others, and a third that Muslim chaplains often have a distinctive focus on law and legal interpretation of the Qur'an, while Christian chaplains are not so concerned about "correct" belief or practice (ibid. 169).

I find that the Muslim chaplains interviewed in a Norwegian context often are asked (by hospital staff) to interpret what is said by laws and written texts, while CofN chaplains more seldom are asked to do the same. It can be considered as two rather different things to reassure a patient that there are no particular faith standards versus interpreting religious "laws" on for example how to fast. But CofN and Muslim interviewees share a rather pragmatic stance. They are eager to interpret the needs of the patient and the needs produced in each situation, such as disagreements on medical treatment. They also share how religious questions and ponderings seem to be close at hand when patients address them – compared to when patients address others among hospital staff. This might be because of the professional capabilities of chaplains – they know the Bible and the Quran, they know rituals and symbols, they know prayers, and patients know that they know. They are religious professionals. But there is more to it. The example of CofN chaplains being asked about texts in the Qu'ran, or about Muslim rituals, illustrates this. When CofN chaplains are asked about Muslim matters, they are asked in their capacity as religious professionals (in a legal capacity), not as an authority managing religious traditions and history. When a Muslim chaplain is asked, he is addressed – or so it seems – as both a professional and a traditional authority on religious matters. More the latter than the former, since legalized professional training as a Muslim chaplain – in line with the training CofN chaplains get – is not possible to achieve in a Norwegian context.

This is an important point to make, because as Gilliat Ray et.al. (2013) underlines, the context, the institutional frames chaplains work "inside" influences their practices and how they understand their role. Muslim chaplains in a Norwegian context are bound to be more dependent on their traditional authority. This is due to their weak legal position in hospital institutions compared to their colleagues from the CofN. Muslim chaplains are in minority and they also lack the legal position CofN chaplains have, since they are engaged in part time positions or as lay chaplains (conversation partners).

Chaplains work in a context and with people who tend to live religion not by the book, but by the needs and existential ponderings in difficult situations. To be trusted as an authority in these relations seem to activate all the three kinds of authority. Chaplains (in my interviews) are hospital employees or part of a formalized group of volunteers at the hospital, and they all have *some* education and formalized training making them professionals. Their legal authority rests on these credentials. Chaplains are also spiritual leaders activating a heritage from their predecessors and carrying along hope but also sacred insights. Their traditional authority is made up of this. Finally, chaplains are persons with their own individual way of relating to people but also with a particular need to train and activate their individual way of relating to others, to hone their ability to be a fellow human being. Their charismatic authority rests on this activation.

To be a hospital chaplain does not rely on only one of these parts of authority, it relies on all three. This goes for Muslim as well as CofN chaplains. But, due to their different possibilities to obtain formal education and qualify as employees, they are given different chances to capitalize on legal authority, a fact making traditional authority more important to Muslim chaplains as part of hospital institutions.

Reference list

Bondevik, Hilde, Ole Jacob Madsen, and Kari Nyheim Solbrække. 2017. "Snart er vi alle pasienter: Medikalisering i Norden fra vugge til grav." In: Hilde Bondevik, Ole Jacob Madsen, and Kari Nyheim Solbrække (eds.) *Snart er vi alle pasienter: Medikalisering i Norden.* Oslo: Scandinavian Academic Press/Spartacus forlag AS.

Boelsbjerg, Hanne Bess. 2013. "Det Hellige Rum. Sjælesorgssamtaler på hospitalet." *Tidsskrift for forskning i sykdom og samfund* 18: 67–86.

Braun, Virgina, and Victoria Clarke. 2013. *Successful Qualitative Research: A practical guide for beginners.* London, Thousand Oaks, New Delhi, Singapore: Sage.

Bråten, Beret. 2019. "Døden – et kirkelig anliggende? " In: Lisbeth Thoresen, and Birgitta Haga Gripsrud (eds.) *Alt som lever må dø.* Oslo: Scandinavian Academic Press.

Cadge, Wendy. 2012. *Paging God: Religion in the Halls of Medicine.* Chicago, London: The University of Chicago Press.

Coble, Richard. 2018. *The Chaplain's Presence and Medical Power: Rethinking Loss in Hospital System.* Lanham, Boulder, New York, London: Lexington Books.

Evensen, Stein. 2017. "Militærhospitalet som ble rikshospital." *Tidsskrift for den norske legeforening* 23/24. DOI: 10.4045/tidsskr.17.0567

Davie, Grace. 2015. *Religion in Britain: A Persistent Paradox.* Oxford: Wiley Blackwell.

Davie, Grace. 2013. *The Sociology of Religion: A Critical Agenda.* London, Thousand Oaks, New Delhi, Singapore: Sage Publications.

Gilliat-Ray, Sophie, Ali Mansur, and Stephan Pattison. 2013. *Understanding Muslim Chaplaincy.* Farnham, Burlington: Ashgate.

Gilliat-Ray, Sophie. 2018. "Afterword: Religion in Public Institutions. Methodological Challenges, Institutional Comparisons, and Key Variables." *Journal of Religion in Europe* 11: 186–194.

Grung, Anne Hege, and Beret Bråten. 2019. "Chaplaincy in the Norwegian context: Towards a process of pluralization." *Nordic Journal of Practical Theology* 2, Special edition on chaplaincy. Oslo: Luther Forlag.

Henriksen, Jan-Olav. 2017 [2012]. "Makt og avmakt bland ledere i Den Norske Kirke." In: Cora Alexa Døving, and Berit Thorbjørnsrud (eds.) *Religiøse ledere: Makt og avmakt i norske trossamfunn.* Oslo: Universitetsforlaget.

Johnson, John M. 2001. "In-depth interviewing." In: Jaber F. Gubrium, amd James A. Holstein (eds.) *Handbook of Interview Research: Context and Method.* Thousand Oaks: Sage Publication Inc.

Kühle, Lene, and Henrik Reintoft Christensen. 2019. "One to serve them all. The growth of chaplaincy in public institutions in Denmark." *Social Compass* 66/2: 182–197. DOI:10.1177/0037768619833310

Kühle, Lene, Ulla Schmidt, Brian Arly Jacobsen, amd Per Petterson. 2018. "Religion and State. Complexity in Change." In: Inger Furseth (ed.) *Religious Complexity in the Public Sphere.* London, New York: Palgrave Macmillan.

Leirvik, Oddbjørn. 2017 [2012]. “Alliansebygging, maktkamp og dialog mellom religiøse leiarar.” In: C.A. Døving, and B. Thorbjørnsrud (eds.) *Religiøse ledere: Makt og avmakt i norske trossamfunn.* Oslo: Universitetsforlaget.
Leseth, Anne, and Kari Nyheim Solbrække. 2011. “Profesjon, kjønn og etnisitet.” In: Anne Leseth, and Kari Nyheim Solbrække (eds.) *Profesjon, kjønn og etnisitet.* Oslo: Cappelen Damm Akademisk.
Liefbroer, Anke I., R. Ruard Ganzevoort, and Erik Olsman. 2019. “Addressing the spiritual domain in a plural society: What is the best mode of integrating spiritual care into healthcare.” In: Anke I. Liefbroer. 2020. *Interfaith spiritual care.* PhD thesis, Vrije Universiteit Amsterdam.
Nordin, Magdalena. 2018. “Blurred Religion in Contemporary Sweden: Health Care Institutions as an Empirical Example.” *Journal of Religion in Europe* 11: 161–185.
NOU 2017:16 *På liv og død. Palliasjon til alvorlig syke og døende.*
NOU 2013:1 *Det livssynsåpne samfunn. En helhetlig tro og livssynspolitikk.*
Okkenhaug, Berit. 2002. *Når jeg ser ditt ansikt: Innføring i kristen sjelesorg.* Verbum Forlag.
Schmidt, Ulla. 2010. “Norge: Et religiøst pluralistisk samfunn.” In: P.K. Botvar, and Ulla Schmidt (eds.) *Religion i dagens Norge: Mellom sekularisering og sakralisering.* Oslo: Universitetsforlaget.
Scott, Richard W. 2008. *Institutions and Organizations: Ideas and Interests.* Third edition. Thousand Oaks: Sage Publications.
Stifoss-Hansen, Hans, Lars Johan Danbolt, and Hilde Frøkedal. 2019. “Chaplaincy in Northern Europe. An overview from Norway.” *Nordic Journal of Practical Theology* 2, Special edition on chaplaincy. Oslo: Luther Forlag.
Stifoss-Hansen, Hans, Anne Hege Grung, Anne Austad, and Lars Johan Danbolt. 2019. “Sjelesorg i bevegelse. Kerygmatisk, konfidentorientert, dialogisk sjelesorg – møte mellom teoretiske posisjoner og et empirisk materiale.” *Tidsskrift for Sjelesorg* 1.
Walderhaug, Marianne Frøystad. 2018. *Filosofiske samtaler med innsatte i fengsel. En fordypning i samtalens form og innhold.* PhD. The University of Bergen.
Weber, Max. 1990 [1922]. *Makt og byråkrati* [Power and Bureucracy]. Oslo: Gyldendal.
Weber, Max. 1995 [1947]. “Fundamental Concepts of Sociology and Types of Authority.” In: Floya Anthias, and Michael P. Kelly (eds.) *Sociological Debates: Thinking about “the social”.* Dartford: Greenwich University Press.
Woodhead, Linda. 2013. “Liberal religion and illiberal secularism.” In: Gavin D’Costa, Malcolm Evans, Tariq Modood, and Julian Rivers (eds.) *Religion in a liberal state.* Cambridge: Cambridge University Press.

Carola Roloff

Buddhist Chaplaincy and Care Practices

Abstract: This article introduces Buddhist chaplaincy and care practices and briefly analyses the field's current state. Taking mindfulness as an example, I discuss what it means to be a Buddhist chaplain or caregiver and argue that Buddhists of different denominations have much in common, while their views and practices may differ.

I give insight into the practices and rituals that are helpful in existential crises, conflict, disease, and death when religious belonging becomes essential, and discuss Buddhist chaplaincy in contemporary societies.

Practices rooted in Buddhist teachings such as mindfulness and meditation strongly influence the development of secular – but Buddhism is far more than that. It not only means transforming our minds, attitudes, and behaviour, but also developing insight into reality and other essential virtues Buddhist chaplains need to cultivate.

Introduction into Buddhist Chaplaincy

Buddhist chaplaincy or Buddhist care is spiritual care that is "Buddhadharma-based", i.e., based on the teachings of the historical Buddha and the three main Buddhist traditions: Theravāda, East Asian and Tibetan Buddhism. Common to these traditions is compassion and "the call to live with death, to look behind the facade of life into the mirror of death" (Heller 2012, 62). The concept of "Buddhist care" as professionalised vocational spiritual care is a relatively young movement that began in the 1950s to 1980s but is present worldwide today.

Buddhist centres and umbrella organizations in Europe are increasingly receiving requests to assist people in difficult life situations. Depending on the tradition, Buddhist spiritual care includes visiting sick Buddhists at home or in hospitals, meditating with them, and accompanying them with prayers or special rituals (*pūjās*). Furthermore, it includes giving instructions for meditation in preparation for the dying process (end-of-life care), organizing Buddhist funeral ceremonies, and to perform after death rituals for the transition to a so-called "pure land" or for a good rebirth. Some Buddhists (lay and monastics) are trained as physicians, counsellors, or therapists. From this context, the question of the Buddhist attitude towards active or passive euthanasia may also arise. We can assume that Buddhists are not all of the same opinion here, and that the de-

 https://doi.org/10.1515/9783110717365-004

cision about euthanasia cannot be tied to any Buddhist tradition either. Within each Buddhist tradition, you will find the full spectrum of opinions.[1]

Another question is, how chaplaincy or spiritual care are understood and defined, what these terms include and how they are limited, for example in contrast to therapy. The boundaries seem to be fluid, especially between systemic counselling and systemic therapy. Next to them there are also three other great traditions, i.e., depth psychology, behavioural psychology and humanistic psychotherapy.

In the following, I will concentrate on traditional Buddhist care and its roots at the time of the Buddha. Then, taking mindfulness as an example, I will discuss what distinguishes Buddhist chaplains from secular chaplains or chaplains of other religious traditions. Which particular skills do they need to counsel Buddhists, i.e., what are the most important teachings, views and tools they need to know and be aware of, when functioning as chaplains? Next, I will investigate the question of what strengths and resources Buddhism can draw from to deal with existential crises and briefly discuss various kinds of Buddhist chaplaincy present in contemporary societies. Finally, I will come to my conclusion and to perspectives for Buddhist chaplaincy raising questions such as: When is belonging to this religious tradition essential? What can interreligious spiritual care learn from Buddhism? What can Buddhism learn from Christian and other religious or secular ways of counselling, and finally, how do I assess the future of interreligious spiritual care?

How do Buddhists traditionally care for each other?

The traditional care for others goes back to the Buddha himself and can be found in the canonical texts of Buddhism. Monks and nuns were active as spiritual caregivers, or spiritual friends (Skt. *kalyāṇamitra/-mitrā*), literally, virtuous or good friend, caring for each other, and their disciples, monastic and lay. But before I go deeper into this, let us first take a brief look at the Buddha and his teaching. He is the main source of trust for Buddhists and gives them orientation throughout life.

---

1 In general, different from the Catholic Church, Buddhism does not have a central overarching hierarchy with a spiritual leader who can speak with one voice for all Buddhist traditions (cf. Roloff 2014, 251) and below.

The Life of the Buddha

The birth name of the Buddha was Siddhārtha Gautama. He was born about 5th century B.C.E[2] at Lumbinī in present-day Nepal as an Indian prince of the Śākya clan, belonging to the Kṣatriya caste, the caste of warriors and nobles. This means he was born as a Hindu. After his enlightenment he became known as Buddha Śākyamuni, the wise of the Śākyas. He married at the age of 16, and left home at the age of 29 to seek spiritual knowledge. At the age of 35, he attained buddhahood or Nirvāṇa through meditation. After his enlightenment, the Buddha gave his first teaching in Sarnath close to Benares. At the age of 80, after 45 years of teaching, he passed away in Kuśīnagar and thus attained *parinirvāṇa*, often translated as final enlightenment. Thus "Buddha" is not a name, but an honorary title, which means "the awakened", or "enlightened". The term derives from the Sanskrit root *budh*, which means to realise, to experience, to wake.

When you visit the Buddha's pilgrimage places, you will find out that his birth, his buddhahood, his turning the wheel of the dharma, and his entrance into Parinirvāṇa are regarded as the major four stages of his life. For our topic Buddhist chaplaincy, however, the most important stage is Siddhārtha Gautama's renunciation of worldly life, or rather, what prompted him to take this step.

The Buddha's encounter with reality: old age, sickness, and death

What caused Siddhārtha's renouncing a life of pleasure? It was his encounter with realities that are familiar to many of us. During four excursions outside his father's palace, he was confronted by the sight of an old man, a sick man, and a corpse, followed by his encounter with a religious mendicant. Siddhārtha wondered why there is this suffering in the world, and decided to seek the truth, to understand things as they are. His desire for release from the suffering in *sāṃsāra*, the endless cycle of involuntary rebirth, is called renunciation.

2 The Buddha's dates are not known with certainty. The current scholarly consensus is that he died between 410–400 B.C.E.

The Buddha's enlightenment and his core teaching

Siddhārtha went to Bodhgayā and sat down for meditation under a Banyan Tree. What did he experience? In a state of deep meditation he obtained three kinds of 'true knowledge': 1. the power to see back into his past lives; 2. the ability to see not just his own lives, but the decease and arising of other beings in accordance with their good and bad *karma*; 3. the insight into the Four Noble Truths, namely into the noble truth of suffering (*duḥkha*), the noble truth of the origin (*samudaya*) of suffering, the noble truth of the cessation (*nirodha*) of suffering, the noble truth of the way (*marga*) leading to the cessation of suffering. (SN 56.13). Thus Siddhārtha awakened, and became a Buddha. He realised *nirvāṇā*, the end of suffering and its causes, and attained liberation (*mokṣa*) from *saṃsāra*. The Buddha's first sermon of Benares after his enlightenment, the "Discourse Setting the Wheel of the Dharma Rolling", Sanskrit "Dharmacakrapravartana Sūtra" (Frauwallner 2010, 13–15), Pāli "Dhammacakkappavatana Sūtta" (SN 56.11), is his core teaching of the four noble truth.[3]

Buddhism posits a basic equality of sentient beings as faced with suffering and in need of liberation (Harvey 2018). It is based on the Vedic Brahmanist and early Buddhist principle that "all beings recoil from pain and desire happiness" (Schmidt-Leukel 2006, 36).

Buddhist practice is mainly concerned with the Eightfold Path

The noble eightfold path, namely, right view, right thought or right resolve, right speech, right conduct or right action, right livelihood, right effort, right mindfulness, and right concentration or right meditation are considered to be the middle way that leads to enlightenment. These are summarised in three trainings (*śikṣā*). In that case, wisdom or insight (*prajñā*) appears at the end, for its final perfection is reached in enlightenment. Morality or ethics (*śīla*) marks the basis of all Buddhist practice and meditative concentration (*samādhi*) is signified by the absorption practices (*dhyāna*), which stand at the pinnacle of Buddhist meditation techniques (Schmidt-Leukel 2006: 136).

When the Buddha entered the *parinirvāṇa*, he did not appoint a successor. This explains, why until today the hierarchies in Buddhism are quite flat and the personal freedom of decision-making of Buddhists is relatively large. This is important to know for Buddhist care, especially when consulted on issues such as organ transplantation, abortion, or euthanasia. A question is, who is en-

---

3 For a detailed explanation see Nyānatiloka (1952, 3–11).

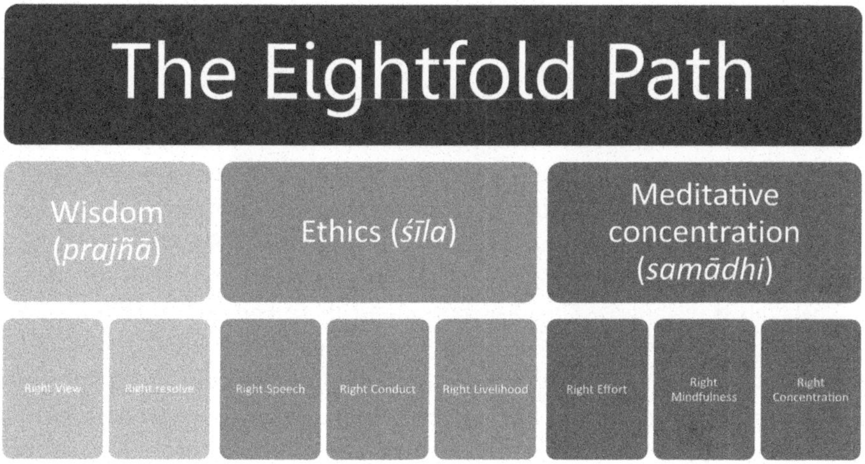

Fig. 1: The Eightfold Path.

titled to appoint Buddhist caregivers in countries where such appointment by a religious community is required by law. The fact that Buddhism does not have a "Christian-style" church does not mean that there is no religious institution in Buddhism. The Buddhist order (*saṅgha*) is traditionally referred to as the central institution of religious virtuosos, and contrasted with lay followers.[4] Four groups (*catuṣpariṣat*) constitute the Buddhist community/ parish: monks (*bhikṣu*), nuns (*bhikṣuṇī*), lay men (*upāsaka*), and lay women (*upāsikā*), whereby the translation "lay" is an unfortunate wording, because there are also professionally trained and Buddhist "lay" teachers and priests.

The Development of Buddhism in India, the Spread and the Varieties of Buddhism (Theravāda – Mahāyāna)

Today exist three mainstreams of Buddhism, which one could compare with three Buddhist denominations. These are: Theravāda Buddhism (3rd cent. BCE), East Asian Buddhism (1st/2nd cent. AD), and Tibetan Buddhism (7th/8th cent. AD). All three base themselves on the "Three Baskets" (Skt.: *Tripiṭaka*,

4 This is also pointed out by Freiberger 2011, 293.

Pā.: *Tipiṭaka*), the Buddhist canon: 1. Vinaya: Legal texts of the order, monastic discipline, 2. Sūtra: Discourses of the Buddha (and his discipleship), and 3. Abhidharma: Higher doctrine/ (systematic) philosophy. Although the label "Tripiṭaka" is the same, the content differs. There are different deliverances in different languages. Theravāda Buddhism is based on the Pāli canon including the Theravāda Vinaya. East Asian Buddhism is based on a Sanskrit/Gāndhārī canon and includes their main text, the Dharmaguptaka Vinaya. And Tibetan Buddhism is based on the Sanskrit Mūlasarvāstivāda canon including the Mūlasarvāstivāda Vinaya. The latter two versions of the *Tripiṭaka* are only complete in Chinese and Tibetan translations. Theories that one of these canonical collections is a kind of original canon, i.e., Ur canon or Ur Vinaya have been criticised and shown to be "almost certainly untenable" (Clarke 2004, 79). There are overlaps, similarities and differences, which makes intra-Buddhist dialogue both difficult and encouraging, as stated by Brahmapundit and Harvey (2017): "To increase awareness among Buddhists of their own rich heritage of religious and ethical thinking as well as to increase understanding among non-Buddhists of the fundamental values and principles of Buddhism" (Brahmapundit and Harvey 2017, vii). In 2017, a first print version of a book has been published that "seeks to strike a balance between what is common to the Buddhist traditions and the diversity of perspectives among them. It consists of selected translations from Pāli, Sanskrit, Chinese and Tibetan, using a common terminology in English of key Buddhist terms" (ibid.)

The common goal of all Buddhists, whether they belong to the Theravāda school, or to one of the major Mahāyāna schools (East Asian or Tibetan Buddhism), is that they seek liberation from rebirth in *saṃsāra* and ultimately want to attain *nirvāṇa*. The understanding what *nirvāṇa* means, partly differs. Theravāda Buddhists, in general, strive for personal liberation as *śrāvaka arhat*, while Mahāyāna Buddhists strive for the ideal of a *bodhisattva* and ultimately for buddhahood. They believe in celestial beings and in pure *buddha* lands such as Sukhāvatī. This leads to different notions of after death, important to understand when trained as a Buddhist chaplain, who wants to serve all Buddhists and not only Buddhists of his/her own tradition.

How is caring based in Buddhist root texts?

The traditional care for others goes back to the Buddha himself and can already be found in the canonical texts of Buddhism. The only canon which is completely preserved in an Indian language is the Pāli canon. Here we find for example the story of one ill, presented in the following section.

How the Buddha cares for a monk suffering from dysentery

Once the Buddha saw a monk lying in his own urine and feces and nobody cared about the sick. Together with his constant companion Ānanda, he washed and bedded him, then he let the order come together and advised them to care for the sick: "Monks, you have not a mother, you have not a father who might tend you. If you, monks, do not tend one another, then who is there who will tend you? Whoever, monks, would tend me, he should tend the sick". (Pli Tv Kd 8)[5]

Five skills of a caregiver taught by the Buddha

At the end of this story we find a list of five skills that a caregiver needs, taught by the Buddha himself: "Endowed with five qualities, monks, is one who tends the sick fit to tend the sick: he comes to be competent to provide the medicine; he knows what is beneficial and what is not beneficial; he takes away what is not beneficial, he brings forward what is beneficial; he tends the sick (from) amity of mind, not in the hope of gain; he does not become one who loathes to remove excrement or urine or sweat or vomit; he comes to be competent to gladden [...] delight the sick from time to time with dhamma-talk" (Pli Tv Kd 8).

Here, a holistic approach becomes evident, early Buddhist communities as well as contemporary communities take care of both the physical and psychological needs of the patient.

The story of Jīvaka, the model healer

In the same portion of the Theravāda Vinayapiṭaka, we also find the story of Jīvaka, the personal physician of the Buddha and the Indian King, who until today figures prominently as a model healer in several Asian countries. Accounts in all versions of the Vinaya tell us that Jīvaka, which means "he who is *alive*", was

5 On the Story of One Ill. Theravada Vinayapiṭaka, Khandhaka (Mahavagga) 8 Robes (Cīvara). The Book of the Discipline translated by I.B. Horner with supplementary translation by Bhikkhu Brahmali. Digital edition prepared for SuttaCentral by Bhikkhu Sujato. Published in 2014 by SuttaCentral, accessed May 1, 2022, https://suttacentral.net/pli-tv-kd8/en/horner-brahmali. For the reading of the original translation see Horner (1951, 433).

born as a foundling of a courtesan. As he grew up, Jīvaka decided to learn traditional medicine and to care for others. It is interesting to know that the Buddhist hospital care in the Vienna General Hospital (AKH) in Austria is named after Jīvaka.[6]

What does it mean to be a Buddhist counsellor, chaplain, or caregiver?

In Europe, especially in Western Europe, an increasing number of people nowadays turn away from churches and other religious institutions (Pollack 2008). In hospitals and hospices, as well as in cases of catastrophes, Christian pastoral chaplains do not only look after Christian church members, but after all people in need, regardless of their denomination. Thus, one may wonder whether it still makes sense to carry out confessional spiritual care. Furthermore, whether it makes sense to establish a new denominational pastoral care for "other" religions following the same model, or whether it would be better to train people from different denominations in interfaith and/or secular spiritual care.[7] In many European countries, the spiritual care is legally adjusted to a co-operation with recognised religious communities.[8] For this reason, denominational caregivers must usually be officially confirmed by religious communities.[9] Depend-

---

6 "Seelsorge und Besuchsdienst im Allgemeinen Krankenhaus Wien, Buddhistische Krankenbegleitung" (Pastoral care and visiting service in the Vienna General Hospital, Buddhist care for the sick), accessed May 1, 2022, https://www.akh-seelsorge.at/buddhistische-krankenbegleitung/.

7 Such approaches are e.g. developed by the society for intercultural pastoral care and counselling (SIPCC) for 25 years (Weiss et al. 2021).

8 Similarly for the United States Cadge et al. (2020, 194) highlight that: "Training in chaplaincy and a degree (either an MDiv or an MA) grants Muslim and Buddhist chaplaincy students legitimacy in civil society and qualifies them for professional religious service." With reference to Seager (1999) they claim that Buddhism has highly developed monastic traditions and a system of passing down wisdom through teaching lineages, but it does not have the kind of ordained or licensed leadership historically required to work in the military or federal prisons as a chaplain.

9 In Germany, the right to pastoral care is guaranteed by the Basic Law Art. 140 GG in conjunction with Art. 141 WRV: "To the extent that a need exists for religious services and pastoral work in the army, in hospitals, in prisons or in other public institutions, religious societies shall be permitted to provide them, but without compulsion of any kind." "Basic Law for the Federal Republic of Germany in the revised version published in the Federal Law Gazette Part III, classification number 100-1, as last amended by Article 1 of the Act of 29 September 2020 (Federal

ing on the legal frame and the concept of the actors in charge, it seems that Buddhist chaplains and caregivers can be found in both fields, in "confessional" Buddhist care as well as in "secular" spiritual care. There seems to be also a number of caregivers who consider themselves bi- or multi-religious, i.e., Christian and Buddhist and thus try to combine the best practices from each. This raises the question to what extent Buddhist care practices can be useful in different areas, in which cases spiritual care indispensably has to be Buddhist care, and how these possible approaches differ.

What makes a caregiver a Buddhist caregiver?

Buddhism is not only a religion. It also has a philosophical and a scientific dimension. Therefore, Buddhism is also increasingly interesting to undenominational Non-Buddhists. Due to the growing interest by psychology and medicine in Buddhist tools or practices like meditation techniques and mindfulness training, a dialogue between the Buddhist traditions and the sciences opened already in the 1980s. One of the largest global research projects that emerged from the International *Mind & Life* conferences[10] has been conducted since 2013 at the Max Planck Institute for Human Cognitive and Brain Sciences in Leipzig, Germany. Among other things, they investigate the effects Buddhist methods of training the mind have on the brain, on health, stress, wellbeing, and social behaviour. Meditation is also said to alleviate early symptoms of dementia and Alzheimer (Russell-Williams et al. 2018).

Before this, in 1979, following a Buddhist meditation technique, the molecular biologist Jon Kabat-Zinn at Massachusetts University developed a programme for stress management based on mindfulness. Clinical studies show that 'Mindfulness-Based Stress Reduction' (MBSR) helps to better deal with diseases, stress, fear, and depression. MBSR is applied in secular as well as confessional spiritual care (Esch 2021).

Spiritual care and hospice work are increasingly important contexts where Buddhists could serve much better and more effective care for Buddhists in need, if the public resources, especially legal entrances, were available. Meditations on death and transitoriness are well-developed Buddhist practices. On the one hand, it is a matter of living everyday as consciously as if it were one's last.

Law Gazette I p. 2048)", accessed May 2, 2022, https://www.gesetze-im-internet.de/englisch_gg/englisch_gg.html#p0825.

10 For observations into this dialogue see Luisi 2010.

On the other hand, many, although not all Buddhists believe in rebirth.[11] Therefore, Buddhist traditions have developed many procedures for accompanying people when they are dying. People should be able to say farewell as peacefully, free of pain, and consciously as possible. In many European countries, we find funeral homes, which offer Buddhist funeral services and/or have acquired special burial grounds to meet the need.

I now return to the question of what makes a caregiver a *Buddhist* caregiver. I would like to illustrate this with the example of mindfulness, an important, though not the only, tool for Buddhist caregivers.

What makes mindfulness a *Buddhist* mindfulness?

An important teaching of the Buddha is that the mind precedes all speaking and acting. Thus, it is said:

> All mental phenomena have mind as their forerunner; they have mind as their chief; they are mind-made. If one speaks or acts with an evil mind, suffering (*dukkha*) follows him just as the wheel follows the hoofprint of the ox that draws the cart.
>
> All mental phenomena have mind as their forerunner; they have mind as their chief; they are mind-made. If one speaks or acts with a pure mind, happiness (*sukha*) follows him like a shadow that never leaves him. (Dhammapada, verses 1 and 2, Daw Mya Tin 1993, 1)

Therefore, Buddhists consider view, intention, and motivation important.[12] In both mainstream traditions of Buddhism, Theravāda and Mahāyāna Buddhism, the practice of mindfulness includes not only introspection, but also working for the well-being of others and one's own well-being. Hence, these are mutually de-

---

11 Garfield (2022, 174) claims that the idea of *karma* which is central to Buddhist ethical thought "is not *essentially* tied to rebirth, although in the Indian and Tibetan Buddhist universe it always is (but not in East Asia, where rebirth does not play such a central role in most Buddhist traditions).

12 As McCormick (2013, 223) points out "[i]ntention plays such a large role in Buddhist ethics that Schlieter (2010) comments that it can be seen as 'intention[al]ist ethics'" Cf. Schlieter 2010, 359. Nevertheless, Jay L. Garfield would not agree to this. He argues that Buddhist ethics is a kind of moral phenomenology. See chapter 3 of his recent publication *Buddhist Ethics: A Philosophical Exploration* (Oxford University Press USA). Garfield shows "that the principal unifying strands in Buddhist moral philosophy – a focus on moral perception and experience as well as an emphasis on a path to moral cultivation and the transformation of character – arise from reflection on interdependence" (Garfield 2022, 3).

pendent. In *Saṃyutta Nikāya* 47.19 the Buddha says: "Protecting oneself [...] one protects others; protecting others, one protects oneself".

This Golden Rule of Theravāda Buddhism is followed by the Golden Rule of Mahāyāna Buddhism: Śāntideva (7/8th cent.) says in his *Bodhicāryāvatāra, Entering the Course Towards Awakening*, Ch. 8 "Perfection of Absorption":

> To calm my own suffering and to calm the suffering of others, I therefore offer myself to others and adopt others as myself. (BCA VIII 136)
>
> "I am connected to others." Assure yourself of that, my mind! Now you may think of nothing other than the benefit of all sentient beings. (BCA VIII 137)[13]

A broad understanding of the term mindfulness is that it refers to an inside and an outside, to 'being aware' as well as 'becoming aware'. Attention to oneself and others leads to an increased form of perception, i.e., seeing what is not obvious, it leads to openness, curiosity and is also an inquiring mind (Knauth and Roloff 2021).

In spiritual care it is important to be sensible when people express a need for religious care or spirituality, especially when it comes to dealing with existential crises, death and dying. Religion gives orientation to many people. When the question of what comes after death – or not – arises, it is difficult to be ideologically neutral and to ignore religion.

For people who have no religion Kabat-Zinn's "secular" approach may be helpful. In his view mindfulness means paying attention in a particular way, to be on purpose in the present moment and without judgment: "I define mindfulness operationally as the awareness that arises by paying attention on purpose, in the present moment, and non-judgmentally." (2013, Kindle, pos. 391)

In Buddhism, being present is considered the greatest gift. However, in addition, mindfulness, is part of the Eightfold path to liberation (see above), i.e., it is a central concept in the Buddha's discourses. Originally mindfulness meant only observing, not intervening, i.e., directing mindfulness to four objects/areas. The name of mindfulness practice is in Pāli "*satipaṭṭhāna*", Sanskrit "*smṛtyupasthāna*". This means "alignment or direction of mindfulness [to four objects/areas]", also translated as the four 'foundations of mindfulness', or the four 'bases' (starting points) of mindfulness (*sati* + *paṭṭhāna*), or better, "Maintaining to make something present" (*sati* + *upaṭṭhāna*), i.e., body, feelings or feeling tones, mind, and mind-objects or phenomena (Nyānatiloka 1999, 203; English version 1980, 307–311).

13 Translation by Ernst Steinkellner and Cynthia Peck-Kubaczek in Schmidt-Leukel 2019, 390.

The fourth step of meditation, directing mindfulness to mind-objects, is clearly linked with Buddhist worldview. But in general, the first goal of Buddhist mindfulness is to be present in every moment and to cultivate healing awareness of one's body, one's feelings, and one's perception. The Buddha speaks not only about mindfulness, but about "Right mindfulness":

> And what, bhikkhus is right mindfulness? Here, bhikkhus, a bhikkhu dwells contemplating the body in the body [...] He dwells contemplating feelings in feelings [...] He dwells contemplating mind in mind [...] He dwells contemplating phenomena in phenomena, ardent, clearly comprehending, mindful, having removed covetousness and displeasure in regard to the world. This is called right mindfulness. (SN 45.8)[14]

In the Buddhist context, mindfulness derives from Pāli "*sati*", Sanskrit "*smṛti*", and means remembrance, not-forgetting, realization, recalling something into memory, and remembering. In the language of Buddhist psychology mindfulness is "a mental factor that does not forget the perceived object and has the function of counteracting distraction" (Asaṅga/Boin-Webb 2001, 209; Ngawang/Spitz 1988–2001, Part 3, sources, 66). Thus, Buddhist mindfulness, being one limb of the eightfold path, is closely linked to the other seven limbs, and to striving for liberation from suffering, i.e., from *saṃsāra*.

Today, the practice of right mindfulness is also closely related to a movement which is called either "Engaged Care" or more generally "Engaged Buddhism", comparable to "Liberation Theology" (Giles/Miller 2012).[15] But there is a difference between the practice of mindfulness and engaged care. As mentioned above, early Buddhist texts show that mindfulness does not intervene, but only observes. The task of directing the mind in an ethically beneficial/wholesome direction lies within the Eightfold Path in the right striving/right effort (Anālayo 2019).

From a Buddhist perspective, it is important to link mindfulness training with Buddhist mind training in love (Skt.: *maitrī*, Pā.: *metta*) and compassion or care (Skt./Pā.: *karuṇā*). This applies to all sentient beings – without exception

---

14 Vibhaṅga Sutta, On Right Mindfulness.

15 Sallie B. King, reflecting the differences of these two categories points out "[P]ondering the similarities and differences between Buddhist and Christian social engagement, it was extremely helpful for me when I discovered those liberation theologians who make it clear that justice is a function of love" (King 2016, 56). See also Roloff (2020a, 83–84): "When dealing with human coexistence, one can therefore rely on the term 'equanimity' or on the Four Immeasurables in total with regard to equality, social justice and gender justice, because the Buddhist mental training in love, compassion, sympathetic joy and equanimity includes all sentient beings without exception and irrespective of their religious affiliation, nationality or gender."

and regardless of their religious affiliation, nationality or gender. This means that Buddhist caregivers, similar to Christian caregivers, if requested, should extend their support to all people in need regardless of their religious affiliation or worldview. But it is vital that when a person is seeking spiritual direction the chaplain refrains from proselytizing and rather supports the patient's own spiritual resources to deal with the situation.

Thus, it becomes clear that the practice of mindfulness can be applied in spiritual care in general as well as in Buddhist care. But the way of practice partly differs: for Buddhists it is a means of gaining liberation from suffering through the Eightfold path. And this includes Buddhist wisdom (view and resolve/intention), Buddhist ethics, and the Buddhist way of meditation to attain Nirvāṇa.

Which skills or competencies are required to counsel Buddhists?

To answer the heading question, we first have to tackle the following question: What defines interfaith or non-denominational chaplaincy, and what specific competencies are *Buddhist* practitioners bringing to the larger field of chaplaincy?

Recent developments have proven that secular and interreligious spiritual care are learning from Buddhist mindfulness practices. Thus, mindfulness is increasingly developing in a kind of ideologically neutral practice. Nevertheless, we should neither deny its Buddhist roots nor the fact that practicing Buddhists need more than mindfulness and meditation.[16] It is an important competence, but not the only one from Buddhism's toolbox. When applying mindfulness practices in a secular or interreligious context, caregivers should understand what is left out or added, and they should understand and reflect upon the reasons for such adjustments as well as its consequences. In particular, Buddhism has much to offer in the care of the dying. As McCormick has shown:

> Buddhism can teach social workers to be humble in the face of death, honest with their own beliefs, and compassionate when working with family members who must make very difficult decisions. With a compassionate approach a social worker can accept the decisions of the family without judgment and provide the care as best he or she can to reduce the suffering experienced with the patient and family. (McCormick 2013, 223)

16 See for example, Rev. Wakoh Shannon Hickey's article "Meditation is Not Enough: Chaplaincy Training for Buddhists" (2012). Hickey is one of the leading American Buddhist Chaplains, and a Spiritual Support Counselor (Chaplain) at the Hospice by the Bay, Sonoma, CA.

I will come back to this below. For now, let us anticipate this much here: Buddhists do not all have the same ideas about what comes after death, nor do all Buddhists have the same ideas about the meaning of Nirvāṇa. Buddhist schools and texts teach different definitions of Nirvāṇa, which caregivers should be aware of. This is one of the reasons why, for example, in the Netherlands, the training in Buddhist spiritual care is not taking place in Buddhist centres and temples of the various traditions only, but also at university.[17] In the frame of intercultural exchange it is important to be aware of and sensitive to the divergent Buddhist concepts.

It is interesting that Sanford and Michon (2019) do not list meditation and mindfulness as Buddhist core competencies (2019, 37). As core competencies Buddhist caregivers need today, they discuss empathy and compassion, listening and responding, interfaith understanding, ritual, and prayer, cultural competencies, and reflection. Depending on the context and legal situation, two different care models are used: intra-religious (i.e. Buddhists of different traditions take care of Buddhists from similar or different tradition) or interreligious-secular (i.e. Buddhists take care of everyone together with caregivers of other denominations or worldviews). As Sanford and Michon point out:

> Distinctions between Buddhist and other forms of spiritual care are based on the care model employed, whether strictly co-religionist (i.e., Buddhists caring for Buddhists) or interfaith (i.e., Buddhists caring for all). In the latter case, professional chaplains (of any religion) are trained to provide spiritual care from the spiritual or religious worldview of the care-seeker. As such, most Buddhist chaplains must possess basic knowledge and competency in many world religions. Nevertheless, Buddhist spiritual care may be distinct in its theory (Dharma-based) and place more emphasis on mindfulness, meditation, and other contemplative techniques to benefit both care-seekers and chaplains. Spiritual care that is "Dharma-based" means based on the teachings of the historical Buddha, Siddhartha Gautama, and/or the Buddhist traditions and teacher who followed him. This includes a broad range of texts and teachings across the Buddhist world. (Sanford/ Michon 2019, 1–2).

A solid practitioner and caregiver will, when understanding the relationship between dependent arising (*pratītyasamutpāda*) and emptiness (*śūnyatā*), be able to develop skilful means (*upāya*), for his or her role as a professional Buddhist chaplain.

17 "Vrije Universiteit Amsterdam, Master's Degree Program Theology and Religious Studies: Spiritual Care", accessed May 1, 2022, https://vuweb.vu.nl/en/education/master/theology-and-religious-studies. For details see chapter 8 in this volume "Spiritual care in an interfaith context: Implications for Buddhist, Muslim, and Hindu spiritual care in the Netherlands" by Anke I. Liefbroer, Stef Lauwers, Pieter Coppens, and Bikram Lalbahadoersing.

Monett rightly emphasises: "[f]or the role of the professional chaplain is not to proselytise a particular dogma but to stand with the patient where they are at and to help the patient utilize their own spiritual views and beliefs as a resource for their own healing" (2005, 58).

Having discussed how Buddhists traditionally cared for each other at the time of the Buddha, how this care is based in Buddhist root texts and how Buddhist caregiving differs from other models of caregiving and which skills or competencies Buddhist caregivers need to develop, let us look at Buddhist chaplaincy in contemporary societies and what important tools it can draw from.

Important tools Buddhist chaplaincy can draw from

As I have shown in my paper "Openness towards the Religious Other in Buddhism" (Roloff 2020, 64): "The readiness to understand, to respect and to appreciate other religious traditions presupposes an open (mental) attitude. For a Buddhist this approach can be facilitated by cultivating an attitude of love, compassion, sympathetic joy and equanimity for all sentient beings." For individual Buddhist practice as well as when caring for others it is central to transform people away from self-centredness towards more love and compassion.

Love and Compassion in Buddhism and their application in spiritual care

Compassion or care (*karuṇā*) is a central ethical attitude of Buddhism. This means not only the wish that all living beings may be free from suffering and the causes of suffering, but also the commitment to helping other people in physically and psychologically painful crisis situations such as old age, illness and death. As mentioned above, the well-being of others and one's own well-being are mutually dependent.

The potential of loving-kindness and compassion meditation for psychological interventions (Hofman et al. 2011) and the role and effectiveness of mindfulness-based interventions (MBIs) and Loving-Kindness Meditation (LKM) in Cultivating Self-Compassion and Other-Focused Concern in Health Care Professionals (Boellinghaus et al. 2014) are being intensively researched from a psychological perspective. These methods are becoming increasingly relevant in the health sector and have not only been introduced in healthcare professionals' training courses and work-based settings, but also into chaplains' training courses.

The Four Immeasurables, Equalizing and Exchanging, Giving and Receiving

As mentioned above the "Golden Rules" of Theravāda and Mahāyāna Buddhism are based on the training of mindfulness. We live in a relational context. As Willa Miller stresses in her article "Listening as Spiritual Care" (2012), even Buddhist "teachers who try to limit their duties to the formal Dharma hall, or to the podium, find themselves – either willingly or not – in relational contexts in which witnessing plays an important role (or should)" (Miller 2012).

The basic Buddhist teaching of developing love and compassion are The Four Immeasurables (*apramāṇas*), also known as the Four Divine States (*brahmavihāras*):[18]

1. *Love*, Loving-kindness or Benevolence (Skt. *maitrī*, Pā. *mettā*),
2. *Compassion* or Care (Skt./Pā. *karuṇā*),
3. *Sympathetic Joy* (Skt./Pā. *muditā*), the opposite of envy or schadenfreude,
4. *Equanimity* or Lack of egocentricity (Skt. *upekṣā*, Pā. *upekkhā*).

In Tibetan Buddhism, daily meditation often starts with the cultivation of equanimity. The point is to develop a sense of equal nearness to all sentient beings, thus counteracting the tendency to discriminate between near and distant, and building upon that, accustoming the mind to new patterns of thought towards love and compassion and a respectful, compassionate, loving, and appreciative attitude towards others.

Founded on the practice of equanimity Mahāyāna Buddhists cultivate not only love and compassion by the so-called sevenfold cause-and-effect instruction,[19] but also great compassion (*mahākaruṇā*) and a sense of universal responsibility:

1. recognizing that *all sentient beings have been our parents* in previous lives,
2. *contemplating their kindness* when they were our parents,
3. wishing to *repay* their *kindness*.

---

18 Cf. Nyānatiloka 1952, 108–118.

19 Tibetan: *rgyu 'bras man ngag bdun: mar shes / drin dran / drin gzo / yid 'ong gi byams pa / snying rje chen po / lhag bsam rnam dag sems bskyed de bdun no.*

These three bring forth

4. *deep affection and heart-warming love* for all beings, which leads to
5. *great compassion [or mercy]* (*mahākaruṇā*). The torment others undergo becomes unbearable to us, and the great compassion arising from that produces
6. *great resolve*, assuming the (*universal*) *responsibility*, also referred to as exceptional attitude (Tib. *lhag bsam*)[20] to work for the welfare of sentient beings. The great resolve is the wholehearted commitment to act to bring about others' happiness and protect them from *duḥkha*.

These six causes lead to

7. the effect, *bodhicitta* – the aspiration to attain full awakening for the benefit of all sentient beings.[21]

From a psychological point of view, however, dealing with one's mother or parents or persons, whom we find difficult, can become unpleasant or – without further explanation or comment – lead to an avoidance attitude. Without a basic embedding, this training may be misunderstood. Therefore, it is important not to teach somebody to practice this meditation without prior discussion on the topic. In my experience, Western people often consider it easier to train in the alternative practice known as "equalizing and exchanging self and others":[22]

---

20 Cf. Roloff 2010, 197.

21 Cf. Dalai Lama & Chodron 2014, 223–224. The arousing of *bodhicitta* marks the beginning of the *bodhisattva* way of life. It is helpful to consider the Tibetan translation of bodhisattva, which is *byang chub sems dpa'* and incorporates the meaning "one who is heroic in his or her intention to achieve enlightenment". Sometimes the term is also rendered as "hero of enlightenment" or "spiritual warrior". In Sanskrit, however, the first component *bodhi* means "enlightenment", deriving from *budh* "to wake". The second component *sattva* has different meanings. First is "sentient being", thus the compound would be understood as "a sentient being seeking enlightenment". The second meaning is "mind" (*citta*) or "intention" (*abhipraya*), so that a *bodhisattva* would be "one whose mind or intention is directed toward englightenment". And third *sattva* means "strength" or "courage", making the compound mean "one whose strength or courage is directed toward enlightenment" (cf. Lopez 1988, 38).

22 We can trace these meditations back to Indian Buddhism in the 7th/8th century. See, for example, Schmidt-Leukel 2019, 375–412. The giving and receiving meditation is a well-known mind training (Tib. *blo sbyong*) practice. It deepens our love, our compassion, and our ability to exchange self and others, and it is also applied helping ourselves and others at the time of death: "Developing a kind heart, generating bodhicitta, and doing the taking and giving meditation at the time of death ... places our mind in a positive and fearless state. Reflecting on emptiness calms grasping and fear, enabling us to peacefully let go of this life" (Dalai Lama XIV and Chodron 2018, 223–224).

This method, in Tibetan Buddhism also combined with a practice referred to as *Tonglen* (Tib. *gtong len*), the practice of "giving and receiving", has been used in Germany for more than 20 years in palliative care in clinics. Christine Longaker, a German pioneer of the hospice movement, describes the secularised form as follows: "In the Tonglen visualisation we receive the suffering and pain of others with a strong, compassionate attitude and give them – with a heart full of tenderness and confidence – all our love, our joy, our well-being and our peace" (Longaker 2009, 117).

One becomes aware that the well-being of others and one's own well-being are interdependent and inextricably linked. One can combine this idea with the observation of one's own breathing. With each inhalation one imagines that one is taking upon oneself the suffering of others together with the causes for it, and with the exhalation one wishes them happiness and passes on to others all the positive causes that one has collected through good actions, one's own good *karma* or merits (Skt. *puṇya*, Pā. *puñña*).[23]

Buddhist chaplaincy in contemporary societies

Buddhism existed and developed in India for about 1,700 years (5th cent. BCE-12th cent.). Indian Buddhism spread at different stages of its development within India into different Asian cultures (cf. above). While in the past, in Asia, we usually found different forms of one and the same Buddhist mainstream tradition in each country, today, especially in the West, we find almost all three mainstream traditions in its various forms in each country, often even in one city.

The European Buddhist Union counts more than 50 Buddhist centers from 16 European countries among its members.[24] Organizations of ethnic Buddhists such as The Unified *Buddhist Church* of Vietnam or the Thai Mahānikāya or Dhammayuttanikāya are not members of the European Buddhist Union, but in some countries members of Buddhist National Unions. For example, the Fo-Guang Shan Temple (Taiwan) has become a member of the German Buddhist Union. In Norway, most of the ethnic-Buddhist temples have become members

23 Auspicious, potent and wholesome deeds of body, speech and mind, which plant seeds or generate good imprints in one's mindstream or mental continuum leading to beneficial and fortunate consequence in this life or lives to come. For further reading on the practice of meritorious action, the transference of merit and the rejoicing in the merit of others see Gethin (1998, 101–110) and Schmidt-Leukel (2006, 40, 71–72, 139).

24 "European Buddhist Union, Our Members", accessed May 2, 2022, http://europeanbuddhism.org/members/.

of the Norway Buddhist Federation (NBF). It seems that memberships also depend on benefits. In Norway, the NBF enjoys governmental support depending on the number of members of the affiliated communities. In other countries like Austria and Germany, members of religious communities need to pay a kind of "church tax", while in Italy, whether a member of a religious community or not, every citizen is subject to a compulsory church and culture tax (*otto per mille*, i.e. 8 ‰, based on gross income tax). The taxpayer can indicate on the tax return which religious community should benefit from the tax or whether it should be given to social purposes or the state.[25]

The European Buddhist Union (EBU), founded in 1975 in Paris, endeavours to establish an international expert's network of Buddhist chaplains in order to offer support, training opportunities and materials for those engaging with Buddhist Chaplaincy. Furthermore, the EBU is trying to identify spiritual and pastoral needs within Buddhist communities to encourage greater community cohesion and social integration. On April 25th 2021, the EBU organised the "1st Meeting of the EBU Buddhist Chaplains".[26] More than 30 European Buddhist chaplains participated. The topics discussed were chaplaincy in hospitals, chaplaincy in the armed forces, a university course in Buddhist Chaplaincy, and chaplaincy in prison. The day before, more than 200 people participated in an EBU online conference on Death and dying from a Buddhist perspective including outstanding keynote speakers like Roshi Joan Halifax, Kirsten DeLeo, and Dario Girolami.

In Asia, similar to the West, as a consequence of globalization and pluralization, non-native Buddhist traditions can increasingly be found in each country. For example, in Thailand, besides the traditional Theravāda tradition, also Taiwanese and Vietnamese Buddhist temples have been established. In Taiwan and Korea, besides the traditional Pure Land and Ch'an or Seon temples, we also find Tibetan Buddhist temples today. In Asia and the United States, professional pastoral/spiritual care is more advanced than in Europe. Buddhist Care Practices are already well established there and, in terms of the standards developed, seem to be comparable to the level of development of Christian pastoral care.

Today, around the globe, many people suffer from loneliness or are facing different kinds of existential crises. The corona pandemic has exacerbated the need for professional support across Europe. The pioneers in professional train-

25 Using the example of religious education in public schools, I have discussed this issue in two book chapters (Roloff 2020b, Roloff 2020c).

26 "European Buddhist Union, Buddhist Chaplaincy", accessed May 2, 2022, https://europeanbuddhistunion.org/activity/chaplaincy. The 1st Meting of the EBU Buddhist Chaplains took place on April, 25th 2021 (online event). For details of the outcome see European Buddhist Union (2021).

ing in Buddhist Chaplaincy are the United Kingdom, the Netherlands, Austria and Norway. The London based organization "The Buddhist Chaplaincy Kalyāna Mitra" offers resources and courses from time to time.[27] Buddhist chaplaincy has increased during the COVID-19 pandemic. In the UK, the Buddhist Healthcare Chaplaincy Trust, the endorsing body for Buddhist Healthcare Chaplains and a charitable trust, is committed to promoting Buddhist Healthcare Chaplaincy. Several Buddhist chaplains are registered with the UK Board of Healthcare Chaplaincy.

In the Netherlands, an ongoing postgraduate course called "Buddhist Chaplaincy" has been available at the Vrije Universiteit Amsterdam (Faculty of Theology) since 2014. Here, an MA in religion, preferably in Spiritual Care, or in Spiritual Care Buddhism is required. In Norway, the University of Oslo, since 2019/2020, for the first time, offers bi-yearly a course on Buddhist care practices.[28] In Austria, since 1983, the Österreichische Buddhistische Religionsgesellschaft is recognised as a corporation under public law. They offer a mobile hospice, pastoral care in the Vienna General Hospital and since 2003 there is a Buddhist cemetery in Vienna.

In Lutheran-Protestant and Roman Catholic Theologies, pastoral training partly belongs to the practical theologies. In contrast, in Germany, Buddhism cannot be studied as a religion at state-funded universities. Buddhist Studies, also known as Buddhology, – unlike theology – is primarily focused on the languages and cultures of Buddhism and is located mainly in the Asian-African sciences (formerly Oriental studies). In Germany, the history of Buddhology dates to the 19th century, but Buddhist practical theology has not been established yet. In Christian theologies, in addition to practical theologies, beginning in the 1920s, Clinical Pastoral Education (CPE), in German Klinische Seelsorgeausbildung (KSA), was developed as a model of in-service theological pastoral care in order to accommodate the contextual differences from the United States (low status of practical theology in academic theology and theology studies) (Pulheim 2006, 137). It was not until the 1970s that psychotherapeutic methods became standard in pastoral care (Hauschildt 2015, 48). Today, European Buddhists can, for example, take Accredited Clinical Pastoral Education at institutes

27 "The Buddhist Chaplaincy Kalyāna Mitra. The Buddhist Society – Founded 1924", accessed May 2, 2022, https://www.thebuddhistsociety.org/page/the-buddhist-society-chaplaincy.

28 "University of Oslo, LES4201 – Buddhist care practices", accessed May 2, 2022, https://www.uio.no/studier/emner/teologi/tf/LES4201/index.html. This course is part of the MA "Leadership, Ethics and Counselling (master – experience-based)" (Lederskap, etikk og samtalepraksis (master - erfaringsbasert – 120 ECTS, with MA certificate), start: August 2019.

such as the New Yorker Zen Center for Contemplative Care in cooperation with the New York Theological Seminary.[29]

This raises the question of relevance of Buddhist chaplaincy, what are the needs of European Buddhists, and what has Buddhism to offer in dealing with existential crises. Today, in general, we find chaplains in schools, hospitals, hospices, companies, universities, and prisons. They provide care during times of crisis and run programs to help deal with grief, anger or depression. Chaplaincy duties include visiting homes, religious services, retreats and celebrations, as well as counselling. They support the spiritual, social, and emotional well-being of care-seekers and help build positive relationships.

When serving in a Buddhist temple in Europe you will need to assist or find yourself responsible for various tasks that spiritual caregivers or spiritual friends (Skt. *kalyāṇamitra/-mitrā*) are expected to provide such as:

- Teaching the Dharma and giving practical advice on how to implement it.
- Giving personal advice in existential crises (life counselling).
- Performing rites of passage (*rites de passage*) for newborn children, for young people of confirmation age, on the occasion of marriage or death.
- Taking care for the sick at home and in hospital including prayers for recovery next to their sickbed, by phone, video call or from afar.
- Spiritual care for the dying / end-of-life care (natural death; different from active/ passive euthanasia) including prayers and death rituals.
- Planning and holding funerals, care for relatives in the event of bereavement.
- Visiting Buddhists in prison or counselling them by letter post.
- Having exchange with military chaplains and soldiers from different denominations.
- Performing prayers and rites in different emergency or tense life situations.
- Counselling of victims or relatives in disaster situations.
- Advice on questions like organ donation, abortion, domestic violence, or sexual abuse.

In spring 2020, under the COVID-19 pandemic, the question arose what Buddhism can offer to people in need during this extraordinary situation.

---

29 "NY Zen Center, Foundations in Contemplative Care, A training program in spiritual caregiving", accessed May 2, 2022, https://zencare.org/education-new/foundations-new/. "New York Theological Seminary, Master of Arts in Pastoral Care and Counseling (MAPCC)", accessed May 2, 2022, https://invent.nyts.edu/prospective-students/academic-programs/master-of-arts-in-pastoral-care-counseling/. For further details see Weilhart (2021).

What has Buddhism to offer in existential crises?

Psychologists call the coronavirus crisis a major life event. It will give our life a new drive. We will ask ourselves: How important is my social life, family, relationship, how reliable?

The term crisis comes from Greek and literally means "difficult situation" (Tib. *nyen kha chen po* – a great danger/risk). Crises can affect a single person or a small group, such as the family. Typical causes of crises are the loss of important resources (for example health, money and housing), the loss of important persons (close relatives or friends), or when demands are placed on you that you cannot cope with. Great crises not only have an impact on the lives of individuals, but can also affect entire countries, continents or the entire world as a global crisis. Crises do not necessarily end in disasters. People who have mastered difficult situations often feel stronger afterwards than before (Burtscher 2014).

What are the Buddhist means for over-coming crises, for crisis resolution? What helps? In his article "Beyond catastrophe: We might all be better people once the Covid-19 crisis has subsided", Jay Garfield (2020) suggests, from a Buddhist perspective, to transform our own minds, attitudes and behaviour, and to cultivate what Buddhist ethicists call the "six perfections"[30], beginning with generosity:

> It is time to be of material, emotional, and social assistance to those around us. By helping family, neighbors, communities, and institutions that find themselves in need, we ameliorate the suffering around us, and reaffirm our membership in these networks that determine our own lives and those of others. (2020)

Garfield also suggests to develop insight in reality, i.e., in impermanence, uncertainty, interdependence. Everything that exists, whether material or mental, depends on many causes and conditions. We are all connected with each other. "By transforming our own minds, attitudes and behavior, we can become part of the solution to the problem of suffering, rather than part of the problem" (Garfield 2020).

Three of the Bodhisattva's six perfections are different from the above-mentioned three trainings (*śikṣā*), i.e., ethics, meditative concentration and wisdom:

30 The six perfections (*pāramitās*) are: 1. *dāna*: giving/surrender/generosity, 2. *śīla*: morality/attentiveness, 3. *kṣanti*: patience/forbearance. 4. *vīrya*: vigor/disciplined effort, 5. *dhyāna*: absorption/mediation/calm, and 6. *prajñā*: insight/wisdom.

Giving (*dāna*), including making one's life a gift to others, patience (*kṣānti*) with a strong connotation of forbearance, and vigour or energy (*virya*) (Schmidt-Leukel 2006, 136-137). All of these are important virtues to be developed by Buddhist chaplains. Other suggestions from Buddhism's toolbox are to use mindfulness in times of crisis, and to tackle corona fears with meditation.

One of the great challenges of Buddhist chaplaincy during the COVID-19 pandemic was that Buddhist chaplains, friends and relatives could not visit the care-seekers in hospitals, hospices, and retirement homes as they would under normal circumstances.. In many places, even visits at home were not allowed. In the following, I will give a few examples from different fields of Buddhist chaplaincy without claim to completeness.

Buddhist chaplaincy in hospitals and hospices

In my experience, Korea and Taiwan seem to be the most developed in the field of chaplaincy. Already in 2004, during the 8th Sakyadhita International Conference in Seoul, I noticed that Buddhist nuns in Korea volunteer in spiritual care by phone and as female "hospital dharma teachers". They describe the following self-image and demands:

> The purpose of hospital Dharma teachers is to take care of the sick with compassion until they are completely recovered. The virtues that hospital Dharma teachers should have are: (1) strong faith; (2) empathy with the patients' feelings; (3) a desire to eliminate disease; (4) continuous effort; (5) thoughtfulness, (6) humility; (7) mindfulness and wisdom; and (8) the wisdom of listening. The duties of a hospital Dharma teacher require a teacher to: (1) have both medical expertise and administrative expertise; (2) be emotionally stable; (3) treat patients as one would treat the Buddha; and (4) be sensitive to patients' cultural values. There are five virtues that caregivers should have. Caregivers should: (1) be well aware of what patients can eat and what they cannot; (2) not feel uncomfortable with patients' bodily fluids; (3) not be arrogant or concerned about personal gain; (4) be committed to their patients' recovery; and (5) make patients happy by sharing the Buddha's teachings with them. (Jihong Sunim 2006, 281).

In Taiwan, in 1998, a "Clinical Buddhist Chaplain" training program was introduced with the help of the Buddhist Lotus Hospice Care Foundation (LHCF) in cooperation with the Palliative Unit of the National Taiwan University Hospital and the Buddhist Dharma Drum Institute of the Liberal Arts. The graduates work in hospices or get involved in their communities. They are obliged to regularly take part in further training (Chen 2017).

Buddhist care for the dying and bereaved

As mentioned above, there are many different ideas about the "afterlife" in Buddhism. Most, but not all Buddhists believe in rebirth, i.e., being reborn in one of the five or six human or nun-human realms within *saṃsāra*, or in the transition to another, better life in a Buddha Land or Pure Land. More generally, they believe in the transition to a "different reality", to a different state of consciousness (nothing material).

What does Buddhism teach about rebirth? Usually, Buddhists do not believe in soul migration or an immutable self (Skt. *ātman*, Pā. *atta*). Buddhists believe in a non-self (Skt. *anātman*, Pā. *anatta*). But this should not be understood in a nihilistic way; the person exists and is morally responsible for his/her action. Buddhism is teaching the middle way, i.e., to avoid the two extremes: eternalism/ unchanging and nihilism/ non-existence. The five constituents of a person (*skandhas*) change and replicate from moment to moment. Body and mind separate at the time of death. Most Buddhists believe in the continuity of consciousness including karmic imprints.[31] Karma influences the connection with a new body. The new and previous person are neither identical nor different from each other.

Tibetan Buddhism teaches according to its Indian Buddhist Abhidharma sources intermediate state (Skt. *antarābhava*, Tib. *bar do*) between death and rebirth, i.e., an in-between state between former and next life. We also find this notion in the Theravāda tradition. The state of mind at the time of death and in the intermediate state is decisive for what will follow next. The intermediate state denotes the state of the continuum of the persons' physical and mental constituents (*skandhas*) between the end of the dying process and the beginning of the new existence, the next birth. The Tibetan Book of the Dead (*Bar do thos grol*), literally states that: "Liberation through hearing in the intermediate state", deals with three phases: dying, death and rebirth.

In some Buddhist traditions, strong faith/confidence is encouraged in order to enter into a pure Buddha land, e.g. in East Asian Amida and Ch'an/Seon/ Thiền/Zen Buddhism (China, Taiwan, Korea, Vietnam and Japan) as well as in Tantric Buddhism (Tibet, Nepal, Bhutan, Mongolia etc.). In Tantric Buddhism during a lifetime, one is trained in daily practice to use the process and subtle stages of dying for attaining liberation by gaining deep meditative insight in

31 On the problem of personal continuity (self as 'causal connectedness') see Gethin (1998, 140–144). Garfield (2022, 175) declines the concept of personal continua that continue after death and thinks that this belief is not necessary for the rest of the Buddhist edifice.

the ultimate truth/reality during the dying process (see chap. 9 "Looking beyond this life" by Dalai Lama XIV and Chodron 2018, 205–229).

What Buddhists of all three mainstream traditions have in common is that they prefer to speak about confidence instead of faith, based on the best kinds of confidence taught by the Buddha, i.e., confidence in the Buddha, in the eightfold path, in the Dharma (especially in dispassion which leads to cessation, and *nirvāṇa*), and in the Saṃgha (AN 4.34).

Especially in the Eastern Amida-Buddhist traditions, also referred to as Pure Land School, Jodo-shin-shu or resp. Jodo-shu, the core of the teaching, as a way to liberation, is trust in one's own Buddha nature, which can manifest in the form of the Buddha Amitābha. Amitābha, also referred to as Amita (Japanese: *amida*) literally means "limitless light" that symbolises compassion and wisdom. Upon entry into the Pure Land, the practitioner is believed to be instructed by Buddha Amitābha and numerous *bodhisattva*s until full and complete enlightenment is reached. This person then has the choice of returning at any time as a *bodhisattva* to any of the five/six realms of existence in order to help all sentient beings in *saṃsāra*, or to stay the whole duration, reach buddhahood, and subsequently deliver beings to the shore of liberation.

According to the tantric tradition, mainly practiced by Tibetan Buddhists, they speak about a clear light consciousness, i.e., a most subtle state of consciousness of a being. It becomes manifest in death in a natural way when all grosser types of consciousness dissolve into this state of consciousness. Then a mere emptiness of great clarity appears. Experienced *yogi*s and *yoginī*s can deliberately evoke this clear light in meditative absorption and link it with the realization of emptiness. In the death process, they stay in this clear light as long as possible to overcome all delusions and all obstacles in their own mind.

In summary, dying care and dying rituals entail accompanying the dying locally and/or from afar. The goal is to assist the dying person to die with a calm state of mind, to develop trust or confidence. This can perhaps be achieved by reminding the dying person of her good deeds and to support her in her daily meditation practice.

Examples of Buddhist approaches to the end-of-life care are explored in part five of the pioneering work of *The Arts of Contemplative Care* (Giles/Miller 2012). Taking the American Upaya Institute's Contemplative End-of-Life Training Program "Being with Dying (BWD)" as an example[32] (cf. Rusthon 2009), Joan Hali-

32 "Upaya Institute and Zen Center, Being with Dying, Professional Training Program for Clinicians in Compassionate Care of the Seriously Ill and Dying", accessed May 2, 2022, https://www.upaya.org/being-with-dying/.

fax Roshi (2012), a Zen priest and pioneer in the field of end-of-life care, provides us with an overall consideration of which challenges caregivers can be faced with:

> The premise of BWD is that in order for clinicians to provide compassionate end-of-life care, it is necessary for them to (1) become self-aware and recognize their own suffering, (2) make a commitment to addressing their own suffering, and (3) develop receptivity, compassion, and resilience through nurturing physical, emotional, mental, spiritual, and social dimensions in their own lives and in relationships with others. (Halifax 2012, pos. 3430).

The training has four components with a focus on the transformation: The caregivers must *first* identify their own worldviews, values, priorities, and knowledge. This gives the clinicians a functional base from which they can work. The *second* focus of the training is to investigate and employ various "contemplative interventions", i.e., to teach the caregivers meditation, including ethical virtues and values that engage in reflective practices that cultivate the mind. Meditation assists creating greater resilience and cultivating prosocial mental qualities, like empathy and compassion. These practices have a profound effect on the well-being of health care providers and this in turn has effect on how the clinician interacts with the patient and how the patient perceives his or her own experience of dying. The *third* area they address in their program has to do with the development of moral character. They explore the moral and ethical basis of what it means to care, and they teach people how to deal with moral dilemmas and moral conflicts. The *fourth* and last area for clinicians that they feel to be very important is to train caregivers in strategies for self-care and how they can support their well-being in a high-stress profession to prevent those caregivers from experiencing burnout.

This training comes down to an exercise from many different perspectives, which opens up to the development of fundamental qualities such as wisdom and compassion to become a sane and reasonable person in the world today.

Now we turn to a completely different area of chaplaincy, namely military and prison chaplaincy.

Buddhist military chaplaincy

For many people, the military and Buddhism do not seem to go together, especially in the West (cf. Harvey 2000, 274; Kariyakarawana 2011). Perhaps because Buddhist converts in their youth have refused military service and/or are in favour of complete demilitarization. The question at stake is, whether and how a

Buddhist chaplain can justify killing as an acceptable reaction when protecting national interests.

In the United States, according to a U.S. Department of Defence report, in 2017, among 3,000 chaplains in the total force there were three active-duty Buddhist chaplains (Wagner 2017). Robert Bosco (2014) discusses how the US military is employing Buddhist chaplains, and highlights some of the difficulties one may encounter.

In Europe, for example, a UK Buddhist chaplain in the HM Forces in London explains that during the past 200 years Nepali Buddhists (Gurkhas who are mainly Buddhists) have been serving in the British Army. Kariyakarawana comes to the conclusion that "[s]erving in the military is no different from serving anywhere else [...] it does not really matter what job you are doing as long as it does not come under the wrong livelihood. What matters is how you do the job and what your intentions are in doing it" (Kariyakarawana 2011, 106).

Bosco puts it differently by pointing out that there is no real analogy between today's American Buddhist soldiers and those of, say, warrior-monks in China, Thailand, or Japan. He even speaks about "the American Buddhist military sangha", who justifies its participation in combat by referring to the protection of the American way of life and the freedoms Americans can enjoy. He quotes a Buddhist Air Force Cadet saying, "we realize that war is certainly a thing that we don't want to have to do, but sometimes it is absolutely necessary, and it requires compassion for your country, your family, and the people that you are protecting. I think Buddhism definitely has a place there" (BMS 11/1/2007), and adds: "Some intentions—defence of one's nation—are the right ones, and can reap positive karmic consequences" (Bosco 2014, 843–844).

As of late, military chaplaincy in the Netherlands also includes Buddhist chaplains. During the EBU chaplaincy meeting in April 2021 Colonel Alie Jimon Rozendal gave some insight into her work. She explained that as chaplains they are *with* the military, not military. The Buddhist Union Netherlands "Boeddhistische Unie Nederland (BUN)" is sending her and can withdraw her endorsement. I understand it to mean that similar to religious teachers at German state schools, who in addition to the Certificate of Educational Competence (Fakultas) from a university, need a certificate of appointment from the religious community, military chaplains must have professional competence and be approved members of the religious community. E.g., when leaving the religious community, this certificate will be withdrawn, which would result in dismissal. Nevertheless, this certainly does not mean that the religious communities interfere in their work with the military. At the time of Alie Jimon Rozendal presentation, in April 2021, Buddhists had only been there for a year. The chaplains are caring for more than 60,000 soldiers. While trying to get familiar with the organization, Buddhist as well as non-Buddhist soldiers are asking her for help.[33]

Buddhist chaplaincy in prisons

Buddhist attitude towards prisoners can be traced back to the Buddha himself. How did the Buddha deal with criminals? The *Aṅgulimāla Sutta* tells us about the Buddha ignoring warnings to venture into the domain of the notorious killer Aṅgulimāla. The Buddha succeeds in converting him to the path of non-violence. After becoming a monk Aṅgulimāla still suffers for his past deeds, but only to a small extent. He uses his new commitment to non-violence to help a woman in labour (MN 86).

One of the most experienced Buddhist prison chaplains in Europe is the Zen priest Dario Doshin Girolami, who is also in charge of the European Buddhist Union's Network of Buddhist Chaplains.[34] Girolami was trained at the San Francisco Zen Center that for decades offered a course in meditation for the prisoners of San Quentin. It was this program that inspired him to propose a course of meditation in the Rebibbia prison of Rome in Italy. According to Girolami, studies show that there is a notable (20%) decrease of criminal recidivism in former inmates that participated in a meditation in prison program. Nevertheless, it took him years of negotiation to get access to the prison in Italy. His presentation seems to correspond with the research results by Irene Becci (2015), who reveals a certain institutional resistance to religious diversity in prisons in Italy, Germany, and Switzerland:

> Issues of equal treatment or equal formal representation of religions in secular prison spaces are today part of a broader process of negotiation concerning the role of religion vis-à-vis the aims of prison institutions. Any possibility of religious activity is weighed against the institution's need to maintain stability. ... The established Christian chaplaincies are in a unique position in this context, because their activity is valued as 'universal'. The 'universalisation' of Christian religion ... leads to a 'neutralisation' of one specific (Christi-

33 Part of her presentation was this film "Diensten Geestelijke Verzorging. 'Omdat je leven betekenis heeft'. Promotie-film uitgebracht ter gelegenheid van 100 jaar Diensten Geestelijke Verzorging. (Services Spiritual Care. 'Because your life has meaning'. Promotional film released on the occasion of 100 years of Spiritual Care Services)", video 6:45, youtube.com/watch?v=yR-toh8OXC-s. "Boeddhistische Geestelijke Verzorging, Team Buddhism", accessed May 2, 2022, https://www.dgv.nl/en/group/1/team.

34 "European Buddhist Union, Prison Chaplaincy", accessed May 1, 2022, http://europeanbuddhism.org/about/activities/ebu-networks/chaplaincy-prison-chaplaincy/.

> an) type of spiritual assistance, which becomes the template for all other religious interaction. (Becci 2015, 17).

But we also find other examples. In 1979, the Israeli government set up a research committee to study the conditions in the local prisons and recommended changes in imprisonment policy. A significant step in this process was the opening of the Hermon prison, a modern rehabilitative facility. In 2006, for the first time, a Vipassana course, based on the teachings of S. N. Goenka, was introduced. This kind of Vipassana meditation is considered an open, nonconditioned spiritual practice, which despite its Buddhist origin does not represent any formal religion. Thus, the decision to conduct such a course at the Hermon prison was easily accepted. A total of 22 male prisoners participated in a 10-day course run by volunteers in the prison. Interviews were conducted with participants before, immediately after, and 3 to 4 months after the course. The findings prove a meaningful impact on the prisoners in rehabilitation (Ronel et al. 2013). However, there seems to be no systematic study that provides and analyses an overview of Buddhist initiatives in this area. Therefore, I can only give some examples from my own experience such as the work of the Buddhist nuns' community of Sravasti Abbey (USA). The abbess, Ven. Chodron, began working with inmates in 1997 when an inmate wrote a letter to the Dharma Friendship Foundation, a Dharma center where she taught, and requested information about Buddhism. Since then the project has expanded. The Abbey produces a quarterly prison Dharma newsletter, which includes transcripts of teachings and inmates' Dharma reflections. Over 350 copies are mailed to individual inmates who share them with their Dharma friends in their respective prisons. The nuns also care for prisoners in the death row.

Buddhist *roshi*, Joan Halifax, also works with people at the last stage of life on death row. She has a doctorate in medical anthropology and lectures all over the world on her workings with the dying. She had become a teacher in Thich Nhât Hanh's school, and still later had been appointed Roshi, i.e., Zen Master, by Bernie Glassman (1939–2018), an internationally well-known American Zen Buddhist roshi and founder of the Zen Peacemakers. He was a pioneer of social enterprise, socially engaged Buddhism and "Bearing Witness Retreats" at Auschwitz and on the streets with homeless people. Roshi Joan Halifax founded the Upaya Zen Center in Santa Fe, New Mexico that offers professional training in end-of-life care and Buddhist counselling (Halifax 2012).

Although prison chaplaincy seems to be especially difficult, Buddhism here has a unique potential currently not being exploited. Buddhist notions of Buddha-nature and the belief in countless past lives in which we may have committed crimes for which we have been convicted, too, enable Buddhists to meet prisoners on an equal footing. Buddhists train in not identifying people with their mistakes. Making mistakes, and doing harmful actions, does not mean that the whole person becomes bad. The Buddha nature, the person's potential for enlightenment, is still there and can be developed when meeting with supportive causes and conditions.

Life counselling

Another important topic that we have not yet discussed is counselling of Buddhists in different emergency, disaster or tense life situations, especially when related to questions such as organ donation, abortion, domestic violence, and sexual abuse.

Let us briefly look into these topics and start with *organ donation*. Do Buddhists want to have organ donor cards? Religion can support, discourage or even forbid to have an organ donor card. In order to make a decision you need to think about death and dying from various Buddhist perspectives. There is no general rejection, but three main questions arise in this context: What is the Buddhist's view on brain death, on organ and tissue transplantation, and on autopsy. Alhawari et al. (2018) analyse from the perspective of forensic medicine ethical and religious argumentation structures when it comes to existential questions of the end of life and the question whether and when a person ceases to exist. In the context of autopsy, the question arises as to how the dead body is dealt with in Buddhism and what religiously motivated objections and reservations may exist regarding brain death. The brain death debate is a relatively new phenomenon within the old world religions. The age of the religion and its geographical distribution both impact the debate. It is not only the religious writings that need to be considered, but also contemporary publications and statements by Buddhist umbrella organizations.[35]

McCormick (2013) notes that ethical guidance for a Buddhist is partly provided by the five basic precepts shared by all Buddhists. The first precept prohibiting the killing of living beings, is the basis for Buddhist approaches to death in clinical situations. But we also need to consider the virtue of compassion, and the goal of a peaceful death. McCormick discusses organ donation, life-sustain-

35 On Buddhism and organ donation see also this BBC website, last modified November 27, 2009, https://www.bbc.co.uk/religion/religions/buddhism/buddhistethics/organdonation.shtml. For a more detailed analysis on organ donation in the context of biomedical applications from a Buddhist perspective, see Schlieter (2003, 31–53).

ing treatment, different situations of assisted death,[36] and palliative and hospice. He gives three examples that illustrate how some Buddhists have struggled with making end-of-life care decisions while being mindful of *ahiṃsā*, the Buddhist principle of not harming. This makes clear that there is not 'one clear Buddhist position' on these questions. Different answers cannot be fixed to traditions. Rather, we find the whole spectrum of different possible answers among adherents of each Buddhist tradition. Ultimately, it is an individual decision that everyone must make for himself or herself. But this does not mean that the interpretation of Buddhism on such questions is arbitrary. As Garfield points out, "Buddhist ethics is both particularist and agent-relative (2022, 165)".

Similarly, you will find different pros and cons on the question of *abortion*. In general, there is no objection against contraception. A possible exception maybe the spiral which prevents the implantation of an already fertilised egg. Buddhists regard life as starting at conception (Roloff 1992; Barnhart 2018). In the Buddhist canonical texts, killing a fetus is already classified as killing. But killing depends on four or five conditions; what is decisive is your own motivation.[37]

Competencies of Buddhist caregivers also include "working with specific populations or problems, such as: alcoholism and addiction, domestic violence, sexual trauma, chronic illness, aging, family conflict, mental illness, and natural and man-made disasters" (Sanford/Michon 2019, 13).

Taking *domestic violence* as an example, despite the basic tenets of love and compassion taught within Buddhism, we know that violence against women occurs. Domestic violence is the most common form of violence against women worldwide. This is the same for Buddhist communities. In the European Union, one fifth to one quarter of all women have experienced physical violence at least once in their lives. Therefore, in 2011, the Council of Europe drew up the Convention on Preventing and Combating Violence against Women and Domestic Violence as an international treaty, which entered into force in 2014. The principle of the Convention in Article 1a is: "The purposes of this Convention is to

---

36 Questions such as why euthanasia should be a moral issue for Buddhists if the patient will soon be reborn can arise. Some Buddhist may think that one has the "right to die" arguing that death is voluntary, and there is no conflict with the Buddhist principle of *ahiṃsā* (non-harming). This raises questions such as whether turning off a life-support machine could ever be the right thing to do for a Buddhist. Cf. Harvey's chap. 7 on suicide and euthanasia (2000, 286–310), and Keown 2018.

37 On further discussion on Buddhism and abortion see Harvey 2000 (chap. 8 on abortion and contraceptions).

protect women against all forms of violence, and prevent, prosecute and eliminate violence against women and domestic violence." To date, 45 of the 47 member states of the Council of Europe have signed the Convention in Istanbul (it has not been signed by Azerbaijan and the Russian Federation). 35 of the member states have ratified it and thus are obliged to put it into practice (including Turkey, who announced its withdrawal from the Istanbul Conventionin on 20 March 2021).

According to Kanukollu and Epstein, "We also know that we do not know enough about this issue within Buddhist communities, nor do we know enough about how best to support and treat victims of VAW [Violence against Women] from Buddhist communities in spiritually competent and relevant ways" (Kanukollu/ Epstein-Ngo 2015, 353). But on a grass root level there is more know-how than we may expect. For example, Buddhist women in Cambodia encourage nuns and lay women to become socially engaged and to become counsellors and Dharma teachers and to engage in conflict resolution and management:

> The practices that the Association of Nuns and Laywomen of Cambodia adopted since 1995 include learning and training in the Dharma, self-development, peaceful mental development, leadership, human rights, promotion of women's rights, conflict resolution, elimination of domestic violence, and care for patients living with AIDS. So far, the nuns and laywomen who are trainers in the association have provided training on how to meditate, cultivate a peaceful mind, and provide counseling to people in crisis, homeless children, and sex workers (Vanna 2006, 20).

In September 2011, the Tibetan Parliament-In-Exile (TPIE) successfully passed a resolution condemning violence against women. After several incidents in the Tibetan exile community, Tibetan women showed solidarity against VAW and founded the organization Acha Himalayan Sisterhood for community service, women's empowerment and ending violence against women and children.[38] Such associations make it clear that domestic violence and other forms of violence against women in Buddhist communities exists and should no longer be ignored.

In Thailand newspapers like Bangkok Post constantly report about child sex abuse which in 2020 nears record high during the coronavirus pandemic. But also before, you can find many reports such as "Two monks arrested for child sexual abuse" (Petcharoen 2015).

---

38 "Acha Himalaya Sisterhood, Community Service, Women's Empowerment and Ending Violence Agains Women and Children", accessed May 2, 2022, https://achahimalayansisterhood.org/.

Although not in accord with Buddhist principles, the social reality proves that it happens that girl trafficking and prostitution in Thailand are justified by outdated Buddhist attitudes toward women. Emma Tomalin (2006) argues "that there is a relationship between the low status of women in Thai Buddhism and the inferior status of women in Thai society," and that "the introduction of female leadership roles in Thai Buddhism could play a role in balancing the gender hierarchies within the tradition as well as in society more broadly" (Tomalin 2006, 385).

Along with the MeToo movement more cases of *sexual abuse* in Buddhism are revealed and increasingly discussed, also in public (see for example, Finnigan and Hogendoorn 2019).

This makes it clear that there is a great need for professional spiritual care and a correspondingly comprehensive and profound education, not only in Asia, but due to increasing pluralization, also in Europe. The question is, where such training in Europe is possible and best connected institutionally.

Conclusion and Perspectives for Buddhist Chaplaincy

As we have seen, Buddhist care practices dating back to the Buddha himself, nowadays require a modern professional training to deal with existential crises and disaster. There is a strong need to care for the sick and dying in hospitals and hospices, for children and adults in schools, high schools, universities and workplaces, as well as for soldiers in the military, for short and long-term prisoners, and in countries like the US, also for those on death-row.

This article has introduced Buddhist chaplaincy with a special focus on Europe and briefly analysed the current state of the field from a Buddhist perspective. I have discussed how Buddhists traditionally care for each other and how such caring is rooted in Buddhist texts. What does it mean to be a Buddhist counsellor, chaplain, or caregiver, and which important Buddhist tools can they draw from, giving examples of Buddhist chaplaincy in contemporary societies, in Asia as well as in the US and in Europe.

Humans are different and therefore we need individual help when we are in need. The training of Buddhist caregivers requires a good understanding of the various traditions of Buddhism, what they have in common and where they differ to be able to develop sensitivity for the different Buddhist paths.

Although Buddhist care practices can be dated back to the Buddha himself, there is no doubt that professional care worldwide has been strongly influenced by Christian chaplaincy. As Irene Becci (2015) has pointed out, the established Christian chaplaincies are in a unique position in this context. Their activity is valued as 'universal'. Similar to the masculine in gender relations, which places men at the center of thinking, pastoral/spiritual care in Europe places Christian concepts at the center of caring, and everyone has to conform to this template, not least to get recognition and financial support.

In our globalised world we now need to identify the strengths of each religious and secular tradition, to learn from each other and to cooperate. Buddhist caregivers take care of non-Buddhist care-seekers, and Christian pastors are interdenominationally active. Furthermore, there are many caregivers with dual or multiple religious belonging, as noted by Liefbroer and Berghuijs: "The combination of Christianity and Buddhism is most common (47% of the total sample), followed by a combination of Christianity and Judaism (38% of the total sample)" (Liefbroer/Berghuijs 2019, 9). During the past years, I was fortunate to teach Buddhism to young adults of different religious denominations and worldviews not only at the University of Hamburg, but also at the Universities of Oslo, Duisburg-Essen, and Mainz and also for about ten days at Smith College in Northampton, Massachusetts. In my personal experience we can observe everywhere a growing number of young adults who grew up in interfaith households. We may take US Vice President Kamala Harris as an example for the common challenges religious education and counselling are facing today. Harris herself is Baptist. Her mother is a Hindu, her father Christian and her husband is Jewish. Every religion has increasingly to deal with its relation to other religions. For Europe, this means that at university we need a structure of a theology of religions or that fits the many theologies of different religions. It is obvious that dialogue needs to be trained during school and high school. At university students should learn to do theology together and how to develop egalitarian difference.

From a Buddhist perspective, Mikel Monnett is describing an interfaith situation such as that which may be found within care institutions in the United States where the Buddhist caregivers will most often find themselves in situations where the caregiver and careseeker do not share their beliefs. Can a Buddhist truly care for a Christian in such a context? Monnett's answer is a resounding yes, as "the role of the professional chaplain is not to proselytize a particular dogma but to stand with the patient where they are and to help the patient utilize their own spiritual views and beliefs as a resource for their own healing" (Monnett 2005, 59).

In view of the limited resources and the importance of community for pastoral/spiritual care, and because there are many common skills to be acquired, it is standing to reason that nowadays part of the caregiver's training should be interreligious and part of it secular. At the same time, it is important to agree on where it is important to call in caregivers who are specialised in a particular religious tradition or worldview, and how to act in the best way for the benefit of the care-seeker when this is not possible.

Acknowledgement

I am extremely grateful to Monika Deimann-Clemens, Helena M. Strandli Schmidt and Anne-Hege Grung for their support in editing and their feedbacks to previous versions of this article.

Abrreviations

AN Aṅguttara-nikāya
Kd Khandhaka
MN Majjhima-nikāya
Pli Pāli
SN Saṃyutta-nikāya
Tv Theravāda

References

Alhawari, Y, M. A. Verhoff, and M. Parzeller. 2018. "Hirntod, Organtransplantation und Obduktion aus der Sicht der Weltreligionen." Part 1: *Rechtsmedizin* 28: 182–190. https://doi.org/10.1007/s00194-018-0243-9. Part 2: *Rechtsmedizin* 28: 272–279. https://doi.org/10.1007/s00194-018-0242-x

Anālayo, Bhikkhu. 2019. "How Mindfulness Came to Plung Into Its Objects." *Mindfulness* 10: 1181–1185.

Asaṅga, and Sara Boin-Webb. 2001. *Abhidharmasamuccaya: The Compendium of the Higher Teaching (philosophy)*. Translated and annotated by Rahula Walpola, English version by Sara Boin-Webb. Fremont: Asian Humanities Press.

Barnhart, Michael G. 2018. "Buddhist Perspectives on Abortion and Reproduction." In: Daniel Cozort, and James Mark Shields (eds.) *The Buddhist Handbook of Buddhist Ethics*. Oxford: Oxford University Press. 592–610.

Becci, Irene. 2015. "Institutional Resistance to Religious Diversity in Prisons: Comparative Reflections Based on Studies in Eastern Germany, Italy and Switzerland." *International Journal of Politics, Culture, and Society* 28: 5–19. DOI 10.1007/s10767-014-9179-6.

Boellinghaus, Inga, Fergal W. Jones, and Jane Hutton. 2014. "The Role of Mindfulness and Loving-Kindness Meditation in Cultivating Self-Compassion and Other-Focused Concern in Health Care Professionals." *Mindfulness* 5: 129–138. DOI 10.1007/s12671-012-0158-6.

Bosco, Robert M. 2014. "Battlefield Dharma: American Buddhists in American Wars." *Journal of Buddhist Ethics* 21: 827–849. http://blogs.dickinson.edu/buddhistethics/
Brahmapundit, Phra, and Peter Harvey. 2017. *Common Buddhist Text: Guidance and Insight from the Buddha*. Ayutthaya: Mahachulalongkornrajavidyalaya University.
Burtscher, Wolfgang. 2014. *Wenn aus der Krise die Katastrophe wird: Situationsgerechte Kommunikation*. Munich. https://www.grin.com/document/273016
Cadge, Wendy, Irene Elizabeth Stroud, Patricia K. Palmer, George Fitchett, Trace Haythorn, and Casey Clevenger. 2020. "Training Chaplains and Spiritual Caregivers: The Emergence and Growth of Chaplaincy Programs in Theological Education." *Pastoral Psychology* 69: 187–208. https://doi.org/10.1007/s11089-020-00906-5.
Chen, Rong-Chi. 2017. "Clinical Buddhist Chaplaincy Training Program: History of the Development of Taiwan's Clinical Buddhism." *Journal of Scientific Discovery* 1.1:1–7.
Clarke, Shayne. 2004. "Vinaya Mātṛkā – Mother of the Monastic Codes, or Just Another Set of Lists? A Response to Frauwallner's Handling of the Mahāsāṃghika Vinaya." *Indo-Iranian Journal* 47.2: 77–120.
Dalai Lama, XIV, and Thubten Chodron. 2014. *Buddhism: One Teacher, Many Traditions* (Boston: Wisdom), Kindle.
Dalai Lama, XIV, and Thubten Chodron. 2018. *The Foundation of Buddhist Practice*. Sommerville, MA: Wisdom.
Daw Mya Tin, M.A. 1993. (Transl.). *The Dhammapada*. Yangoon, Myanmar: Department for the Promotion and Propagation of the Sāsana.
Esch, Tobias. 2021. "Meditation in Complementary and Integrative Medicine: Taxonomy of Effects and Methods." *Complementary Medicine Research* 28.3: 185–188. DOI: 10.1159/000516849.
European Buddhist Union (ebu). 2021. "Death and dying from a Buddhist perspective." *The European Buddhist Magazine* 7: Retrievable from: http://www.ebumagazine.org/wp-content/uploads/2021/09/EBU_Autumn_2021_Magazine.pdf
Finnigan, Mary, and Rob Hogendoorn. 2019. *Sex and Violence in Tibetan Buddhism: The Rise and Fall of Sogyal Rinpoche*. Portland OR: Jorvik Press.
Frauwallner, Erich. 2010. *The Philosophy of Buddhism* [Die Philosophie des Buddhismus]. Translated by Gelong Lodrö Sangpo with the assistance of Jigme Sheldrön under the supervision of Professor Ernst Steinkellner. Delhi: Motilal Banarsidass.
Garfield, Jay L. 2020. "Beyond catastrophe: We might all be better people once the Covid-19 crisis has subsided." *iai news. Changing How the World Thinks. An online magazine of big ideas* (September 29, 2020). https://iai.tv/articles/impermanence-interdependence-buddhist-reflections-covid-19-auid-1386.
Garfield, Jay L. 2022. *Buddhist Ethics: A Philosophical Exploration*. New York: Oxford University Press.
Gethin, Rupert. 1998. *The Foundations of Buddhism*. Oxford, New York: Oxford University Press.
Giles, Cheryl A., and Willa B. Miller (eds.). 2012. *The Arts of Contemplative Care: Pioneering Voices in Buddhist Chaplaincy and Pastoral Work*. Foreword by Judith Simmer-Brown. Preface by Pat Enkyo O'Hara (Sommerville: Wisdom Publications), Kindle.
Halifax, Joan Jiko. 2012. "Being with Dying: The Upaya Institute Contemplative End-of-Life Training Program." In: Jonathan S. Watts, and Yoshiharu Tomatsu (eds.) *Buddhist Care for the Dying and Bereaved*. (Boston: Wisdom Publications), Kindle.

Harvey, Peter. 2000. *An Introduction to Buddhist Ethics: Foundations, Values and Issues.* Cambridge: Cambridge University Press.

Harvey, Peter. 2018. "The Buddhist Just Society." Daniel Cozort, and James Mark Shields (eds.) *The Buddhist Handbook of Buddhist Ethics*. Oxford: Oxford University Press. 375–406.

Hauschildt, Eberhard. 2015. "Kommunikation und Seelsorge zwischen religiösen und kulturellen Welten." *Interkulturelle Theologie. Zeitschrift für Missionswissenschaft* 41.1: 45–59.

Heller, Birgit. 2012. *Wie Religionen mit dem Tod umgehen: Grundlagen für die interkulturelle Sterbebegleitung* (PalliativCare und OrganisationsEthik 22). Freiburg: Lambertus Verlag.

Hickey, Wakoh Shannon. 2012. "Meditation is Not Enough: Chaplaincy Training for Buddhists." In: Cheryl A. Giles, and Willa B. Miller (eds.) *The Arts of Contemplative Care: Pioneering Voices in Buddhist Chaplaincy and Pastoral Work* (Boston: Wisdom Publications), Kindle.

Horner, Isaline Blew. 1982. *The Book of the Discipline.* Vol. 4. Sacred Books of the Buddhists 20 (Reprint 1982). Oxford: The Pali Text Society 1951.

Jihong, Sunim. 2006. "Volunteer Activities of Korean Buddhist Nuns." In: Karma Lekshe Tsomo (ed.) *Out of the Shadows*. Delhi: Sri Satguru Publications. 281–284.

Kabat-Zinn, Jon. 2013. *Full Catastrophe Living: The Program of the Stress Reduction Clinic at the University of Massachusetts Medical Center* (Revised Edition) (New York: Random House Publishing Group), Kindle.

Kanukollu, Shanta Nishi, and Quyen Epstein-Ngo. 2015. "Violence Against Women Through a Buddhist Lens." In: Andy J. Johnson (ed.) *Religion and Men's Violence Against Women.* New York: Springer Science+Business. DOI 10.1007/978-1-4939-2266-6_21.

Kariyakarawana, Sunil. 2011. "Military careers and Buddhist ethics." *International Journal of Leadership in Public Services* 7.2: 99–108. https://doi.org/10.1108/17479881111160087.

Keown, Damien. 2018. "Euthanasia." In: Daniel Cozort, and James Mark Shields (eds.) *The Buddhist Handbook of Buddhist Ethics*. Oxford: Oxford University Press. 611–629.

King, Sallie B. 2016. "Through the Eyes of Auschwitz and the Killing Fields: Mutual Learning between Engaged Buddhism and Liberation Theology." *Buddhist-Christian Studies* 36: 55–67.

Knauth, Thorsten, and Carola Roloff. 2021. "Achtsamkeit und dialogisches religionsbezogenes Lernen. Konzeptionelle Überlegungen und Schlussfolgerungen für die praktische interreligiöse Zusammenarbeit." In: Telse Iwers and Carola Roloff (eds.) *Achtsamkeit in Bildungsprozessen*. Wiesbaden: Springer. https://doi.org/10.1007/978-3-658-30832-2_2

Liefbroer, Anke I., and Joantine Berghuijs. 2019. "Spiritual Care for Everyone? An Analysis of Personal and Organizational Differences in Perceptions of Religious Diversity Among Spiritual Caregivers." *Journal of Health Care Chaplaincy* 25.3: 1–20. https://doi.org/10.1080/08854726.2018.1556549.

Longaker, Christine. 2009. *Dem Tod begegnen und Hoffnung finden: Die emotionale und spirituelle Begleitung Sterbender*. Munich: Piper Verlag.

Luisi, Pier Luigi. 2010. *Mind and Life: Discussions with the Dalai Lama on the Nature of Reality.* New York: Columbia University Press. https://doi-1org-100c00emb044e.emedien3.sub.uni-hamburg.de/10.7312/luis14550

McCormick, Andrew J. 2013. "Buddhist Ethics and End-of-Life Care Decisions." *Journal of Social Work in End-Of-Life & Palliative Care* 9: 209–225. DOI: 10.1080/15524256.2013.794060.

Miller, Willa B. 2012. "Listening as Spiritual Care." In: Cheryl A. Giles, and Willa B. Miller (eds.) *The Arts of Contemplative Care: Pioneering Voices in Buddhist Chaplaincy and Pastoral Work* (Boston: Wisdom Publications), Kindle.

Monnett, Mikel. 2005. "Developing a Buddhist Approach to Pastoral Care: A Peacemaker's View." *Journal of Pastoral Care & Counseling* 59.1–2: 57–61.

Ngawang, Geshe Thubten, and Christof Spitz (Trans.). 1988–2001. *Systematisches Studium des Buddhismus*. Part 3: *Cittamātra-Lehrmeinung* (vols. V-VI, transcript 1-270, sources 1-125). Unpublished manuscript, widely circulated against course fee. Teaching material of a seven-year study programme on Buddhism consisting of the edited transcripts of all teachings by Geshe Thubten Ngawang 1988-1996 and the German translation of the related Tibetan sources with the respective references. Hamburg: Tibetisches Zentrum e.V.

Nyānatiloka. 2009 [1952]. *The Buddha's Path to Deliverance* (eBook version). Onalaska, Washington USA: BPS Pariyatti Editions.

Nyānatiloka. 1980. *Buddhist Dictionary: Manual of Buddhist Terms and Doctrines*. Fourth Revised Edition. Kandy, Sri Lanka: Buddhist Publication Society.

Nyānatiloka. 1999. *Buddhistisches Wörterbuch*. Stammbach-Herrnschrot: Verlag Beyerlein & Steinschulte.

Petcharoen, Rarinthorn. 2015. "Two monks arrested for child sexual abuse." *Bangkok Post* (March 5, 2015). https://www.bangkokpost.com/thailand/general/489630/two-monks-arrested-for-child-sexual-abuse.

Pollack, Detlef. 2008. "Religious Change in Europe: Theoretical Considerations and Empirical Findings." *Social Compass* 55.2: 168–186.

Roloff, Carola. 2020a. "Openness towards the Religious Other in Buddhism." In: Douglas Duckworth et al. (eds.) *Buddhist Responses to Religious Diversity – Theravāda and Tibetan Perspectives*. Sheffield, Bristol, UK: Equinox eBooks Publishing. 63–96.

Roloff, Carola. 2020b. "Dialogue with Buddhism and Developments towards a Buddhist Theology at the University of Hamburg." In: Wolfram Weisse, Julia Ipgrave, Oddbjørn Leirvik, and Muna Tatari (eds.) *Pluralisation of Theologies at European Universities*. Muenster, New York: Waxmann. 163–186.

Roloff, Carola. 2020c. "Dialogical Theology – Doing Theology Together. A Buddhist Response to the Challenge or Religious Pluralization." In: Anna Körs, Wolfram Weisse, and Jean-Paul Willaime (eds.) *Religious Diversity and Interreligious Dialogue*. Cham, Switzerland: Springer Nature. 281–295.

Roloff, Carola. 2010. "Women's Rights in the Vajrayāna Tradition." In: Carmen Meinert, and Hans-Bernd Zöllner (eds.) *Buddhist Approaches to Human Rights. Dissonances and Resonances*. (eds.) Bielefeld: transcript. 195–210. https://library.oapen.org/handle/20.500.12657/22585.

Roloff, Carola. 1992. "Kostbare Menschengeburt? Zur Position des Buddhismus zum Schwangerschaftsabbruch." In: Andrea Hauner, and Elke Reichart (eds.) *§ 218: zur aktuellen Diskussion*. Munich: Knaur-Verlag. 108–113.

Ronel, Natti, Noa Frid, and Uri Timor. 2013. "The Practice of Positive Criminology: A Vipassana Course in Prison." *International Journal of Offender Therapy and Comparative Criminology* 57.2: 133–153.

Russell-Williams, Jesse, Wafa Jaroudi, Tania Perich, Siobhan Hoscheidt, Mohamad El Haj, and Ahmed A. Moustafa. 2018. "Mindfulness and meditation: treating cognitive impairment and reducing stress in dementia." *Reviews in the Neurosciences* 29.7: 791–804. https://doi.org/10.1515/revneuro-2017-0066.

Sanford, Monica, and Nathan Jishin Michon. 2019. "Buddhist Chaplaincy." *Oxford Research Encyclopedia of Religion*. 1–37. DOI: 10.1093/acrefore/9780199340378.013.641.

Schlieter, Jens. 2003. "Ein Gutachten erstellt im Auftrag der ‚AG Bioethik und Wissenschaftskommission' des Max-Delbrück-Centrums für molekulare Medizin, Berlin-Buch." 2nd revised version https://www.academia.edu/1765203/Die_aktuelle_Biomedizin_aus_der_Sicht_des_Buddhismus (accessed May 5, 2022).

Schlieter, Jens. 2010. "Charles Goodman, Consequences of compassion: An interpretation and defense of Buddhist ethics." New York: Oxford University Press [Book Review]. *Religion* 40: 358–359.

Schmidt-Leukel, Perry. 2006. *Understanding Buddhism*. Edinburgh: Dunedin Academic Press.

Seager, Richard Huges. 1999. *Buddhism in America*. New York: Columbia University Press.

Tomalin, Emma. 2006. "The Thai bhikkhuni movement and women's empowerment." *Gender & Development* 14.3: 385–397. DOI: 10.1080/13552070600980492.

Tsomo, Karma Lekshe (ed.). 2006. *Out of the Shadows. Socially Engaged Buddhist Women. Contributed articles presented at the 8th Sakyadhita International Conference on Buddhist Women held in Seoul, Korea from June 27 to July 4, 2004*. Delhi: Sri Satguru Publications.

Vanna, Peou. 2006. "The Quiet Movement of Buddhist Women in Cambodia." In: Karma Lekshe Tsomo (ed.) *Out of the Shadows*. Delhi: Sri Satguru Publications. 19–21.

Wagner, Don. 2017. *Buddhist chaplain serves all spiritual needs*. U.S. Department of Defense Section 508. August 4, 2017, https://www.army.mil/article/191733/buddhist_chaplain_serves_all_spiritual_needs.

Watts, John S., and Yoshiharu Tomatsu (eds.) 2012. *Buddhist Care for the Dying and Bereaved*. Boston: Wisdom.

Weilhart, Regina. 2021. "Warum wir in Deutschland eine buddhistische Seelsorge brauchen." *Buddhismus aktuell* 35.3: 8–9.

Weiss, Helmut, Karl H. Federschmidt, Daniël Louw, and Linda Sauer Bredvik (eds.). 2021. *Care, Healing, and Human Well-Being Within Interreligious Discourses*. Afrian Sun Media, SUN MeDia. https://doi.org/10.2307/j.ctv2bgz3js

Naveed Baig

The Islamic theology behind spiritual care and hospital chaplaincy

Abstract: Over the last two decades Muslim chaplaincy in general has emerged into a distinct field of discussion, practise and study at the institutional level in the Nordic countries. There is no identifiable 'canon' of original sources that identifies and traces the theology behind Muslim chaplaincy. I argue that a large portion of that theology is derived from the primary and secondary sources of Islam- the Quran and Sunnah. I explore the salient features of spiritual care in Islam and equate them with a Muslim chaplaincy practise that is exemplified through chaplains' own reflections.

Introduction

At present there is little systematic mapping and investigation within Islamic theology available that addresses spiritual care and hospital chaplaincy. In this contribution I aim to identify and make accessible Islamic theological reasoning behind spiritual care and its use in hospital settings. Furthermore, based on Islamic literature I will give examples of practical spiritual care seen through the lens of Muslim chaplains working in hospitals. I have also used my own work, primarily drawing on my experiences, teachings and written recommendations as a Muslim hospital chaplain for 16 years in a hospital from Denmark, to illustrate the dynamics and complexities of spiritual care.

The whole human being

Everything in Islam is 'spiritual'. To understand this it is important to dissect the word 'spirit' and its understanding from the viewpoint of Islamic tradition. The word *ruh* (spirit or breath of life) has its basis from the Quran where the root of the term is mentioned 19 times (Osama 2005). The term *ruh* is used in the Quran to refer to many metaphysical beings like angels, Archangel Gabriel, revelation and divine inspiration. But often it connotes the most inner essence of humans. Quran commentators have used various meanings for the word *ruh*. For example the Quran-exegetist Al-Zamakhshari (d.1144) interprets it as divine inspiration that gives life to the hearts (heart as an organ of perception and not a psychical

 https://doi.org/10.1515/9783110717365-005

entity) that were dead in their ignorance, and points out that the *ruh* has the same function for the body as the soul (Ansari 2006). The human in Islamic psychology consists of: self, heart, intellect and soul (Rassool 2016).

The relevance of Islamic spiritual care, its content and definitions cannot be understated since their theological foundations, that go back to Islam's early history, are brought into dialogue with prevalent practices and social sciences of today in a variety of ways. It is commonly known that the essence of Islamic spiritual care is based on theology founded on the Quran and the sunnah, (the words, actions, approvals/disapprovals of the Prophet Muhammad) albeit the resources of social sciences such as grief theory, developmental theory and gender studies have a correlation to Islamic spiritual care (Isgandarova 2016). Therefore a ' backstage' look at the Islamic theology of care can give new opportunities for engagement in and with other fields of knowledge.

In this section it is imperative to describe and distinguish between the Quranic terms self, heart, intellect and *ruh,* for the sake of clarity.

1. The self or *nafs*, the humans innate nature has several interchangeable states varying from the animalistic, to the self at peace and the pure angelic form. Therefore, in its untrained state, the self is appetitive and only through *mujahadah al nafs* (combatting the self) can it be refined and advance. Keshavarzi and Haque, 2013 translate *nafs* as 'behavioural inclinations'. The word *nafs* originates from *nafees* meaning valuable and precious but also from *nafas* denoting breathing.
2. The heart or *qalb* is described in detail later in this chapter as 'the spiritual heart' which is the receptacle of all health and pathology (Keshavarzi, Khan, Ali & Awad 2021). This understanding of the heart in Islam, makes it an organ of illumination and wisdom, that is, if the other components of the human work towards that end, otherwise the heart risking decay. The word is derived from the verb *qalaba* which means to tilt, turn, and transform. According to Sufi understanding the heart must constantly rotate around its Creator and be ready to return upon the physical death (Haeri 1997).
3. Intellect or *aql* is a rational faculty by which humans may attain knowledge and reasoning. Derived from the root verb *aqala* , it has different meanings as, 'to confine', 'to understand', 'to restrain a camel by tying its forelegs'. The implication is that true rationality can be cultivated alone by constraining the base and animalistic *nafs* (Haeri 1997). This faculty is necessary for ethical and moral accountability and it allows the human to distinguish between right and wrong.
4. The physical body also called *jism* in Arabic is the biological 'shell' of the faculties of the human. The body and soul are normally seen as opposites

but while the body is material it is also the manifest condition of humans which is seen as a gift from and trust of God (Baig 2010).
5. Spirit or *ruh* is the 'Divine spark' within humans and is limitless. Its origin lies in the realm of non-time and non-space. It is the infinite within and at death it will depart from the body and be imprinted with the 'image' of the body (jism). The *ruh* transcends the limits of the intellect (aql) albeit the importance of rationality in this world is undeniable (Haeri 1997).

Even though the Quran has scant information about the *ruh* it does nevertheless, mention humankind being gifted a special position in the universe containing a 'Divine spark': *When I have fashioned him (Adam) and breathed into him of My spirit, fall you down in prostration unto him* (Quran, 15:28 – 29).

According to Al-Ghazali, the *ruh* is a special faculty for acquiring knowledge and gnosis (Winter 2005). It was a capacity that was given after God fashioned humans physically and biologically. God then announced his decision to create Adam: *Behold thy Lord said to the angels: I will create a vicegerent on earth* (Quran, 2:30). Alongside the characteristic of knowledge given to the *ruh*, there is also the aspect of God consciousness: *Am I not your lord, they said Yes, we testify* (Quran, 7:172).

The above-mentioned verse relates to the primordial event where all souls according to the Quran took a pledge to God acknowledging him as their Lord. Since human beings are 'beings of spirit' according to Islamic teachings, all activities in life have a spiritual value and significance. Although the Quran does not venture into any metaphysical discussion about the spirit it does in detail explain other aspects of the psyche that are more directly related to the human behaviour and its relation to society (Ansari 2006). *Qalb* (heart) has the independent ability to either turn its direction towards the divine unity and order prevailing inside the self and universe at large, or to remain bounded by and into the 'random stimuli' (Ansari 2006). His point is that if the heart is predominantly occupied with the sensory and lower self-inclinations like gluttony, lust, arrogance and the likes, they will ultimately override the faculties and make the human a slave of sensual pleasures. The Prophetic saying 'there is a certain organ in the body, if its wellbeing is secured the whole body is sound, that is the heart', establishes the basis for the heart's unique capacity for a deep spiritual life (Choureif 2011).

Khidmah as an integral culture

Khidmah from the Arabic language, literally means servitude and implies service to humanity (Zaman 1986). The Christian equivalent, as I understand it, is *diakonia*, a Christian theological term from Greek that encompasses the call to serve the poor and oppressed. [1]

Care or caring for oneself, parents, family and community is an obligation in Islam (Gilliat-Ray, Ali & Pattison 2013). The concept of viceregency and its functions cover this. Islam's family system brings the rights of the husband, wife, children and relatives into an equilibrium as the decrees of the family are clearly stated in the Quran and hadith literature (Rassool 2014). Moreover, Islamic values attach special importance to the family, and extended family structures are encouraged to maintain and guard the needs of the young and elderly specifically (Rassool 2014). The words used for family in Arabic are *usra* (to bond) and *aa'ila*. (to have needs) (Gilliat-Ray, Ali & Pattison 2013).

The practice of *Khidmah* goes beyond the nuclear family, widening the circles of blood ties, which the Quran calls 'relation of the womb' (*silhah rahm*). The word womb, *rahm* in Arabic, is derived directly from Gods name *Al-Rehman*, the most compassionate. (Bukhari 5988) God has filled the mother's womb with His qualities of compassion and mercy and because of these attributes members of families bond with each other (Gilliat-Ray, Ali & Pattson 2013). Besides the family, Muslims see themselves as part and parcel of a global community in faith, the *ummah*. The word *ummah* in Arabic is derived from the word *umm*, meaning mother, denoting values like unity, warmth, compassion and tenderness. While the word *ummah* suggests an 'intra-Muslim fraternity' there is also 'human fraternity' in Islam which encompasses all of humanity. According to Prophet Muhammad's famous words from his farewell sermon: "All people are equal like the teeth of a comb. You are all from Adam and Adam is from dust. There is no superiority of white over black, nor of Arab over non-Arab except for God-consciousness" (Musnad Imam Ahmad 19774 and Hathout 2008 p.82).

Likewise, the Prophet mentioned that the most beloved to God are those most caring to God's creation (al-Muʿjam al-Awsaṭ 6026) and after belief in God the best deed is benevolent love towards people (Choureif 2011). This type of care and benevolence transcends ethnic, cultural and religious boundaries.

Also providing care to other creatures than humankind, including the mineral and plant worlds including the vast nature in general is a recommended

1 "Diakonia's History: About us," Diakonia Sweden, accessed 01, July, 2021, https://www.diakonia.se/en/About-us/Organization/History/.

duty for Muslims (Baig 2007). Hence this concept of 'theological humanitarianism' is embedded in the Islamic sources and can be equated with the concept of *khidmah*. The concept of *khidmah* impedes the logic of dependency and reciprocity since – in material terms at least – nothing is expected in return from the *khadim*, literally meaning the service giver (Mittermaier 2014). The thinking behind on a broader level implies that everyone is dependent on God and therefore 'poor' or a *faqir*, meaning 'poor toward God' – a Quranic term (Quran, 35:15).

An example of *Khidmah:* Visitation of the sick

Visiting the sick or iyaddah is a social obligation for Muslims although the visit should be considerate to the patient. (Mazrui 2005). There is a wide range of hadith literature that emphasizes visiting and consoling the sick. Some of the views of sickness in the Islamic tradition are:

1. God's nearness to the sick person.
2. Sickness as inner purification for the affected – erasure of sins and elevation of one's 'spiritual' rank.
3. The sick person's prayers being answered by God.
4. The high religious merits of visiting the sick and dying (Fareedi 2008).

Attending to the sick, whoever they might be, is known by Muslims to have high spiritual value (Kowalski 2009). This type of practical spiritual care is engraved in the daily Muslim cultural practise. There are certain dilemmas as well. Can there be too many visitors at hospital wards? How do the families deal with a situation when visitors from the periphery want to come and visit?

During my work at Rigshospitalet, a Copenhagen hospital as the Muslim chaplain, I once encountered a group of 5–6 young practising Muslims outside my office who had some questions. They informed me about their desire to visit the patients at the hospital and wanted access. As they said, we want to console and talk religion with all the patients and give them advice. I had in my mind some considerations and wanted to communicate it to the enthusiastic volunteers.

Since we already at the hospital had an organised and operationalized volunteer corps, I informed them that they could write and sign up to be part of the team which visits minority patients who have cultural, spiritual or religious needs. In addition, I told them that it is always the patients, that summon people of this character from outside if they desire. I also told them that I, even as an employee and chaplain, do not go around the wards freely but visit on request of the patients/relatives.

After they left, many questions emerged in my mind. Firstly, what type of qualifications are needed for supporters/visitors? Who is legible to visit patients in the first place? Are there any human traits and features that are a prerequisite for supporters/visitors to have before visiting? What place does *dawah* (propagation of Islam) or missiology for that sake, have at public, state financed institutions? Secondly questions relating to patient autonomy and 'protection' were imminent. What services and information are offered (and how) to the patient through hospital staff? Who decides what services are offered? How does one avoid 'spiritual abuse' directed towards patients and relatives?

At one occasion I was called to ICU where a patient was on a life-saving respiratory machine. There were about 35–40 relatives and friends present in and around the ICU. Some were waiting outside and reading the Quran. The doctors had just notified the family members about the irreversible brain death condition of the patient, and family members were very troubled and emotional. Some of them were very vocal in their disapproval over the fact that the respiratory machine would have to be turned off soon. Others were quiet and in sorrow. One family member asked me what the Islamic position was on stopping the respiratory machine since the imam they consulted from a country in the Middle East (over the phone) was of the opinion that it was the heart-death criteria that was to be followed and not the brain-death (hence turning off the machine would not be valid Islamically since the patient was 'only' brain dead). This created a lot of confusion amongst the relatives and family members who had different approaches to this ethical dilemma. I informed them, amongst other things, the brain-death criteria to be a valid position in Islamic thinking, and that in the end it was always the physicians' decision from the ICU to make.

In my reflections after this counselling session there where many central questions. What different roles do relatives play in visiting their loved ones? What is life and its definition? How to help- if possible- relatives and family during their bereavement?

The two cases illustrate different perspectives on visiting the sick including how significant a practise it is in the daily Muslim life. The cases also show that apart from visitation and volunteering (case 1), making important decisions on behalf of the patient (case 2) is considered part of the visiting responsibility. Even though there was controversy over the doctor's decision in case 2, it was very clear that the relatives wanted to be involved actively in the decision-making process. The thinking behind being, that we exhausted all means, as relatives, to save our dear ones' life. Also, the collective grief culture in case 2 highlights the importance of being together in times of distress and hardship. There is a 'doing' function along with the 'being'. Thus, visitation of the sick, can also be viewed within the framework of *Khidmah*, and plays a pivotal role in a hospital setting having implications for patients, relatives, staff, administration and their inter-relations.

The Prophet and spiritual care

Apart from giving Prophet Muhammad meta-physical attributes and qualities, the Quran and hadith literature illustrate a human picture of him. The Quran refers to the Prophet as 'most kind', *rauf* and most merciful, *raheem* (Ayad 2008). Several other names of God are used to refer to the Prophet Muhammad as well. The Quran describes the Prophet's morals as of highest stature and his advent as a "mercy to all worlds" (21:107). His interpersonal and pedagogical skills are numerous, and Islamic traditions record how people were drawn towards his person through his compassion and non-judgemental behaviour. His spiritual care was directed to everyone, his family and friends, followers and adversaries, Muslims and non-Muslims, animals and nature (Quran, 21:107).

There are many stories in Hadith about the caring attitude of the Prophet crossing different boundaries: A bird, belonging to a son of one of the companions of the Prophet, died. The son known as Abu Umayr was upset and when the Prophet found out he visited the boy and consoled him by repeating the words " O Abu Umayr what happened to *al-nughair* (little bird)?" In Arabic this is a play on words because Umayr rhymes with *nughair.* (Sunan Abu Dawood 4969).

A funeral procession was once passing and the Prophet stood up out of respect for it. He was then told that it was a Jew, whereupon the Prophet said: " Was he not a human?" (Ṣaḥīḥ al-Bukhārī 1250)

The *Ta'if* episode: After being stoned and ridiculed by opponents in the city of *Ta'if* who were dissatisfied with the Prophets message of the new faith, his shoes covered with blood, he said the following prayer:

> O Allah! I complain to You of my weakness, my scarcity of resources and the humiliation I have been subjected to by the people. O Most Merciful of those who are merciful. O Lord of the weak and my Lord too. To whom have you entrusted me?
>
> To a distant person who receives me with hostility. Or to an enemy to whom you have granted authority over my affair? So long as You are not angry with me, I do not care. Your favour is of a more expansive relief to me. I seek refuge in the light of Your Face by which all darkness is dispelled and every affair of this world and the next is set right, lest Your anger or Your displeasure descends upon me. I desire Your pleasure and satisfaction until You are pleased. There is no power and no might except by You (Mubarakpuri 2002).

This critical incident demonstrates amongst other things how to react to crisis situations and afflictions. This reaction to offensiveness from one's enemies is a type of 'care' where one does not talk badly or curse but instead directs one's attention towards God through prayers and God-talk. Prayers, God-talk and other practises/rituals can be described as 'religious coping' or 'coping strategies' that are particularly defined in the scientific field of psychology of religion. These strategies can be both positive and negative (Pargament 1997).

Once a person approached the Prophet and asked him:

> I have committed a grave sin, is there forgiveness for me? The Prophet replied: is your mother alive? The man said: no. Is your aunt alive the Prophet inquired? The reply was yes, to which the Prophet said: do well to her (Sunan Tirmidhi 1904).

Substituting a bad action with a good one is a recommended practice in Islam since it removes the evil (Quran, 11:114) deeds, and the Prophets advice in the above-mentioned story, clearly encourages 'meaningful action' and goodness to others. The Prophet is non-judgemental and does not ask of the man's grave mistake but focuses on what can be done to restore his self-worth and dignity.

At one of the cancer wards at Rigshospitalet, I was called by a male patient for a visit as a chaplain. The middle-aged man was on his death bed and the doctors could not give any curative treatment anymore. The patient was very inward and expressed fear of dying because of his past mistakes and what they would mean for his afterlife. He recited the *astaghfaar* (formula of repentance to God) he told me and gave away money for charity hoping that he would be forgiven by God. He was alone and had no family members that could visit him. Since he was troubled by his past mistakes and was hit by shame and guilt, I spoke to him about his image of God- how did he ultimately perceive Allah? Gods all-encompassing mercy became the center point of our conversation very quickly and he began to narrate different Prophetic stories elucidating Gods infinite mercy and love whilst being touched emotionally. During the end of the session he kept on saying that he loved Allah and his Prophet and that he was "ready to go". He died later that day.

Making God personal: spiritual care through remembrance of God's names

In Islamic theology, health beliefs are along with other doctrines based on the concept of *tawheed* or oneness of God (Rassool 2014). Fundamental to Islamic teachings are the connections between knowledge, health, holism, the environment and the Oneness of Allah, the unity of God in all spheres of life, death and the hereafter. Rassool explains: "*Tawheed* requires that a Muslim lives in a way that reflects the unity of mind and body with Allah; and implies that there is no separation of physical and spiritual dimensions of health. Muslims have a spiritual obligation to maintain health" (Rassool 2014).

Intimately connected to *tawheed* is the term *dhikr*. The Quran encourages few practices to the same degree as '*dhikr Allah*' (Remembrance of God). The word *dhikr* does not only mean remembrance (mentally) but also mentioning (verbally) and reminding that can be done standing, sitting and lying, meaning at any time and place (Murata & Chittick 2005). Practising Muslims remember God through daily prayers, recitation of the Quran and through many other rituals and practises (Rassool 2016). Strictly speaking, remembering God does not require a specific ritual or practise but it can make it easier. The mental form of remembrance of God which consists of a persons' recollection, that God observes all acts and thoughts, has many stages. (Murray 2016) This type of 'lived mindfulness' is also illustrated in the hadith of Gabriel where the Prophet answers thus to the definition of *ihsaan* (to act beautifully and in excellence): "Excellence is to worship Allah as if you see Him, for if you do not see Him, He surely sees you " (Sahih Muslim, 8).

The spiritual heart

"Blessed are the pure in heart, for they shall see God." (Jesus, son of Mary, Matthew 5:8)

The heart *(al-qalb)* has a variety of meanings in the Arabic language and its Quranic usage. (Baig, 2007) There is a vast literature in Islamic history dealing with the heart and its intellectual and spiritual significance. There are over 130 references to the heart in the Quran and plentiful traditions of the Prophet relating to this subject matter. (Cutsinger 2002). Al-Ghazali points out in his magnum opus that the heart 'denotes two things, the physical heart and the 'ethereal spiritual sort' (Al-Ghazali 2010). He mentions that the 'spiritual heart' is the essence of man, the potential seat of God's illuminations and serenity, to be kept sound for the physical body to operate optimally (ibid).

The Prophet Muhammad explained: "Surely in the breasts of humanity is a lump of flesh, if sound then the whole body is sound, and if corrupt then the whole body is corrupt. Is it not the heart?" (Ṣaḥih al-Bukhari 52, Ṣaḥih Muslim 1599). This statement underlines the fact that the heart can become unhealthy with various 'diseases' like lust, anger, jealousy, hate and its remedy is also mentioned by the Prophet: "Verily, everything has a polish and the polish of the heart is the remembrance of Allah Almighty" (Shu'ab al-Imaan 503).

The Quran like other scriptures associates knowledge and understanding with the heart and the blindness of the heart with loss of understanding (Cutsinger 2002). This loss of understanding is also associated with 'hardness' and veiling of the heart. The heart can, however, be softened and veils removed through the help of God 'who is aware of what is in your hearts' (33:51). As explained above, divine remembrance, *dhikr*, is one way of attaining a pure heart. This remembrance, in the Islamic spiritual tradition – also called Sufism, is the highest level of prayer of the heart and by the heart. It is not only to invoke, but to live at the heart-center which is an abode of spiritual meaning (Cutsinger 2002).

In the daily Muslim prayer life, training oneself in increasing one's faith, is through the *dhikr* of God's beautiful names (asma' al- husna). 'And Allah's are the most beautiful names, so call on Him thereby...' (Quran, 7:180)

Al-Jilani (d.1166 AD), the founder of the Qadiriyya sufi order writes regarding remembrance:

> The way to free the heart, to purify it, is to remember God. At the beginning this remembrance can only be done outwardly, by repeating His divine names, pronouncing them aloud so that you yourself and others can hear and remember. As the memory of Him becomes constant, remembrance sinks to the heart and becomes inward, silent. Allah says:
>
> Believers are those, when Allah is mentioned, feel a tremor in their hearts, and when they (see and) hear his manifestations their faith is strengthened (Al-Halveti 1992, Page 41).

Tremor here signifies awe, fear and love of God, according to Jilani. In the same treatise he

concludes that when one reaches inner purity, as a result, he/she is beautified with the best of

character and manners. Hence purification of the heart leads to outer change and a reformation of one's morals (Al-Halveti 1992). Additionally, remembrance of God also gives peace of heart because the heart embraces the love of the divine (Al-Halveti 1992).

God's attributes

How can these attributes assist the human being in his/her daily life? The answer to this question (which will follow) would lead us to approach a practical theology of God's attributes. Qualities such as the Patient (as-Sabur), the Giver of serenity (as-Salam), the Protector (al-Muhaymin), the Protecting Friend (al-Wali), the Pardoner (al-'Afu), the Clement (al-Haleem), the Merciful (ar-Rahman), the

Subtle (al-Latif), the All-embracing (al-Wasi'), the All-responsive(al-Mujeeb), the One Who expands (al-Basit), the Loving (al-Wadud) to mention a few, indicate how significant these immeasurable attributes are and what potential the human has to offer humanity. Here, it should be said, that only God has the 'patent' to these names in absolute terms since God and creature 'never combine' hence no incarnationism in Islam (Winter 2008). Humans can contemplate upon and enrobe these qualities but cannot 'own' them in their entirety. The qualities are already implanted in the human *fitrah* or natural disposition as it is often translated. The word *fitrah* originates from *fatara* meaning 'to split, 'to originate', 'to create'. This alludes to an original blueprint so that this 'bringing into being' may take place (Haeri 1997).

These qualities have to be explored, discovered, identified and polished in the self (nafs) according to the Quran:

> By the nafs,
> And the proportion and order
> Given to it,
> And its inspiration
> As to its wrong and its right;
> Truly he succeeds
> That purifies it,
> And he fails
> That corrupts it.
> (Q 91:7–10)

It is God's attributes that are implanted in the self, but they have to be 'known.' A well-known example of this discovering and reflection is the example of Adam who is given knowledge of all the names. (Q 2:30). But to comprehend these at a higher intensity he had to repent, redress and reflect over his actions after the fall. So, the human being through the example of Adam is encouraged to ponder over and actively come to terms with the inner tribulations in order to learn valuable and untold information about the self.

The more divine names and their remembrance fills the individual instead of the daily distractions, usual inner confusion, opinion of others, the more one may begin to experience the breath and pattern of remembrance. Just as God is the Ever-Living, the divine names are understood to be alive and spiritually inexhaustible and are transferred from the tongue where the remembrance initiates, to the mind, deeper levels of the personality and arrive and encompass entirely, the inner being. (Helminski, 1999)

The names of God, which are just one form of *dhikr Allah*, have a spiritual connotation in the Muslim mind. It acts like a *wird* (invocation) where reciting and hymning the names of God can give patients solace and spiritual soothing. (Isgandarova, 2018) The 99 names, *asma al husna* (minimum 99, the total unknown) refer to the one God in multiple ways (Kowalski 2009).

Muslim theologians and Sufis have written exhaustively on the names of God. In the process they frequently describe the effect that each name may have on the selves that remember them (Al-Ghazali 1999). In practical terms, using Gods names gives Muslims guidance and personal image of God. In his introduction Al-Halveti writes:

> The beautiful names of Allah are proof of the existence and oneness of Allah. O you who are burdened and troubled with the weight and suffering of the material world, may Allah make His beautiful names a soothing balm for your wounded hearts. Learn, understand and recite Allahs beautiful names. Seek the traces of Allahs attributes in the skies above, on the earth below and in what is beautiful in your being[...] (Al-Halveti 1983).

For one in need of spiritual care, Al Ghazzali and Al-Halveti's manuals can be regarded as means to retrieve immanence of God into the heart by 'adorning' themselves with the names of God. The names of God are attributes that patients can contemplate upon and make Gods personal in their experience of suffering and crisis. Patients having anxiety of death can for instance call upon *Al-wadud*, the all-loving, *Ar-Raheem*, the most merciful and *Al-qareeb*, the most near. They function, as solace-bringing practises and 'personalized rituals' for patients and relatives where prayer beads are used for recital.

A nurse from a neonatal ward calls me on phone and asks for a set of prayer beads for a mother with Muslim background who is hospitalized alongside her sick daughter pre-maturely born and weighing much under the average. I visit the ward the same day with the beads and some days later have a counselling session with the mother. She tells me that she has been chanting the names of Allah, *Hafeez* (protector), *al-Hayy* (the ever living) and *Malik-ul Mulk (*The owner of all creation) constantly. I ask her what this practice meant to her and she said that holding a prayer bead gave her something to hold on to physically, and the invocations of those particular names gave her a feeling that God would protect and give life to her baby.

I pondered afterwards on how hospital wards could store/make room for religious and spiritual 'merchandise' from different religions and life stance communities. It could be of countless interest to know what impact it had on staff-patient relationship if the nurses/doctors knew more about how their patients struggled and coped in times of tribulation.

A liver patient, once said to me during a counselling session: "In the beginning of my sickness, I thought a lot inside of myself, wrestled with Allah, complained to Him. I asked "why me?" Then I thought I was the cause of my sickness. I had committed an offense. So, I sought forgiveness from friends and family and called everyone. That gave me a feeling of satisfaction. I had a direct line to Allah. I didn't think about anyone else. Read a lot of *Istaghfaar* (reciting the repentance formula)". The patient also mentioned that he recited the Qur'an with translation daily and prayed and recited the *asma al husna* (names of Allah).

The liver patient actively uses the religious practises during hospitalization and makes God personal by using terms as 'wrestling with God' and asking questions directly to God. This form of religious and spiritual practise highlights the importance of finding meaning and significance during calamity.

Until now we have investigated the theology and important concepts behind spiritual care in Islam, concentrating on the holistic human construction, the idea of *khidmah*, the motivation behind visitation of the sick alongside the more practical lived religious rituals as remembrance and its theistic connection. The sections above, even though theoretical in character, give background information and the rationale behind the thinking of spiritual care in Islam. My personal anecdotes from the hospital chaplaincy work illustrate practical and operational spiritual care.

In the next section the focus will be on chaplaincy, its institutionalization and an examination of an American female chaplains' work.

Muslim Chaplaincy in the West- from theory to practise

Dr. Attaullah Siddiqui in his meticulous report' Islam at Universities in England-meeting the needs and investing in the future' written for the Minister of Higher Education in 2007 expounds these qualities of the Muslim chaplain/advisor:

1. *A good knowledge of Islam, preferably some kind of formal Islamic qualification.*
2. *Understanding of British society and university culture.*
3. *Understanding of other faiths and willingness to engage with them positively.*
4. *Communication and counselling skills and willingness to listen and be approachable.*
5. *Being open to all denominations within Islam. (Siddiqui 2007 p. 53)*

Even though there is a consensus, according to this study about the five qualities needed of a Muslim chaplain, it still leaves the reader pondering over the central question, what is Islamic chaplaincy? How do we define the concept and content of Muslim chaplaincy practice and is it compatible with secular institutions?

These questions are pertinent for discussions pertaining to Muslims and Islamic theology in public institutions also because of the increased interest in care services to citizens with Muslim backgrounds at predominantly monocultural Scandinavian countries.

On 8 November 2020, the world of British Muslim Studies lost one of its most thoughtful founding scholars. Dr. Ataullah Siddiqui worked at the Islamic Foundation in Leicester and its sister institution, Markfield Institute of Higher Education (MIHE), for some 40 years. Dr. Siddiqui was for a period responsible for the Islamic chaplaincy program at MIHE. His vision was very clear as he wanted a comprehensive and holistic alim/alima/imam role in the UK where the chaplaincy function plays a vital role in giving interpersonal skills and theological reflection to this function. His boldness can be exemplified by the fact that other faith chaplains taught at the Islamic chaplaincy program including Catholic and Anglican representatives. Dr. Siddiqui understood that Christian chaplaincy with its long tradition and grounded institution in the UK, could serve as an inspiration and resource for upcoming Muslims working in secular public institutions with inter-faith spiritual care settings, prevalent in the UK. He also understood the intricate and sensitive relationship that Muslim chaplains could have with chaplains with other faiths/life stances and had experience in dealing with that qua his interfaith work and relations.

Dr. Siddiqui mentioned once to me the importance of highlighting the theological spectrum of Islamic chaplaincy which too has its justification. The background information pertaining to 'Muslim practise' at hospitals is something which is implored by hospital staff. Why do Muslims do such and such? There has been keen interest from hospital staff in the West, especially in the area of palliative care, thanatology, end of life rituals, mental health issues, view of sickness, bereavement issues, domestic violence, sexual abuse for many years (Ahmed & Amer 2012, Baig 2019). This is also true for other religions and life stances. In this section I will attempt to give the rationale behind Islamic chaplaincy theology; navigating through the theological tunnel of Islamic care and how it is understood today.[2]

The word chaplain is English and comes from the Latin *cappellani*, which has different meanings. One of them is cloak. The word shows back to a tale of St. Martin, who was a Roman soldier (A.D. 316–397). After one day having

2 In my ongoing PhD work at the University of Oslo entitled 'Muslim patients with COVID-19 at Nordic hospitals- the role of faith and spirituality during times of sickness and tribulations', I will also investigate the theology behind hospitalization of Muslim patients and its significance. "Naveed Baig: Ph.D. projects," University of Oslo, accessed 01, August, 2021, https://www.tf.uio.no/english/research/phd/phdprojects/Baig/index.html.

helped a poor freezing man by tearing his cloak in two and covering him with one, he had a dream. In the dream he saw Jesus wearing that particular robe, and this vision led to a 'life conversion', through which he devoted his life to God and service of humanity (Farmer 2019).

A 'chaplain' is therefore a person who 'gives a part of himself' to a needy person.

The term chaplaincy is used in English-speaking countries for the employees who provide religious and life stance services at public institutions. These types of services are value based and include, among other things, existential conversations, spiritual support, religious rituals, counselling and often teaching and guidance to staff on ethical and existential issues -also in cross disciplinary settings (Snorton 2020).

Chaplains work closely with institutional leadership to ensure that religious and general services delivered by the institution are culturally sensitive and representative of the diversity of the patients/relatives that the hospital serves. Chaplains are also included on hospital ethics committees, advising on the complex biomedical ethical issues, teach and train hospital staff in topics related to religion, culture, ethics, spiritual care and the interplay between these. Chaplains also counsel patients, families/friends and staff as ethical decisions are considered and made for instance on abortion, ceasing respiratory machines and fasting during the Islamic month of Ramadan (Baig 2019).

The chaplaincy title is used today in English-speaking countries across religion and beliefs, and employees may therefore be Muslims, Catholics, Buddhists, etc. and are named after them: Buddhist Chaplain, Humanist Chaplain, etc. Chaplaincy is a specialist function within spiritual and existential care with special competency requirements (Gilliat-Ray et al. 2014). The Nordic countries do not currently have a similar concept or common word for this type of position called chaplain. Words like *sjælesorger* (soul carer / pastoral care worker) *koordinator* (coordinator), imam and more recently *muslimsk* samtalepartner [3] (Muslim counsellor) are used in different contexts for care givers with Muslim backgrounds. (Baig 2019).

Norway, Denmark and Sweden have a deep-rooted and historical connection to their respective Lutheran churches – Protestant Christianity being the majority religion since the reformation. In Sweden, church and state are separated, but at the institutional level including hospitals, there is close cooperation. In Denmark, the Lutheran pastors are the only religious representatives who are formal-

3 "En historisk ansettelse: News," Oslo University Hospital, accessed 01, August, 2021, https://oslo-universitetssykehus.no/om-oss/nyheter/en-historisk-ansettelse

ly employed at public institutions apart from a few exceptions and according to the Danish constitution, § 4, "The Evangelical Lutheran Church shall be the Established Church of Denmark, and as such shall be supported by the State". [4] In Norway, there is today a formal separation between church and state[5], but in terms of the historical pastoral services at hospitals for instance, the church still has a marked presence and organizational structure intact. True for these Scandinavian countries is that the church is embedded in chaplaincy services at most of the hospitals in this region (Baig 2019).

Fields of Islamic spiritual care and its understanding

Even though Islamic spiritual care as we have seen, is an independent discipline, it is related to other forms of care and formation in Islamic theology like bildung (*tarbiyyah*), preaching (*dawah*), ethics (*ikhlaaq*), spiritual purification (*tazkiyyah*) and prophetic medicine/healing (*tibb un nabawi*). Islamic spiritual care has many forms and levels to help individuals strengthen and reflect upon their life convictions and abilities to face personal, relational, or public challenges which may include grief and loss, emphatic listening, parenting etc. Islamic spiritual care is more than clerical responsibility. The main goal is healing, sustaining, guiding and reconciling (Isgandarova 2014).

Although there is no tradition of institutionalized chaplaincy that goes back to the early formative years of Islam there is an implicit theology that supports and inspires what can be paralleled to Christian pastoral care. Moreover, the long history of organizing and systematizing pastoral care in the West has not been seen in the Islamic theological history (Baig, 2010). There are three primary reasons for that:

1) there is no single authority that can define the word of God. The imam role is decentralized and there is no 'imamhood' in Islam.
2) The family role is superior.
3) Social conditions have been changing (Gilliat-Ray et al. 2013).

---

4 "The constitutional act of Denmark: Publications, " The Danish Parliament, accessed 25, August, 2021, https://www.thedanishparliament.dk/-/media/pdf/publikationer/english/the_constitutional_act_of_denmark_2013,-d-,pdf.ashx.

5 "Norway Ends 500-Y-O Lutheran Church Partnership, 'Biggest Change Since the Reformation: News," Christian Post, accessed 25, August, 2021.https://www.christianpost.com/news/norway-ends-500-year-old-lutheran-church-partnership-biggest-change-since-reformation-172480/

The changing religious demography (Islam being the largest religious minority in all Scandinavian countries) has had consequences for public institutions across Western Europe serving a 'mixed population' stemming from a wide range of cultures and faith groups (Swift et al. 2016). Today, the facilitation of religious diversity (or the lack of it), the local context of the institution and national socio-economic/political circumstances are determining the degree of recognition of multi-faith chaplaincy in many European countries including Scandinavia.

It is a paradox that chaplaincy – even though a liminal area in religious practise – has had powerful significance on how it's viewed on legal, political, educational and religious grounds in Nordic countries (Sw ift et al. 2016). An example of this is The University of Oslo's (UIO) new Master program in Chaplaincy including Buddhist, Muslim and Humanist modules that made headlines in the press and its launch reception attended by notables including Crown Prince Haakon Magnus of Norway, something quite unique, for University academic programs in Norway.[6]

Spiritual care through institutional chaplaincy

One of the complexities that institutionalized Muslim chaplaincy faces today is the task of excavating and polishing the vast theological material into the chaplaincy services that meet the 'everyday Muslims' living 'ordinary lives' in vulnerable situations.

An American study led by the University of Michigan Health System, finds positive aspects in Muslim hospital chaplaincy (Padela et al. 2011). The study that was published in the Journal of Religion and Health argues that four major types of roles for religious leaders in the healthcare setup emerged in their thematic analysis. They are as follows:

1. Encouragement of healthy behaviors through religious based messages in Friday sermons and lectures.
2. Performing rituals around life events, illnesses and death
3. Advocating for Muslim patients and delivering cultural sensitivity training in hospitals
4. Assisting in healthcare decisions for mosque congregants

6 " Kronprins Haakon deltar når UiO åpner masterprogram for imamer og andre religiøse ledere: News," University of Oslo, accessed 26, August, 2021, https://www.uniforum.uio.no/nyheter/2019/03/kronprins-haakon-deltar-under-apningen-av-nytt-stu.html.

But participants in this study also identified several areas of cultural conflict and challenges for imams. For example, limited medical knowledge, clinical uncertainty, lack of accessibility and availability of imams are some of the barriers that the study finds.

The American findings strengthen the perception that there is a clear need of addressing the issue of involving and integrating Muslim religious figures in health care related matters. But this involvement requires prerequisites such as education and confidence building measures between health care institutions and religious care-givers.

Also, the study elucidates on the taxonomy of imams and describes the categories of imam as sermon-giver (khateeb), spiritual guide (shaykh/imam), Islamic law expert (shaykh/imam), director of mosque(shaykh/imam). The term imam is fluid and imams are not like clergy in Christianity, often having more diffuse, varied and informal roles (Rassool 2016). These types of discussions and classifications are essential for what is in a word? In this case very much. The word imam has a certain connotation but is also understood very differently (for example between shia's and sunni's) and can be a hindrance in employment for Muslim women who wish to work at hospitals and cater for patient needs for instance. The study highlights primarily ritual and educational focused functions of Muslim leaders not addressing the potential roles of counselling, chaplaincy and pastoral care, including its dilemmas in healthcare institutions.

"Musings of a female Muslim chaplain" – a case study

What is clinical pastoral care seen from a Muslim chaplain's lens?

One of the most complex and intrinsic tasks for contemporary Muslim theology is recovering its tradition from that past and making it available for the present. How do Muslim spiritual caregivers extract from the past texts and deliver in the present? In 2003, I was invited to deliver a lecture around the topic of Islamic spiritual care at the Islamic-Christian Study Centre in Copenhagen. I was a novice and had made a power-point presentation with religious quotes primarily from the Quran and *ahadith* literature with some help from colleagues. But I was entangled in the following questions: How to deliver spiritual care in specific clinical situations? How to communicate with patients by bed side? Is there an Islamic equivalent to the Christian pastoral/spiritual care?

In the following pages I have used an example of an American female chaplain who reflects on her chaplaincy work (gives answers to my above mentioned queries) and lays a foundation for a praxis of contemporary Islamic chaplaincy based on theology.

Sondos Kholaki, an American-Muslim chaplain working at a hospital in Southern California describes her encounters in diary form collecting her entries which she posted on social media between the years 2016–2019. It became a publication titled 'Musings of a Muslim Chaplain' (Kholaki 2020). She earned her Master of Divinity degree in Islamic chaplaincy from Bayan/Claremont School of Theology and completed her Clinical Pastoral Education residency at a hospital in Southern California.

Kholaki has divided her diary into themes and the book has 8 chapters with headings such as 'chaplaincy', 'heart work', 'community', 'Gods plan' and 'children'. Her writings give readers substantial insight not only into her own abilities and concerns but takes the reader into the deep abyss of patients' 'meaning making' processes. She describes scrupulously her own uncertainties giving the reader an intimate experience of her encounters with patients, colleagues and staff.

One of these concerns is what Kholaki calls 'leaning into the discomfort' alluding to the difficulties addressing patient's hardships and aligning oneself with them. Here she emphasizes her clinical training program (CPE), supervision, clinical experience and self-awareness shaping her to attain competencies and subsequently foothold. Another concern was focusing on 'being' instead of 'doing' – understanding the importance of holding back from giving advice and offering 'clear cut' solutions to patients. Kholaki describes an attribute of the Prophet Muhammad as, 'being absorbed in the narrative of other' as an existential tool in her work. Her active use of the Prophetic example as described earlier in this text is not uncommon amongst Muslims – laymen and theologians alike.

Kholaki describes her own God talk and connection to God in a daring experiment. Using Sufi terminology (*Dost* for friend) she explains that Sufis have an unfiltered and candid conversation with God wherein they have the freedom to express their deepest emotions just as friends do. She exposes herself and tells of her own transformation from formal and memorized prayers to more open and frank prayers to God. Due to the emotional pressure from her chaplaincy work she needed to verbalize her pains and longings to a 'comforting presence', with 'a knowledge that someone is a witness to your unbearable pain' (Kholaki 2020).

Community and colleagues

For Kholaki, community is not only her Muslim network and congregation but her co-workers, the chaplains and neighbours. The intra-chaplaincy spiritual connection and cooperation between Kholaki and her colleagues is mentioned profusely, and one senses the deep respect and humility she has for her seniors and educators especially from her clinical education program. Some studies have reflected upon the role of the majority church in cooperating and engaging chaplains from other faiths. In one Scandinavian study it was established that all Muslim chaplains (employed and volunteers) had close cooperation with their Christian counterparts at many levels. But it was not just left to cooperation. Muslim chaplains explain that much of their practical pastoral and counselling skills were either learnt from, or inspired, by Christian chaplains (Baig, 2019). Until recently there was no Islamic chaplaincy education in Scandinavia and that can be one of the reasons for this approach and desired learning from Christian pastoral care givers. One Christian chaplaincy manager at a Norwegian Hospital explained that cooperating/working with Muslim chaplains enabled the chaplaincy team's multicultural and multi-faith image to take flight, alluding to the chaplaincy services getting recognition from the institution and society in large, in return (Baig, 2019). Bearing in mind the character of the secularized Scandinavian institutions, it could also prove to be strategically smart to 'join forces' with other faith groups to prove chaplaincy's legitimacy at public institutions.

Kholaki also has a chapter on chaplaincy where she presents five 'whats' of Islamic pastoral care in condensed form. She emphasizes hospitality as a central tenet which involves creating a welcoming environment, using presence, active listening, compassion and connection regardless of the care-seekers faith background. In the chaplaincy team where Kholaki works it is expected that chaplains can speak and chaplain everyone. With hospitals becoming more professionalized and specialization being the trademark at many places, the chaplaincy domain is also under pressure to adopt and 'perform'. The central question today is what are the essential chaplaincy functions and what are their effectiveness? What are professional chaplaincy skills and how do they differ from psychotherapy, trauma psychology, nursing care etc.?

Not only does this diary publication give a starting language to Muslim chaplaincy in a modern setting but it introduces albeit in note form, an Islamic care theology. It's a rare publication that sheds light on the core issues of practical care immersing from a chaplain's mind and heart. Kholaki does not have much theory in her musings but leans on her self-reflection and deep contemplations. This makes the entire booklet very personal, which was the intent. However, it does not give a theoretical exploration of Islamic chaplaincy.

The finest form of theology is that which critically recovers the theology from the past only to constructively renew it for today's needs. Recovering theology is a beautiful, demanding and skilful act that requires insight and knowledge just as much as it requires seeing the world through lenses of the present. It is the interplay of the past and present that stimulate a new language and knowledge and broaden our horizons. Theology has its relevance for its users, if it manages to give the individual a meaningful understanding of the world and inspiration for a 'caring engagement' in the world.

Concluding remarks

Hospital chaplaincy done today has its base, inspiration and legitimacy from Islamic theology and practice. Also, Islamic pastoral care, as seen in the case of Kholaki is contextual, practical, reflective and patient-centered. The interdependency of classical Islamic theology and the contextual lived reality of humans cannot be underestimated. As I have tried to establish in the first section of this chapter, theological humanitarianism as enshrined in the concept of *khidmah* puts the human being in the center of affairs. The whole human being is sacred and needs full attention during times of need and crisis. The humans physical, psychological, social and spiritual needs all must be catered for to bring equilibrium in life.

Here it is necessary for institutions which have the responsibility of delivering care and comfort see the whole human being. Hospitals are places where hospitality flourishes for the sick and their relatives. From decorated and personalized rooms for children at intensive wards, to hospital art exhibitions and gardens at premises, many hospitals are moving towards a more holistic approach to person centered care where the physical, psychological, social and spiritual needs are all part and parcel of the hospital culture and policy. Not surprisingly the Scandinavian word for hospital is *sygehus /sjukehus* meaning a home for the sick. If chaplaincy wishes to stay relevant it must recall exactly that. To make patients feel at home – being hospitable and concerned for them and their wellbeing.

If Islamic chaplaincy wishes to be present and be relevant at hospitals and other public institutions for that sake, it must too address patient needs and ponder over its own raison d'être. The process of individualization in the West has forced minority religious traditions- including Muslims, to find way and means to deliver spiritual care in settings where earlier, families partook that function. This institutionalization has resulted in, amongst other things, a kind of renewed and systematic understanding of spiritual care- getting inspiration from the long Christian history and practise of chaplaincy.

Islamic spiritual care is the Muslim term to describe religiously based spiritual care offered by religious and spiritual leaders to congregations and individuals. Its essence is founded on the Qur'an and the Sunnah as we have discussed earlier in this chapter. Even though Islamic spiritual care is an independent discipline, it is related to other forms of Islamic care such as Islamic education, preaching, ethics and spiritual healing. It has many forms and levels to help Muslim patients to broaden their understanding of life and abilities to face the personal, relational or public challenges, which include grief and loss, emphatic listening, parenting, etc. Islamic spiritual care today is more than clerical responsibility since it is a specialized and professional field where training, research, inter-faith, administration, teaching staff and other responsibilities are part of the daily work. Subsequently, there is a challenge ahead, for congregations, hospitals, practitioners, academia and most of all society at large to define the what, who and how of spiritual care. This chapter tried to assess and define the what of Islamic spiritual care and partially the how. These pertinent questions will remain and their importance will increase in the diverse and multireligious societies we are living in.

References

Ahmed, Sameera, and Mona M. Amer. 2012. *Counselling Muslims: Handbook of Mental Health Issues and Interventions*. Milton Park: Routledge.

Al-Ghazali, Abu Hamid ibn Muhammad, Hamza Yusuf, and Walter James Skellie. 2010. *The Marvels of the Heart: Science of the Spirit* (*Ihya' Ulum al-Din/The Revival of the Religious Sciences*). Louisville: Fons Vitae Publishing.

Al-Ghazali, Abu Hamid ibn Muhammad. 1999. *The Ninety-Nine Beautiful Names of God*. Translated by David and Nazih Daher. Cambridge: Islamic Texts Society.

Al-Halveti,Tosun Bayrak al-Jerrahi. 1983. *The Most Beautiful Names*. New York: Threshold books.

Al-Jilani, Hadrat 'Abd. 1992. *The Secret of Secrets*. Interpreted by Shaykh Tosun Bayrak Al-Jerrahi Al-Halveti. Cambridge: Islamic Texts Society.

Ansari, Zafar Afaq (ed.). 2006. *Quranic Concepts of the Human Psyche*. Dehli: Adam Publishers and Distributors.

Ayad, Amira. 2008. *Healing Body and Soul: Your Guide to Holistic Wellbeing Following Islamic Teachings*. Riyadh: International Islamic Publishing House.

Chourief, Tayeb. 2011. *Spiritual Teachings of the Prophet*. Louisville: Fons Vitae.

Baig, Naveed. 2012. "Counseling in the Health Service." In: Jørgen Nielsen (ed.) *Islam in Denmark*. Lanham: Lexington Books. 219–230.

Baig, Naveed. 2019. "Omsorgsarbejde for muslimer på hospitaler i Sverige, Norge og Danmarkam." *Report for the University of Oslo*, https://www.tf.uio.no/forskning/forskergrupper/interreligios/fagrapporter/fagrapport-naveed-baig.pdf

Bayrak Al-Jerrahi Al-Halveti. 1992. (Golden Palm Series) Foreword by Syed Ali Ashraf. Cambridge, England: Islamic Texts Society.

Cutsinger, James. 2002. *Paths to the Heart: Sufism and the Christian East*. Bloomington: World Wisdom.

Fareedi, Rasheed Ahmad. 2007. *Virtues and Etiquettes of Visiting the Sick.* Isipingo Beach: Madrasah Taleemudeen. https://www.muslim-library.com/dl/books/English_Virtues_and_Etiquettes_of_Visiting_the_Sick.pdf

Farmer, Sharon. 2019. *Communities of Saint Martin: Legend and Ritual in Medieval Tours.* Ithaca: Cornell University Press.

Gilliat–Ray, Sophie, Mansur Ali, and Stephen Patterson. 2013. *Understanding Muslim Chaplaincy.* Surrey: Ashgate.

Happold, Frederic Crossfield. 1963. *Mysticism: A Study and an Anthology.* Westminster: Penguin Books.

Hathout, Hassan. 2008. *Reading the Muslim Mind.* 9th Edition. Indianapolis: American Trust Publications.

Helminski, Kabir. 1998. *The Knowing Heart: A Sufi Path of Transformation.* Boulder: Shambhala Publications.

Isgandarova, Nazila. 2019. "Muraqaba as a Mindfulness-Based Therapy in Islamic Psychotherapy." *Journal of Religion and Health* 58/4.

Isgandarova, Nazila. 2014. "The Evolution of Islamic Spiritual Care and Counselling in Ontario in the Context of the College of Registered Psychotherapists and Registered Mental Health Therapists of Ontario." *Psychology & Psychotherapy* 4/3: 143.

Isgandarova, Nazila. 2016. "The Correlational approach to Islamic Spiritual Care." *Tidsskrift om Islam og Kristendom* 1: 15 – 28.

Keshavarzi, Hooman., Fahad Khan, Bilal Ali, and Rania Awaad. 2021. *Applying Islamic Principles to Clinical Mental Health Care.* Milton Park: Routledge.

Kholaki, Sondos. 2020. *Musings of a Muslim Chaplain.* Independently published.

Kowalski, Mumina. 2009. "Names of God: Practical Theology For Muslim Chaplains in CPE." *Reflective Practice: Formation and Supervision in Ministry* 29: 178 – 187.

Leeming, David. A. (ed). 2020. *Encyclopedia of Psychology and Religion.* New York: Springer.

Mazrui, Al-amin bin Ali. 2005. *The Content of Character: Ethical Sayings of the Prophet Muhammad.* Sandala.

Mittermaier, Amira. 2014. "Bread, Freedom, Social Justice: The Egyptian Uprising and a Sufi Khidma." *Cultural Anthropology* 29/1: 54 – 79.

Mubarakpuri, Safiur Rahman. 2002. *Ar-Raheeq al Makhtum.* Riyad: Darussalam Publishers.

Murata, Sachiko, and William C. Chittick. 2005. *The Vision of Islam.* London: I.B. Tauris.

Osama, Syed Muhammad. 2005. *The Encyclopaedic Index of the Quran.* New Delhi: Goodword Books.

Padela, Aasim, Amal Killawi, Michele Heisler, Sonya Demonner, and Michael D. Fetters. 2011. "The Role of Imams in American Muslim Health: Perspectives of Muslim Community Leaders in Southeast Michigan." *J Relig Health* 50/2: 359 – 373.

Pargament, Kenneth I. 1997. *The Psychology of Religion and Coping.* New York: The Guilford Press.

Rahman, Fazlur. 1997. *Health and Medicine in the Islamic Tradition.* New York: Crossroad.

Rassool, G. Hussein. 2016. *Islamic Counselling.* Milton Park: Routledge.

Rassool, G. Hussein. 2014. *Cultural Competence in Caring for Muslim Patients.* London: Palgrave Macmillan.

Renard, John (ed.). 2014. *Islamic Theological Themes.* Oakland: University of California Press.

Siddiqui, Ataullah. 2007. “Islam at universities in England: report submitted to Bill Rammell MP, Minister of State for Lifelong Learning, Further and Higher Education.” *Journal of Beliefs & Values* 28/3: 331–341.
Swift, Christopher, Mark Cobb, and Andrew Todd. 2016. *A Handbook of Chaplaincy Studies.* Milton Park: Routledge.
Winter, Tim J. 2005. *Al-Ghazali on Disciplining the Soul: breaking the two desires.* Cambridge: The Islamic Texts Society.
Winter, Tim J. 2008. *The Cambridge Companion to Classical Islamic Theology.* Cambridge: Cambridge University Press.
Zaman, S. M. 1986. “Place of Man in the Universe in the World- View of Islam.” *Islamic Studies* 25/3: 325–331.

Jussra Schröer

Development of Muslim spiritual care (Seelsorge) in Germany Challenges and perspectives

Abstract: In recent years, the debate about Islamic spiritual care in Germany has expanded. For a long time, politicians have been pushing for the training of Muslim chaplains. Underpinned by socio-political developments, a process of realisation has taken place. Since the winter semester 2016/17, it is now possible to study Practical Islamic Theology for Chaplaincy and Social Work at the University of Tübingen. Many students have taken up the degree programme primarily out of interest. At the same time, the uncertainties and indeterminacies regarding the graduates' professional perspectives are omnipresent and rather unclear. This chapter gives an overview of current developments in the master's programme and discusses the current requirements and challenges within this field.

Introduction

The Muslim community in Germany is changing. Family and community care, which is shaped by religion and culture, is reaching its limits due to people's living, and working conditions. Long-term migration to Germany of Muslims and their families also requires professionalization and qualification of Spiritual care.

The practice of spiritual care for Muslims, however, is still done on a voluntary basis and takes a different form in Germany than in Catholic or Protestant in the country. This is because among the major churches in Germany, pastoral care in public institutions is a common field of cooperation between the state and religious communities. The decisive foundations for this are the constitutional right to freedom of faith, conscience, and confession (Art. 4 GG), the German constitutional law on religions and the federal and state laws based on it. In Article 140 in conjunction with Article 141 of Weimar State Constitution, the Basic Law guarantees religious communities a right of access to state institutions insofar as there is a need for worship and spiritual care in armed forces, hospitals, prisons, or other public institutions. [1] This is not the case with Muslim spiritual

1 https://www.gesetze-im-internet.de/englisch_gg/.

 https://doi.org/10.1515/9783110717365-006

care. Muslim spiritual counsellors help after accidents, in prisons and hospitals. They are needed, but mostly work on a voluntary basis. Unlike Christian chaplains, very few Muslim spiritual counsellors are employed in paid, full-time positions. Most Muslim spiritual care projects also rely on funding from Christian or government organizations. Although the number of projects is growing, the projects often rely on great commitment of individuals and are poorly networked among themselves. In addition, there is a lack of uniform training standards for Muslim spiritual counsellors (Aslan et al 2015, Aslan et al 2017, Hauschildt & Uçar 2010, Ceylan 2012)

To the principal question of self-understanding and the mission from which Muslim spiritual care and counselling can draw theologically and academically there is no uniform answer. Research and publication on this issue is still in its infancy in Germany and in other German-speaking countries. The most common publications are mainly practical reports on training and further education, anthologies on conferences and short reflections on the topics of chaplaincy and counselling in the Qur'an and in the traditions about the Prophet Muḥammad (Lemmen et al 2011, Wenz & Talat 2012, Ucar & Blasberg 2013, Begić et al 2014). Other contributions inform about the current development of training Muslim volunteers for Islamic chaplaincy and counselling (Badawia et al 2020) Cultural, legal and religious contexts as well as cooperation between Muslim and Christian partners are discussed (Hauschildt & Uçar 2010). Only a few studies, however, provide empirical research results in this area (Akca 2019, Aslan et al 2015, Aslan et al 2017, Rückamp 2021, Yanık-Şenay 2018, Şahinöz 2018). This could be due, firstly, to the fact that the sources and data on which the political statements of the Islam Conference and the research studies are based are incomplete and still raise relevant research issues. Secondly, further research challenges also arise from the fact that this is a highly politicised field and the people who are classified as Muslim spiritual care givers are not infrequently skeptical about research studies themselves. This chapter provides an overview of current developments in the Master's programme and discusses the current demands and challenges in the field. It draws on preliminary results from a survey of spiritual care professionals and Master's students during the study and practice phase. In the first part, I will explore the question of how Islamic spiritual care and counselling may be understood. In the second part, I will ask how Islamic spiritual care and counselling is discussed in the context of research studies. The third part is based on expert interviews, in which I will present aspects of Islamic spiritual care and counselling in the context of practice. In the concluding part, the following question will be discussed: What are challenges and opportunities associated with discussions on establishing Muslim spiritual care and counselling in Germany?

Spiritual care, counselling in context of university Islamic theology

The initiation of German Islam Conference by the federal government in 2006 shows that the government has recognized needs for Islamic spiritual care and counselling in Germany. Since then, the government has supported the development of university-based Islamic theology. The German Islam Conference supports the goal of establishing institutionalised cooperation between the state and Islamic organizations and religious communities in Germany on the basis of the German constitutional law on religion. In principle, this also enables Islamic organizations to comprehensively exercise the rights of religious communities if they fulfil the constitutional requirements.

German constitutional law on religions provides for a variety of forms of cooperation between the state and religious communities. Among other things, they concern the area of education, such as religious education at public schools or theology at public universities. The German Islam Conference has already been able to provide important impulses in this area.[2] Since 2011, the Federal Ministry of Education and Research (BMBF) has been funding centers for Islamic theology in Tübingen, Frankfurt (with Gießen), Münster, Osnabrück and Erlangen-Nuremberg, and since 2019, institutes for Islamic theology have also been established at the Humboldt University in Berlin and at the University of Paderborn. According to BMBF, the locations of these centers reflect diversity of Muslim faith and life in Germany, and thus the academic system is responding to the growing plurality of religious currents in Germany by establishing a university-based Islamic theology. The teachers and academic staff in university Islamic theology have different regional, ethnic, and academic educational backgrounds. According to a survey commissioned by the Academy for Islam in Research and Society (AIWG) at Goethe University Frankfurt, there are currently about 2,500 students enrolled in bachelor's and master's programs at these centers.80 per cent of the students are female. They state that they either want to teach as teachers in schools, work in social and spiritual care or stay in scholarship. All of them want to be actively involved in society. This social motivation of students of Islamic theology is often associated with the current discourse on Islam in society. One of the reasons given by the students in the surveys "Who studies Islamic theology?" (Dreier/Wagner 2020) was that the image of Islam

2 https://www.deutsche-islam-konferenz.de/SharedDocs/Anlagen/DE/Ergebnisse-Empfehlungen/20170314-la-3-abschlussdokument-seelsorge.pdf?__blob=publicationFile&v=7.

in society and the structures in Muslim organizations should be changed. Some students describe their experiences in the mosque as the motivation to study and to do things differently as future chaplains. In this respect, the motivation is also connected to the will to change – a change to which the students hope to contribute through their studies. A further motivation to change society through study lies in the way Islam is practiced in Germany and represented by "false" or self-appointed experts. Therefore, a concrete career perspective is an important factor for a successful graduation. However, due to the unclear career prospects for Muslim theologians, students rarely see specific perspectives to follow, even after graduation. Many graduates therefore orient themselves in the direction of the field of education. (Dreier/Wagner 2020).

In the winter semester of 2016/2017, a master's program- Islamic Practical Theology for Spiritual Care and Social Work- also started at the Centre for Islamic Theology (ZITH) at the University of Tübingen, which is unique in Germany. The examination of diversity and faith in the context of migration and social work are core components of the degree program. This will prepare students in four semesters to work as spiritual and religious counsellors in hospitals, prisons, refugee work, in military, in schools, in elderly care or in mosque congregations. In addition to pedagogical and legal basis of spiritual care and social work, as well as theory and practice of Islamic rituals, the degree program has an intensive practical orientation through compulsory internships. During the study and internship phases, students develop individual professional competences and form their professional identity.

Islam, Spiritual Care and Counselling Contemporary First Interview Results

The following results are based on first analyses of interviews within the framework of an empirical study on Islam, spiritual care and counselling.This study focuses on Muslim spiritual counsellors and allows them to comment on the topic of "Muslim spiritual care and counselling" in Germany. Within this framework, fifteen Muslim spiritual care givers and imams were interviewed in the time from 2019 to 2020. In the context of this study, I asked: How do chaplains in spiritual care and social work deal with the religious diversity of Muslim people seeking advice and with the diverse forms of living that have developed in the context of a plural society? In individual and group interviews, they talked about their understanding of "Muslim spiritual care" and about demands and challenges they face in practice. The respondents were working as imams, hospital, and prison Muslim spiritual counsellors when the survey was conducted. Also, this study is currently in the publication phase and is part of one of my post-doctoral research projects.

The analysis revealed five "categories of spiritual care". In the following, the categories are presented in short form to gain an insight into the practice of Muslim spiritual care and counselling in Germany.

1 Being close to human beings

> I'm just here for you right now, everything else doesn't matter (Muslim spiritual counsellor 1, 28 years old. She studied Islamic theology in Germany, works as teacher in a primary school and part-time as Muslim counsellor in several hospitals).

Some of the Muslim spiritual counsellors, who were interviewed, describe their task as an effort to help people out of critical situations by assisting them. The major concern here is to help suffering people by giving comfort and strength. In this context, spiritual care can simply mean consolation and does not have to have a solution or immediate answer:

> Working with people, working with people, yes? .... I can speak badly in categories, I have those here, especially in spiritual care, who have fallen into the debt trap. Then I have those who are drug addicts, who have a drug problem or another addiction. But I see each person individually. So, every person stands for him/herself, has his history, has his past, has his present, has his future, and has just as well his (sadness grief), his happiness and the way in which one shows his happiness and the way in which one shows grief. Exactly (Muslim spiritual counsellor 2, 31 years old. She studied Islamic Theology in Germany, works as Muslim counsellor on a part-time basis, in cooperation with the Christian pastoral and supports male prisoners and their families).

2 Living faith

Muslim spiritual care also means accompanying people in questions of faith and life, in crises and conflicts, in illness, death and grief. Spiritual care is the energetic proclamation and tells in its own way of the *Qur'an* revelations. The return to *Qur'an* and to traditional Muslim values can gain importance in crises. Without recitation of the *Qur'an*, something would be missing in spiritual care. For many Muslims, recitation is an essential form of faith lived in the Islam. Spiritual care can also be defined by ritual. It happens out of an attitude of mindfulness, and it is based in hope of God's mercy and acts out of mercy:

People are afraid that they will die. Furthermore, when you talk so openly about death and recite a few *Qur'an* verses, people feel comfortable. The recitation is the most effective. I think that recitations of the *Qur'an* are very helpful. For example, as I said before, 50 percent of counselling is just listening. I think maybe 30 percent, I guess now, is that you are reciting something from the *Qur'an*. Then maybe 20 percent, as they say. Of course, that is important, how you say that and how people take it. But I think the recitation you do and how you perform is very important (Muslim spiritual counsellor 3, 28 years old, born in Germany. After graduating from school in Germany, he studied Islamic theology in Turkey. Today he works as an Imam for a Muslim community in Germany).

3 Religious guidance

Spiritual care can be experienced as a religious experience. Some of those interviewed understand spiritual care as trust in life through trust in God, it gives hope where despair torments. In this sense, spiritual care means for them to show people the "right way", whereby this understanding is based on revelations and traditions of the Prophet: With us, for example, spiritual care is from the Sunnah, with verses, with patience, etc. What does that mean? (...) A person is exhausted, he needs help, and another person offers it, but the problem is, with what does he offer it? With religious values, that is different to other help, but different than the others, because in psychology for example it is not religious. Spiritual care is an act between two people, one in a state that needs help, the other is, not giving, but offering, someone in that state who offers help, with what? With religious symbols, meanings, traditions, and values (Muslim spiritual counsellor 4, 52 years old, born in Turkey. He studied Islamic theology in Turkey. Since 2005 he has been working as a religious affairs advisor at the Turkish-Islamic Union for Religious Affairs (DİTİB; German: Türkisch-Islamische Union der Anstalt für Religion e.V.; Turkish: Diyanet İşleri Türk-İslam Birliği). He also trains Muslim spiritual counsellors.

One Muslim spiritual counsellor who belongs to one of the major Islamic religious communities in Germany, argues that a theological justification for Muslim spiritual care can only be established in an Islamic community:

Spiritual care is also a challenge. All Muslims in our mosques come and benefit from us, not only Turkish people, and if in the future we are recognized as we wish and can professionally train and lead Muslim spiritual counsellors, we will also address the other Muslim communities, not only Turkish ones (Muslim spiritual counsellors 4).

This demand that spiritual care may only be offered as a task of Muslim communities can be interpreted differently in this context. It meets the long-standing demands for recognition of Islamic religious communities as contact persons for Muslims in Germany. Article 4 (Freedom of faith and conscience) of the Basic Law for the Federal Republic of Germany and Article 140 (Law of religious denominations) of the Basic Law in conjunction with the following Art. 141(To the extent that a need exists for religious services and pastoral work in the army, in hospitals, in prisons or in other public institution ns, religious societies shall be per mitted to provide them, but without compulsion of any kind) protect the freedom of faith, conscience and freedom. Article 137, (1) Weimar Constitution, there shall be no state church and (2) The freedom to form religious societies shall be guaranteed. Stand for the fundamental separation of church, religion and state as well as for the guarantee of religious freedom. From both results a fundamental duty of neutrality of the state towards the different religious communities. Religion can play a role in public life. In Germany, the state provides religious communities with opportunities for social action (e. g. religious education in state schools, hospital and prison chaplaincy). The state must not privilege any religion over others; rather the state must maintain a uniform attitude to all religions.

Muslim communities have existed in Germany for many decades. One of the ways in which religious communities can be recognised in Germany is through the status of a "public corporation". This status comes with some special rights, such as the collection of membership fees by the state tax authorities, the maintenance of civil servant-like employment relationships or the operation of their own cemeteries. They are also automatically responsible for youth welfare. The Protestant and Catholic churches as well as the Jewish community were already granted corporate status in the Weimar Republic when the Basic Law came into effect. Religious communities must submit an application to be recognised as a religious community by the respective federal government. For example, in 2013, the religious community of the Ahmadiyya Muslim Jamaat in Hessen was recognised for the first time as an Islamic community with corporate status. The main challenge for Islamic applicants now is to prove membership. Some associations are in the process of changing their statutes, drawing up membership lists and forming regional associations in order to meet the requirements. In addition, consolidated structures, competences and resources have to be built up in order to be able to take on the tasks they are aiming for, such as in youth and senior citizen work. However, in order to be able to practice Islamic spiritual care, a legal recognition is necessary, because it provides access to participation and equal rights. It would certainly help to strengthen Muslims' trust, sense of belonging to Germany and thus their participation.

This interview shows that mistrust of some Islamic religious communities towards the state influences the cooperation with the government, but also with Christian communities:

> There are always attempts to subordinate Muslim spiritual care to Christian spiritual care, attempts are often made by churches or federal states, both unacceptable to us. This work must be given to one hand, something belongs to us, and something belongs to you. By hand giving I mean religiously and from the welfare association, thus a Muslim welfare association on federal level (...) the politicians and the churches are trying to regulate, so that they can do everything themselves according to the motto, we do not need Muslim spiritual care, they have *Qur'an* Apps on their mobile phones or whatever, but for us this is unacceptable (caregiver 4).

Islam is not hierarchically organized and does not know church and membership. Nevertheless, the state always demands that Muslims should found a kind of church (Uçar /Blasberg-Kuhnke 2013, Ceylan 2012). In addition, the major Islamic religious communities in Germany would like to have the role as "legal representation of all Muslims" in Germany:

> Muslim plurality is also a challenge for us and the society. We always try to cooperate and work in a friendly way with other communities, e.g., the Bosnian and Albanian communities have signed brotherly agreements in a friendly way (...) we also try to integrate other Muslim nations and open the doors to our activities (Muslim spiritual counsellor 4).

But it is above all important that in every model of state cooperation for the establishment of Muslim spiritual care the range of Islamic influences is presented. Both Muslim spiritual counsellors and those seeking advice want to recognize their religion in everyday life and do not want to have a unified church.

4 Prevention

Spiritual care can fulfill a protective function, as prevention, in the sense of care. This includes the early identification of risks before problems can arise and can be used to prevent violence and radicalism.

> So, to speak, this is also a prevention, that one deals with people in advance in such a way that they do not reach this stage, that they need spiritual care. (Muslim spiritual counsellor 3).

Spiritual care as prevention also means that Muslim spiritual counsellors gain insight to difficult themes through their conversations and consultations, so-called taboo issues, which primarily concern and affect young people. This content that is reluctantly spoken to parents and family because young people feel ashamed, do not feel understood or are afraid of an unpleasant reaction from the person they are talking to. There are social themes in life, such as questions of faith and questions about sexuality, which are also asked in spiritual care:

I'm always open to everything. And in my mosque tours, I also always like to mention that there are *Qur'an* verses that call to use the mind. And then I say: "Please ask everything, ask all questions. You have the opportunity here to ask a Muslim, whether he is an Imam or not, all the questions. I am not omniscient, but as far as possible I will try ... Because I confess myself as a Muslim, therefore I believe in all this. You have the opportunity to really ask anything". That is what I do in my conversations. That is why there is no issue for me to talk about so called taboos. And when someone says, "I did *Zinā*", then he sinned. (The term "Zinā" in the Qur'an refers to forbidden sexual relations, adultery. (Qur'an 24:4).

I sin too. Of course, we do not do it ... We do not want to do it, but we are weakly created, we also sin every day. So, when you talk like that and they think, "Okay, I've done something wrong, but he still does see me as a Muslim". Then you start talking. So far, I have never blocked anyone on any topic, But I can imagine that other Imams have some taboo topics (Muslim spiritual counsellor 3).

1 "Living-world orientation"

Spiritual care also means perceiving the reality of people's lives. In this context, spiritual care is interested in how people live, what shapes people and what this means for the mission of Muslim spiritual counsellors in Germany.

> If I go in, I do not know what makes the family tick now, do I? May have a Turkish migrant context, but that does not mean anything. And can be more atheistic, more secular. That is why I just go in and see how the family welcomes me, whether the family wants me to help or not. And I try then, yes, just to be there, to support them, just give the signal I am here whenever they need to talk. That is perfectly okay. And then when it comes: Can you do that? ... That was the case with another colleague who then said that the family itself said: We cannot read the *Qur'an* at all, can you? Would you say a prayer? Then we will do it. But no other way. Well, there must be a need from the family. Nothing is being put over there. And when the family says: "I don't need it" – it is okay too (Muslim spiritual counsellor 5, 48 years old. She studied Islamic Studies and Pedagogy in Germany and works in family counselling and part-time in emergency spiritual care).

In interviews, it is often said that spiritual care always focuses on people in its counselling and would develop appropriate support and help along individual experiences, needs and drafts of people seeking advice:

> To say so I understand you and that's okay the way you're acting right now. And do not come with your finger and say, "Oh, oh, you can't say that". No. Very, very important: Ability to be patient and tolerant! Yes, I do (Muslim spiritual counsellorn 5).

The living world that is meant here contains the subjective construction of reality (Grunwald &Thiersch 2016).This world of people seeking advice is direct, individual, and is according differently for children or adults, for men and women, for people with and without migration biographies, for religious and non-religious people:

> You don't know how religious the family is or so. It does not matter. I am not giving any tips from *Qur'an* or anything like that, but rather that one really gives comfort as human being to human being. That as a human being you simply hold hands and comfort each other (Muslim spiritual counsellor 5).

But even within respective groups of people and families in structurally comparable situations, the living world of the individual people are subjectively not comparable. The world in which Muslim family, the fourth generation of which lives in Germany, lives is subjectively completely different from that of a Muslim family that has just immigrated to Germany. The world in which we live is an expression of the individuality of each person:

> Usually, I come in and the person is irritated or pleasantly surprised. And I am not saying I am a Muslim spiritual counsellor! But I say: I wanted to visit you, I work here on an honorary basis, how are you? I am already starting the conversation a little. Rarely, but it happens that I come in and the person starts crying and immediately starts talking. These are exactly the conversations where I am very grateful that I visited the patient because I realized that he or she was waiting for a person to give him or her attention (Muslim spiritual counsellor 1).

Some interviewees understand the term spiritual care as a process of sensitive interaction between people. Spiritual care is communication, empathy, and a kind of help in life, in sense of help for self-help, where being human is in the center. In this context, the functions of counselling, conversation, and communication, also the religious sensibility play an important role (Nauerth et al 2017).

Other interviewees understand spiritual care as a religious guidance given by the spiritual Muslim counsellors. Spiritual care is also situation-dependent and the boundaries between religious and helping counselling in conversation can be fluid. In spiritual care there are people who need help to get out of their situations or crisis. The extent to which religion is effective in the setting of counselling and when and how the category "religion" is updated or called up in spiritual care and counselling depends on person seeking advice but also on mission and guiding principles of Muslim communities of spiritual care.

It is not the case that a Muslim understanding of spiritual care in Germany has to be imported from Islamic majority countries. One of the interviewees stated that "it is not necessary to reinvent the wheel" and that Muslim spiritual care can benefit from the previous experience of Christian spiritual care in an inter-religious context.

The results of the interviews show that there are different possibilities of practice. Thus, the implementation of Muslim spiritual care is linked to a certain independence in the context of a plural society in Germany. Particularly regarding Muslim diversity in Germany, this can also open possibilities for establishing a kind of "care" that considers the realities of the lives of those affected. The reality is that Muslims in Germany are very diverse, also due to migration.

Accordingly, spiritual care and counselling must start from a position that accepts diversity. Spiritual care must assume that all people have the right to their own understanding of religion and that they have the right to be cared for adequately. In the Muslim spiritual care, it is often mentioned that diversity is wanted in Islam and in the *Qur'an*. This is also the case, but in reality, it is often much more complicated. The situation in Germany has led Muslims to identify new common interests, all of which revolve around the question of equality with the other religious communities and the desire to be able to live Muslim religious life here on an equal basis and without discrimination. These issues were, and still remain, about mosque construction, religious instruction, the headscarf, and spiritual care. As a result, Germany-wide spiritual care services have come into being.

However, it is apparent that Muslim diversity is often perceived as a challenge in spiritual care. One reason for the challenge in dealing with Muslim diversity is certainly the uncertainty caused by the realities of life in a plural society. This also means, as the interviews show, that traditionally taboo subjects are not discussed in the families. One of these taboos is the topic of sexuality. Here, there seems to be the least room for necessary questioning of traditional values and beliefs that dominate and burden the daily lives of many, sometimes unconsciously, sometimes involuntarily.

Considering this context, it is important for Muslim spiritual care to give space to people who long for a way of life that is not controlled and ruled by the heteronormative constraints and has its own space outside this norm. In this sense, Muslim spiritual care and counseling should be open to all people, regardless of age, gender or sexual orientation, and also regardless of membership in a Muslim religious community.

Discussion
Muslim Spiritual Challenges and Perspectives

Age, gender, and education play an important role in the context of Muslim spiritual care. According to some Muslim spiritual counsellors, these factors can influence the effectiveness of spiritual care. The following part states an overview of challenges and perspectives in Germany:

1 Professional stress among Muslim spiritual counsellors and Imams

The results show that Muslims often seek the advice of religious scholars or Imams after praying in the mosque or between times of praying in communities. In this context, those seeking advice come to scholars with many questions and expect some form of support on the questions and problems they experience throughout life. The purpose of counselling can range from providing information on theological issues to counselling which requires professional support in different situations. Depending on the subject which the advice is directed to, such as a legal or health issue, different professions are necessary, which require not only theological knowledge but also different methods and approaches in human and social sciences:

> So, I can tell the way I experience it in mosque community. People, no matter what, if they do not find a place to go, come directly to the Imam and expect that he can do everything, to cover all their needs. Whether they are looking for a job, whether they have a problem with their wife (...) And that is what happens every day when people come to the mosque. Moreover, if these Imams do not have a counselling training or further education, then of course it is more difficult. What I also said bevor, that it is already a part of their tasks, because they are preachers. They try to follow the tradition of the prophet as much as possible (...) Sometimes solutions are simple, but you must listen to the people until the end, patient listening without teaching, or it will not do any good. They will think that the Imam, he could not listen properly, he cannot help! That is why you must take the time and have the intention to be there for all as Muslim spiritual counsellors (Muslim spiritual counsellor 3).

People consider spiritual care in the form of counselling when they cannot make progress with solving problems within their family. Consultation usually takes place within the framework of mosque offers and an Imam or a theologian usually carries them out.

Spiritual care in mosque communities happens in contexts of crises and unforeseeable experiences, which are often connected to emergencies. In some situations, both theologians and Imams may not be able to solve the problems. A referral of people seeking advice by professional counselling institutions seems essential, e.g., in case of acute psychological problems, suicide or traumatic experiences; However, spiritual care can reach its limits:

> A topic that overtaxed me, but that was also such an extreme example again, it was about a 14-year-old Muslim young girl who was brain dead. She was in the intensive care unit, the family did not want to accept this, because she was still at the devices and her heart was still beating through the devices. That means I had a very difficult situation. I had a family who could not handle it, who did not want to accept it, and a staff who finally wanted to convey that she was dead. And first, this acceptance of brain death was an issue for me where I noticed ... We had it in training, but brain death is like death when two doctors confirm it. But I had the feeling that the family thought I was on the side of the doctors. Well, I noticed right away that they could not take me on yet. And then there's organ donation. So, the doctor wanted to talk about this. And that was too much for me. To addresses this topic with this family was an unbelievable overload for me because I knew, they cannot even cope with death, the organ donation, that will not be an issue now. I felt between the two chairs in this case and did not feel free at all. So, I had the feeling that the doctor absolutely wants me to be there, that I somehow want to clear up topics for him. In addition, a family who misunderstood my role at the beginning because her mother thought I was coming [...] She saw me and said, "Ah, I've been waiting for you. I am like, um, okay. She thought I could talk to the doctor and prevent the devices from being turned off. Well, that was one of those situations where I realized my role was not clear here. So, I am being pulled from both sides. And certain topics ... I did not have the self-confidence to address certain topics that way either. Organ donation. I said organ donation was allowed. But I was also totally afraid of the reaction. Well, that was very overwhelming for me (Muslim spiritual counsellor 1).

From time-to-time questions can arise within the framework of Muslim spiritual care, for which a cooperation between psychological counselling, Muslim and Christian spiritual care would be a more suitable method. Many Muslim spiritual counsellors would like to work together in an interreligious or interfaith network. They would like to work in cooperation with Christian spiritual care on site. They have the opinion that they would benefit from the experience of Christian spiritual care and psychological counseling a lot:

> When I came from Turkey as Imam, they just asked me to do everything. And I had never actually done many things before and had never known many things either. And there was an expectation that I could do just anything. And there I was ... Just like a non-swimmer in a sea, I found myself. Of course, I learned quickly and a lot. If, for example, you need counselling, then you simply go to Imam, because he can do that easily. If someone, for example ... My first (break) burial was already interesting because I could not do it. I just ... In theory,

> I had that. Well, I do not want to say fortunately now, but fortunately my grandpa died two years ago. So, where I got there, it was the first time I experienced how to do it. I then introduced it to my ... like Imams have prayed, and then I could do it myself, exactly. For example, shortly afterwards I had already buried a baby who had died at the age of four weeks. You do not know anything, and you expect everything from the Imam. And I do not know if there is going to be a ceremony. So, in theory, what you must do, like, towards graves, I do not know. You probably know everything, but you think there has got to be some sort of process. Since this was missing, I invented something myself, I said: Okay, now this, let us do this and that. Exactly ... I think one could learn a lot from Christian chaplaincy, because a lot also appears there ... But this does not work for these Turkish mosque communities because they simply do not speak German. That is why these dialogues do not exist. I am sorry for this (Muslim spiritual counsellor 3).

2 Taboos and controversial subjects

In spiritual care, themes such as education, relationship problems, psychological problems, or burnouts as well as problems within families or between young people are often mentioned. Interestingly, in spiritual care there are also inquiries that explicitly deal with social issues or taboo topics. The elderly generation of Imams und Muslim spiritual counsellors is confronted with challenges of responding to questions on both social and theological issues. Regarding social issues, Imams try to find out what a theological response to issues might look like. In this context, the attitude towards competence in consulting is particularly stressed:

> I'm always open to everything, in my mosque tours; I may always mention that there are Qur'an verses that call for using the mind. And then I say: Please ask everything, ask all questions. You have the opportunity here to ask a Muslim, whether it is an Imam or not, all the questions. I am not omniscient, but as far as possible I will try ... Because I confess myself as a Muslim, therefore I also believe in all this. You can really ask anything. That is what I do in my conversations. That is why there is no issue for me what's taboo. And when someone says, "I did Zinā". Then he sinned. I sin too. Of course, we do not do it ... We do not want to do it, but we are weakly created, we sin every day (Muslim spiritual counsellor 3).

He also responds to the question of whether young women would also receive advice from him during a crisis as follows:

> We also try to support women. However, there are many things that women want to talk about only with women. One woman has lost her child; another has experienced physical violence through her husband. It is better for them to seek advice from a sister in our mosque community (Muslim spiritual counsellor 3)

He remarks self-critically in the interview that the men in spiritual care still have a lot to learn about dealing with women. At the same time, he asks for understanding:

> It is not necessarily easy for men in Muslim communities to deal with women as a matter of course (Muslim spiritual counsellor 3).

His opinion is that gender should not be played off against each other. Women are very important for the communities:

> If women today stopped working in Muslim communities, the community would collapse (Muslim spiritual counsellor 3)

3 Gender issues

Gender in counselling can have an important meaning in the context of Muslim spiritual care. For example, those seeking advice may feel uncomfortable while discussing intimate and sensitive issues with Muslim spiritual counsellors of a different gender.

The results of interviews show that there is no fixed rule in counselling situations of spiritual care, only a sensitivity about when and on which topics people seeking advice might feel uncomfortable:

> And when I look at it this way: "Okay, the woman also needs comfort in the sense that she gets hugged, just when she has this need to cry, and when I just offer her my shoulder, just hug her, that is okay with a Muslim woman when I do that. But it could be difficult when a male emergency counsellor is there, and she has this need, and he cannot do that at that moment. Or the other way around, if there is a man there now whom I would also like to hug and where it does not work out like that right now, then it would be good male / male, female / female (Muslim spiritual counsellor 5).

Clearly, the question of gender in some contexts depends on culture and age. The results of the interviews confirm the conclusion that it is very unusual, mostly in Muslim contexts, to discuss any kind of personal issue with persons of other gender. Many Muslim spiritual counsellors feel overwhelmed and left alone in this situation:

> From my own experience, I can say it plays a role, definitely. I have personally experienced, at least with my peers, with men who are a little younger, in middle age, as a young woman, that access is simply not there. So, I did not always feel respected or taken seriously. And after some bad experiences, I decided that I would not do that anymore. So that I only visit

> male patients from a certain age, who are perhaps also seriously ill, emergencies. But otherwise, up to a certain age I have decided for myself ... And I have noticed that it is generally the case that women have issues that they can only discuss with women. And men have issues they can only discuss with men. And so, gender plays a role. But this does not mean that one should close oneself off to the opposite gender, only that each one must decide for oneself to what extent one can open oneself. There are some who say, "I don't mind the patient just hitting on me. They are not all like that. But there are some like me who, after a few experiences, then, to avoid that again, decide for themselves: We're not doing this again. So, this is it (Muslim spiritual counsellor 1)

There may also be situations where gender issues can be important, for example when giving and taking of Muslim spiritual counsellors and seekers are very different. For example, in a crisis. It may be helpful to check whether the assistance offered corresponds to current crisis of person seeking:

> We had one, he had just been on emergency call. He then wrote to the WhatsApp group about rape, about death by rape, and he is male ... And then he said: "I think it's better if one of the sisters goes somehow than if I go now as a male Muslim spiritual counsellor. And there went another emergency spiritual counsellor (Muslim spiritual counsellor 5).

The aspect of gender in spiritual care and counselling does not necessarily have to be a problem: On the one hand, Gender can influence spiritual care context and the further use of counselling services by people in crisis situations. Often female Muslim spiritual counsellors report that spiritual care can be influenced by gender variables, both in communication and in counselling settings. However, this does not necessarily lead to the failure of the consultation. For example, Janna, who works with Muslim men in prison, is confident that gender bias can influence spirituality. She pleads for gender sensitivity, which can often lead to successful consultation:

> So, with men in Prison, I had the feeling that ... Well, for one thing, they looked at me with big eyes: There's one I know from my culture, my religious context, yeah? I know a covered woman, one who wears a headscarf. What is she doing in an institution like this now? For one thing. But then also the openness and of course the acceptance, because in the end the prisoners took part in my group lessons and partly came to talks. Of course, there are also prisoners who want to test this in their own way, yes? To what extent does my counterpart bring theologically sound knowledge? This is not only possible in terms of gender, but above all in terms of age. So, the younger you appear, the more implausible it might seem. And the whiter hair you have, the wiser the counsellor will be (Muslim spiritual counsellor 2).

She shows here that gender is partly constructed by social expectations. The results of interviews also show that gender differences can be time- and culture-dependent. The low proportion of women in the practice of Muslim spiritual care in prison shows how much role assignments are subject to social change. She does not consider her role as a "Muslim spiritual counsellor in men's prison" to be unusual. She believes that according to Islamic understanding, women can also work with men. Even then, at the time of the Prophet, the role of women in society was very diverse. Women were nurses, teachers and even allowed to preach as Imams. There is a collection of the Prophet's traditions that make it clear that women had many and different roles in society. She argues: When Muslims today discuss whether a woman as an Imam can do the prayers, including the Friday prayers in the mosque or in prison, there is a clear answer from me: yes, we can! In addition, this is confirmed by the Islamic tradition (Muslim spiritual counsellor 2).

4 Spiritual care and age

Sometimes challenges can be a question of age. Young counsellors may be perceived as inexperienced and less competent in counselling. For example, a patient in hospital may have doubts about the ability of a younger counsellor.

> I also have the problem, I am 28, I look like 18. The moment I enter the room – and I have experienced this before – they are still looking for the Imam (Muslim spiritual counsellor 3).
>
> In the same way, a young person seeking advice may feel that the Muslim spiritual counsellor is too young to understand his or her life situation.
>
> I once had a situation where a female relative saw me and was disappointed. She said: Ah, I was expecting an older gentleman. I wanted my mother to have her recited from the Qur'an. I told her I could do that, too. Then I took my Qur'an and I recited it. And I think she was a little ashamed of it and she was also very grateful. So, this picture of her: It must be an elderly gentleman with a beard reciting the Qur'an (Muslim spiritual counsellor 1).

Like gender characteristic, age differences in spiritual care and counselling are not necessarily an obstacle, but they can make spiritual care more difficult depending on context.

5 Education and employment

A special challenge in spiritual care and counselling is the characteristics of theologians trained "in Germany" or "abroad". The results of interviews show that Muslim community continues to prefer Muslim Imams who are trained in their home countries and then sent to Germany to teach and preach.

The communities fear that their faith could be deformed by the "institutional science" in Germany. Furthermore, some Muslim communities do not agree with the contents of Islamic theology at German universities. In their opinion, teaching of a Muslim theological education at a German state university is not equal to teaching at Turkish universities. Until today, the major Muslim communities in Germany support training of their Imams and theologians at the theological universities in Turkey:

> Theological basic training is a must, either at a recognized institution or in Turkey ... At the moment we cannot prevent that the education today and now in Germany is so different, we have only experience with agreed religion commissioners, here in the mosques, who complete their theology studies in Turkey, come back and are hired here, after cooperation it is decided to also support them, but are then hired by religious communities, paid by Turkey, they are German-speaking, born here, but studied in Turkey... I can only say that they have much more luck here than the others, are more accepted... Those who have studied in Turkey, if they are employed, will be accepted more positively than the others, also by the communities. This week we have organized a one-week training in Turkey, it is all internal students who have studied in Turkey, and 150 students are now in Ankara (Muslim spiritual counsellor 4).

Despite numerous efforts to further expand the training of Imams in Germany, according to a study published by the Konrad Adenauer Foundation almost 90 percent of Imams working in Germany come from abroad. The Imams come mainly from Turkey (Jacobs/Lipowsky 2019).

Since 2016, the first of the approximately 2.500 students currently enrolled at German universities have completed their studies in Islamic theology. Only a few have managed to find employment in spiritual care or as an Imam (Dreier/ Wagner 2020). The reasons for the lack of prospects in the profession are manifold. Besides the lack of acceptance by the mosque communities, the theologians fail because of open legal questions and institutional difficulties. This is also since Muslims are not organized as corporations under public law and do not have the financial means to adequately pay Muslim spiritual counsellors, teachers, and Imams. Another problem with the integration of graduates into the existing structures of spiritual care is, according to the Adenauer Foundation, the headscarf. Most students are women and many of them wear the headscarf. However, this is exactly what teachers and educators are forbidden to do in most federal states in Germany (Jacobs/Lipowsky 2019). A further point is that also the Muslim communities in Germany today can hardly imagine hiring a woman for public spiritual care or as Imam (Borchard/ Ceylan 2011).

Conclusion

This contribution shows that the academic foundations for the training of Muslim chaplains have been laid in Germany. For some years now, models for the training, financing and employment of Muslim spiritual counsellors have been discussed and tested at various institutions. Since 2016, the Centre for Islamic Theology at the Eberhard Karl University of Tübingen has been offering a master's program in Islamic Practical Theology for Spiritual Care and Social Work. The first graduates have already completed their studies.

Furthermore, the article identifies current challenges and requirements for establishing Islamic spiritual care and counselling in Germany. Firstly, the increasing religious plurality means that people of different religions are also seeking spiritual care and counselling. For Muslim counsellors, this means clarifying whether and how they can provide spiritual care to accompany religious diversity. As mentioned, the *Qur'an* and the tradition of the Prophet represent, among other things, the theoretical content of Islamic spiritual care and counselling. Clearly, a normative approach is often used to justify spiritual care and counselling in scholarship. Furthermore, the empirical studies show that both Muslim spiritual counselling and Muslim counselling are always a voluntary offer.

A further aspect is that Muslim spiritual counsellors also represent religion, a concrete religion, and they have a clear Islamic religious position from the outset and fill this position with their faith in the encounter and in the conversation. Spiritual counsellors may also encounter people who have different religious positions or no religious position at all, or who have different ideas about questions of meaning and faith. For example, in daily life situations, the topic of conversation may not be about God and faith, but rather about the challenges and demands of everyday life. It can be deduced from this that counselling or spiritual care settings do not have to be viewed only from a religiously based perspective. Rather, context and cause of encounter always determine what happens in spiritual care or counselling, in what forms it takes place and what is to be understood by Muslim spiritual care, and what is not. It also becomes obvious here that a Muslim spiritual counsellor must be prepared to consider the religious diversity in society. The issue of religious diversity is playing an increasingly important role in the discussion of Islamic spiritual care. In Islam, religious diversity is also evident not only in the large denominational currents of Sunnis, Shiites and Alevis, but also with regard to local traditions and personal preferences. This diversity can be legitimized with verses from the Koran. Many Muslims see the diversity of Islamic ways of thinking and living as something positive that distinguishes Islam as a religion without cultural boundaries. According to Hundhammer (2020), the main challenge, however, lies in those areas where normative scriptures of Islam primarily provide restrictive or simply no answers, such as in questions of homosexuality and transgender. As Hundhammer points out, methods of deductive norm derivation, such as the "maqāṣid aš-Šarīʿa" can offer solution models here, but only if a certain minimum textual basis can be drawn upon. However, examples from practice – such as Muslim hospital spiritual care and brain death question – show that there are cases in which normative texts remain silent (Hundhammer 2020). Furthermore, Tittus-Düzcan emphasises that the Qur'anic revelations consider humans' own neediness towards God and that the Islamic image of humans in relation to the soul is, however, by no means negative or pessimistic. He assumes that the image of human beings is decisive for spiritual care. According to this, Muslim spiritual care is characterised by the fact that it is based on the Islamic view of human beings and considers the God-human relationship as the basic building element of its help (Tittus-Düzcan 2020). Tittus-Düzcan affirms that religiosity, spirituality, and ritual acts, as found in the Qur'an and in the Prophet's traditions, can become a decisive effective factor for healing mental suffering. In particular, the strengthening of spiritual resources is shown to be a necessary field of action for spiritual care. For this reason, Islamic theological knowledge must be an important precondition in counselling work with Muslims. However, it is important to examine the extent to which Muslim counselling seekers are open to spiritual and religious elements in crisis situations. The fact that a person calls himself a Muslim does not necessarily mean that spirituality is of great importance to him as a coping strategy. Therefore, the request here is that trained Muslim spiritual counsellors should always be aware that the need for help for those affected can vary greatly (Tittus-Düzcan 2020, 148).Moreover, the legal basis and financial support from the state are still considered to be the main challenges for establishing Islamic spiritual care and counselling in the lack of such support As mentioned before, there is a so-called representative institution for religious and faith communities, such as the representative institutions of the two large Catholic and Protestant churches in Germany, to be able to appoint chaplains to public state institutions. Until these representative institutions are officially recognized by the state, they are not allowed to appoint Muslim spiritual counsellors. They are only able to appoint when they have been officially recognized. Likewise, the question of whether and under what conditions Muslim communities or umbrella organizations can be religious communities in the future is still one of the most challenging questions of religious constitutional law, and which remains unanswered. This means that those who have completed their studies can work at hospitals, prisons and in the military, but cannot be appointed to serve as chaplains. This situation means that the profession of Muslim spiritual counsellors in Germany is not in an attractive and active status.

The point to be made here is that Muslim spiritual counselling is always interwoven with the lives of those seeking advice and that both life and practice are indispensable as productive sources for spiritual counselling. Accordingly, both spiritual care and counselling have a mandate to work for the benefit of people in a wide variety of life situations. To realize this mandate, they need to know about the scope of methods and concepts in the context of theology and the realities of Muslims' lives. Ultimately, spiritual care and counselling have the task of developing ways of helping and coping with new social issues. For this, they need access to knowledge through research. It involves basic research to elaborate the diverse lifeworlds of Muslims in Germany. How the practical implementation of Muslim spiritual care in Germany develops, remains to be seen. However, one must not forget that it is about people who need spiritual care and counselling in certain situations in the here and now. To make this possible, spiritual care needs to be located within the institutional and legal framework in Germany. For example, cooperation between the state, churches and Muslim religious communities can offer opportunities for establishing Muslim spiritual care in Germany. This also raises the question of what alternative spiritual care formats are available if Islamic spiritual care is not available. For example, possibilities for interreligious spiritual care can be considered, that is, spiritual care by Muslims, for Muslims and for all, to be close to all people.

References

Akca, Ayşe Almıla. 2019. *Moscheeleben in Deutschland: Eine Ethnographie zu islamischem Wissen, Tradition und religiöser Autorität.* Bielefeld: Transcript.

Aslan, Ednan, Jonas Kolb, and Erol Yildiz. 2017. *Muslimische Diversität: Ein Kompass zur religiösen Alltagspraxis in Österreich.* Wiesbaden: Springer Verlag.

Aslan, Ednan, Magdalena Modler-El Abdaoui, and Dana Charkasi. 2015. *Islamische Seelsorge: Eine empirische Studie am Beispiel von Österreich.* Wiesbaden: Springer Verlag.

Badawia, Tarek, Gülbahar Erdem, and Mahmoud Abdallah. 2020. *Grundlagen muslimischer Seelsorge: Die muslimische Seele begreifen und versorgen.* Wiesbaden: Springer Verlag.

Begić, Esnaf, Helmut Weiß, and Georg Wenz (eds.) *Barmherzigkeit: Zur sozialen Verantwortung islamischer Seelsorge.* Neukirchen-Vluyn: Neukirchener Verlagsgesellschaft.

Begić, Esnaf. 2014. "Islamische Grundlage der Hilfe für Menschen." In: Esnaf Begić, Helmut Weiß, and Georg Wenz (eds.) *Barmherzigkeit: Zur sozialen Verantwortung islamischer Seelsorge.* Neukirchen-Vluyn: Neukirchener Verlagsgesellschaft. 53–68.

Borchard, Michael, and Rauf Ceylan. 2011. *Imame und Frauen in Moscheen im Integrationsprozess: Gemeindepädagogische Perspektiven.* Osnabrück: V&R unipress.

Ceylan, Rauf. 2012. *Islam und Diaspora: Analysen zum muslimischen Leben in Deutschland aus historischer, rechtlicher sowie migrations- und religionssoziologischer Perspektive.* Frankfurt am Main: Peter Lang.

Dreier, Lena, and Constantin Wagner. 2020. "Wer studiert Islamische Theologie? Ein Überblick über das Fach und seine Studierenden." https://aiwg.de/wp-content/uploads/2020/03/Wer-studiert-islamische-Theologie_Expertise.pdf

Grunwald, Klaus, and Hans Thiersch. 2016. *Praxishandbuch Lebensweltorientierte Soziale Arbeit.* Weinheim: Beltz Juventa.

Hauschildt, Eberhard and Bülent Uçar. 2010. "Islamische Seelsorge in Deutschland im Aufbruch." *Pastoraltheologie* 99/6: 256–263. DOI: https://doi.org/10.13109/path.2010.99.6.256

Jacobs, Andreas, and Janosch Lipowsky. 2019. "Imame – made in Europe?" https://www.kas.de/documents/252038/4521287/Ausbildung+und+Besch%C3%A4ftigung+von+islamischen+Geistlichen+in+Deutschland+und+Frankreich.pdf/c52f425e-22f4-e9bd-d1ba-4747b4e9cc1a?version=1.1&t=1553679831106

Lemmen, Thomas, Nigar Yardim, and Joachim Müller-Lange. 2011. *Notfallbegleitung für Muslime und mit Muslimen: Ein Kursbuch zur Ausbildung Ehrenamtlicher.* Gütersloh: Gütersloher Verlagshaus.

Hundhammer, Marianus. 2020. "Der Begriff 'nafs' im Koran und seine Interpretation – Anwendungsmöglichkeiten im Kontext islamischer Seelsorge." In: Tarek Badawia, Gülbahar Erdem, and Mahmoud Abdallah (eds.) *Grundlagen muslimischer Seelsorge: Die muslimische Seele begreifen und versorgen.* Wiesbaden: Springer Verlag. 89–106.

Nauerth, Matthias, Kathrin Hahn, Michael Tüllmann, and Sylke Kösterke. 2017. *Religionssensibilität in der Sozialen Arbeit: Positionen, Theorien, Praxisfelder.* Stuttgart: Kohlhammer.

Rückamp, Veronika. 2021. *Alltag in der Moschee: Eine Feldforschung jenseits von Integrationsfragen.* Bielefeld: Transcript Verlag.

Şahinöz, Cemil. 2018. *Seelsorge im Islam: Theorie und Praxis in Deutschland.* Wiesbaden: Springer Verlag.

Tittus-Düzcan, Rabia. 2020. "Spiritualität in der islamischen Seelsorge." In: Tarek Badawia, Gülbahar Erdem, and Mahmoud Abdallah (eds.) *Grundlagen muslimischer Seelsorge: Die muslimische Seele begreifen und versorgen.* Wiesbaden: Springer Verlag. 137–152.

Ucar, Bülent, and Martin Blasberg-Kuhnke (eds.). 2013. *Islamische Seelsorge zwischen Herkunft und Zukunft: Von der theologischen Grundlegung zur Praxis in Deutschland.* Frankfurt am Main: Peter Lang Edition.

Uçar, Bülent, and Martina Blasberg-Kuhnke. 2013. *Islamische Seelsorge zwischen Herkunft und Zukunft: Von der theologischen Grundlegung zur Praxis in Deutschland.* Frankfurt am Main: Peter Lang Verlag.

Wenz, Georg, and Talat Kamran. 2012. *Seelsorge und Islam in Deutschland: Herausforderungen, Entwicklungen und Chancen.* Berlin: Verlagshaus Speyer.

Yanık-Şenay, Aylin. 2018. *Familienberatung in muslimischen Migrantenorganisationen.* Wiesbaden: Springer VS.

Online Sources

Fachtagung muslimischer Seelsorge: http://www.deutsche-islam-konferenz.de/DIK/DE/DIK/01_UeberDieDIK/01_Aktuelles/04dik2016fachtagung-seelsorge/dik-2016-fachtagung-inhalt.html? nn=8660654

Islamische Praktische Theologie (Seelsorge) (Master of Arts): https://uni-tuebingen.de/fakultaeten/zentrum-fuer-islamische-theologie/studium/studiengaenge/islamische-praktische-theologie-seelsorge/

Islamische Seelsorge: www.deutsche-islam-konferenz.de/DIK/DE/DIK/01_UeberDieDIK/07_DIK_2014-2017/05%20Arbeitsausschuss/13_Arbeitsausschuss/13-arbeitsausschuss-node.html

Nazila Isgandarova

Female voices in Islamic spiritual care: Tensions and achievements

Abstract: With the aim of contributing to current debates on the role of Muslim female spiritual caregivers, this paper aims to explore the current state of the voices of Muslim female caregivers in Islamic spiritual care, in order to contribute to a better understanding of their role. The purpose is to identify ways that enable them to collectively improve an egalitarian vision of Islamic spiritual care, and to provide the potential to strengthen in a holistic manner the commitment of the practitioners of Islamic spiritual care to the well-being of the community, and to social justice and social change.

Introduction

Islamic spiritual care currently provides positive space for Muslim female leadership in many settings, including a public setting and in a co-educational context (Khoja-Moolji 2011; Gilliat-Ray, Ali, & Pattison 2013). Nevertheless, gender disparity still continues to be one of the central categories of analysis in Islamic spiritual care practice. In addition, as an academic and professional discipline, Islamic spiritual care does not adequately reflect the voices of Muslim female spiritual caregivers along with other marginal voices within the community, which is evident from the lack of the research to support and develop the role of Muslim female spiritual caregivers in their profession.

As a helping profession, Islamic spiritual care helps the sick find the sacred and holy by exploring meaning and purpose to life using traditional Islamic resources and social sciences. Effective Islamic spiritual care helps the person integrate his/her physical, mental, spiritual and social dimensions. The benefit of such a service can protect the client from feeling isolated and give the person a sense of companionship. Furthermore, Muslim spiritual caregivers play significant roles as public spokespersons, religious service facilitators, advisors, counselors, advocates, teachers, and administrators to address the spiritual and mental issues that Muslims face in varous settings. Thus, the theoretical and practical issues that Muslims face on a daily basis create and hold space for the voices of Muslim female spiritual caregivers. However, we need to address barriers that prevent the establishment of an egalitarian space for Muslim female spiritual caregivers.

 https://doi.org/10.1515/9783110717365-007

Why is it important to talk about the perspectives of Muslim female spiritual caregivers? Is there a need? My answer to this question is a resounding "Yes!", because there is a need to open up academic and professional spaces for the voices of Muslim female spiritual caregivers in order to identify the structural issues and factors that impact and inform their practice on a daily basis. Further, my reflection on the voices of Muslim female spiritual caregivers comes from my own personal and professional reflexivity on women's issues for more than ten years.

Islamic spiritual care, as with all spiritual care practices, demands that the practitioner practice reflexivity; this implies that we must acknowledge that "all knowledge is affected by the social conditions under which it is produced and that it is grounded in both the social location and the social biography of the observer and the observed" (Mann/Kelley 1997, 392). Through my practice of reflexivity, I intend to provide critical reflections on the challenges faced by Muslim female spiritual caregivers with the intention of creating a new praxis: to develop new awareness, knowledge and collective action.

This paper has two goals: first, to identify issues that Muslim female spiritual caregivers face in their practice of Islamic spiritual care; and second, to provide a tool for bringing these issues to light. I try to draw a roadmap to show how it is possible to transform Islamic spiritual care practices in order to bring Muslim female spiritual caregivers to the centre of the production and reproduction of Islamic spiritual care. Such a claim may sound ambitious in its intent and scope. Nevertheless, I realize that there is fertile ground to engage female issues in Islamic spiritual care, which strikingly remains behind in multidisciplinary discussions and explorations of spiritual care research. Also, the everyday challenges that Muslim female spiritual caregivers face make it essential to address issues of power, authority, and ethics as we still live and function within a male-dominated paradigm that still strongly shapes and guides our lives. Therefore, androcentric bias in society affects and limits the representation of Muslim female spiritual caregivers in Islamic spiritual care practice.

This paper provides a context for the issue by highlighting personal accounts, and it discusses gender disparity in Islamic spiritual care by pointing out the various accomplishments, tensions, and development of the voices of Muslim female spiritual caregivers in the practice of Islamic spiritual care. I particularly examine patriarchal approaches to Islamic spiritual care and argue that such approaches create various tensions and stresses for Muslim female spiritual caregivers. I also discuss some challenging and practical issues for Muslim female spiritual caregivers by presenting the dilemma of leading mixed-gender congregational prayers and reciting the Qur'an in public in the context of Islamic spiritual care. Finally, I discuss egalitarian steps to solve these challenges for

Muslim female spiritual care givers. The goal is to create a space for the accomplishments and developments of female voices in the Islamic spiritual care profession.

The context of the issue

The main task of Muslim spiritual caregivers is to respond to and address human crises and existential questions, especially of those who are on a quest to find out why they suffer (Isgandarova 2008; Isgandarova/O'Connor 2012). Islamic spiritual care aims to help them understand and address emotional and spiritual aspects of their suffering, their sense of estrangement and isolation, and to facilitate healing by bringing clarity to polarities and contradictions in order to allow them to regain their health. Islamic spiritual care practice supports a client in the direction of liberation from evil, or the destructive forces of trauma, and the re-establishment of personal communication with the Creator and the self. It is the process of contributing to human development and spiritual maturity through helping people achieve the moment of enlightenment. This process is achieved by reviewing a living human document and capturing the moment of truth by providing different lenses to see it (VanKatwyk 2008). The duty of the Muslim spiritual caregiver is to help the client see their problem differently and transcend it through creative imagination or theological reflection. In addition, they need to facilitate relief as the Prophet Muhammad instructed Muadh b. Jabal before appointing him as his representative in Yemen: "make life easy for people and not difficult and give people good news and not difficult news".

Although research in the area of gender disparity and challenges of Muslim female spiritual caregivers lags behind, the struggles of Muslim female spiritual caregivers can be understood from a gendered discourse in Islamic feminist Muslim literature. Such a discourse emerged in the early 1990's and is grounded in re-readings of the Qur'an and other fundamental sources of Islam (Badran 1999).

Muslim feminist scholarship takes a critical approach to the ways of patriarchal Muslim and non-Muslim societies where power and social inequalities distort a healthy image of gender, and where females have limited access to opportunities and do not have enough space to excel in their profession. Such writings emphasize the importance of moving beyond the traditional methodological approach to Islamic texts. Instead of feeling comfortable with their 'knowledge' of the sources of the misogynistic practices against women, these writings pioneer and implement new methodologies to reveal the misogynistic interpretations and 'restore' the egalitarian messages of the Qur'an. By doing so, they do not limit themselves to religious or theological sources only, they also use the humanities and social sciences, and apply post-structuralist principles of intertextuality (using references within the structure of the Qur'an) and intratextuality to the Qur'an (applying secondary references to understand the Qur'an) (Mernissi 1987; Wadud 1999; Barlas 2002; Barazangi 2006; Shaikh 1997; Bakhtiar 2011; Ali 2006; Chaudhry 2013).

Being inspired by Islamic feminism scholarship and activism in Islamic spiritual care practice, many authors such as Sophie Gilliat-Ray, Mansur Ali and Stephen Pattison (2013), Shenila Khoja-Moolji (2011), Sajida Jalalzai (2016), etc. draw attention to the dynamics of gender in the work of Muslim spiritual caregivers. For example, in her meticulous research, Khoja-Moolji (2011) points out that although Islamic spiritual care now offers women more opportunities than in the past, challenges within the field still exist. Sophie Gilliat-Ray, Mansur Ali, and Stephen Pattison (2013) also highlight gender disparity in Islamic spiritual care in the United Kingdom. Their research particularly reflects the controversies in the debates on Muslim females leading the Friday or holiday prayers, reciting the Qur'an in public and other existing gender tensions and lack of voices of Muslim spiritual caregivers in the Islamic spiritual care profession. They conclude that the traditional Islamic organizations limit women's capacity to emerge as leaders and reach society. Whereas the active leadership of Muslim female spiritual care givers in multifaith prayer services still challenge beliefs in the community that the "ideal Muslim female" should not be visible in "male" public spaces, especially in leading mixed congregations in the prayer, for many traditional Islamic organizations, a woman should stay within her domestic private space or at least in "female" public space.

An in-depth reflection on the challenges within the Islamic spiritual care profession demonstrates that one of the challenges for Muslim female spiritual caregivers is the misinterpretation of the "ideal Muslim female" image in many Muslim communities that prevent many Muslim female spiritual caregivers, especially those who work for religious organizations, from taking more leadership roles in this area of care. For example, Sajida Jalalzai quotes from Dr. Nevin Reda from Emmanuel College of Victoria University in the University of Toronto, who once expressed her frustration that "the imam told his congregation that females were forbidden from speaking to men without the permission of their husband or father" (Jalalzai 2016, 239). This observation suggests that the sense of alienation for some Muslim women is real, as some Muslim women have virtually no voice within their own mosques.

Furthermore, research also indicates that the gender disparity has become especially visible since the active presence of Muslim females in spiritual care in the 2000's. For example, by reflecting on her journey in Islamic spiritual care, Mary Lahaj (2011, 174), a Muslim woman chaplain in the UK, states that the main motivation in pursuing a career in this profession was her "long desire to connect deeply with individuals [...]", her comfort in "standing before an audience giving a speech [...]", practicing Islam in her "every day work," and "the deep listening and compassionate response [...] to visit the sick, comfort families, and be present with those grieving, suffering a loss, or experiencing dying or death," etc. In order to do so, she concludes that she needed to possess "a softer heart and deeper love of God and His Creation [...]" (Lahaj 2011, 174). Although Lahaj had also been encouraged by two male imams to pursue chaplaincy training, she acknowledges that she "spent a lot of time" claiming a leadership title other than "imam" to which Muslims could relate in Islamic spiritual care. Also, despite the fact that she was confident that her "authority as a staff member at the hospital sufficed," she indeed faced uncomfortable questions such as "Who are you? What is a chaplain? Can a woman do it?" (Lahaj 2011, 175). Lahaj probably did not respond to these questions in a more assertive manner because she preferred to accept a non-agitating role in these arguments. Her passive stance might also be explained by her perspective that an imam is the best resource in some crisis situations because of their role as a "traditional authority figure with expert knowledge of the religion". She also believes that "imams with legitimacy, education, and status in the community can bring more comfort to Muslims and strengthen their faith" (Lahaj 2011, 177).

Similarly, Doha Hamza (2009), a Muslim female chaplain at Stanford Hospital and Clinics and Lucile Packard Children's Hospital, also reported that her presence as a chaplain evoked surprise among some Muslims. Hamza (2009) explains it with the fact that the Muslim community is not fully familiar with the spiritual care profession, as it is a new and evolving field since historically, spiritual care was provided within one's family. Nevertheless, she is confident in her role as a female chaplain because of the joy spiritual caregivers bring to the lives of the patients, "but also a big part of it is the profound lessons one learns about his or her own life" (Hamza 2009, 145). Hamza calls the spiritual care profession "the blessing" of her life as it "has taught" her a lot of the reality of life, the fragility of life, the preciousness and sacredness of life, the importance of sound relationships with others, humbleness, and appreciation of the traditional notion of visiting the sick. Also, as a Muslim female chaplain she plays an active role in tackling Islamophobia by providing a good example of "a different face of Islam [...] on a very deep level, a humane and intimate level" (Hamza 2009, 144).

In my professional experience, although my authority in ethical issues was accepted initially, I also had to explain the role of spiritual care to my fellow Muslims who asked questions about the role of Muslim women as a spiritual and religious leader and advisor. I also had to explain my reasoning to non-Muslim staff who asked me to replace the imam to read the *khutba* (sermons) or lead the Friday prayers in one institutional setting which, like Lahaj, I had to reject. My refusal did not imply that I endorse the claims that Muslim female spiritual caregivers should not lead the mixed-gender prayers; rather, I support the idea that Islamic spiritual care must go beyond theological and religious arguments and should take into consideration the lived experience of the diverse and vulnerable populations in institutional settings. This implies that as a spiritual caregiver, the goal is to meet the spiritual and emotional needs of clients by going beyond prayer and reading the Qur'an.

The challenging aspects of Islamic spiritual care

As mentioned earlier, Islamic spiritual care should not be limited to reading the Qur'an and leading the prayers only. However, these two functions of Islamic spiritual care among the others present the most challenged aspects to Muslim female spiritual caregivers. Therefore, based on the examples from the literature of Islamic spiritual care and my personal experience, this section explores two theological controversies that create tensions/challenges for Muslim female spiritual caregivers in Islamic spiritual care practice.

Who Should Lead the Prayer in Islamic Spiritual Care?

The Islamic traditions not only play an important role in shaping the experiences of Muslim female spiritual caregivers' daily lives but also their practice. Muslim female spiritual caregivers who choose to lead both male and female Muslims in Islamic rituals might be seen as challenging traditional or cultural ideas about female behavior and appearance in the Islamic tradition (although this may also vary from culture to culture). For example, if a Muslim female spiritual caregiver is asked to perform the functions of imam, i.e., lead the Friday prayer, what would be her response? The answer to this question depends on that Muslim female spiritual caregiver's theological and gender understanding. However, these perspectives also redefine their identity in Islamic spiritual care within different contexts, including economic, political, cultural and ethnicity factors that shape the experiences of Muslim female spiritual caregivers. Nevertheless, it should be noted that in situations when Muslim female spiritual caregivers are requested to lead the congregational or funeral prayer and read the Qur'an loudly and in melody in a mixed gender audience, tension arises and many Muslim female spiritual caregivers choose either to challenge the dominant view on who should do these "priestly" tasks, or embrace a "conservative approach" as they do not want "to be used" against the traditional understanding of Islam. Many still believe that with respect to worship, following the footsteps of the Prophet Muhammad is important (Mattson 2005), despite considering who "legitimizes" and "interprets" these footsteps.

Furthermore, Muslim religious authority is still considered of "[...]the office of the imam, who is also expected to perform multiple, distinct functions for the community" (Mattson 2005, 260). These functions include leading prayers, delivering Friday sermons, drafting marriage contracts, adjudicating divorces, organizing youth and adult education, governing prayer spaces, distributing charitable donations, and representing the Muslim community in larger communal settings. A majority of Muslim scholars still believe that women can only lead their own households or female-only congregations in prayer. For example, a prominent Muslim scholar Yusuf al-Qaradawi points out that:

> [...]the currently extant juristic schools agree that it is not permissible for women to lead men in the obligatory Prayer, though some scholars voice the opinion that the woman who is well-versed in the Qur'an may lead the members of her family, including men, in Prayer on the basis that there is no room for stirring instincts in this case (Qaradawi 2005, https://islamonline.net/archive).

In brief, a misogynistic approach to women's religious and spiritual leadership is a major factor limiting women's opportunities as spiritual caregivers and further hampers the full exercise of their abilities as spiritual caregivers. Therefore, many Muslims do not welcome women's reading the Qur'an and leading prayers outside of their home, particularly in organizations and groups where men are present.

The consequences of this approach resulted in various responses among Muslim female spiritual caregivers who still find themselves behind "curtains." For example, some prefer a more conservative approach by maintaining certain norms about the relational and contextual requirements of prayer leadership in an attempt to follow the Prophetic tradition and endorse inactive involvement in the profession, rather than as a leader and advisor (Jalalzai 2016; Gilliat-Ray, Ali, and Pattison 2013; Khoja-Moolji 2011). Conversely, some Muslim female spiritual caregivers support performing the functions of imams in institutional settings and argue that the term "imam" holds potential for Muslim female spiritual caregivers, even though it contains controversial interpretations within the Muslim community. These women bring forth examples from Islamic history that suggest that in the past, some Muslim women also assumed the leadership role, including in prayer and other forms of devotion and meditation and teaching the tradition, especially in the Sufi traditions around the Muslim world (Ahmed 1992; Stowasser 1999; Hill 2014; Frede and Hill 2014; Hill 2010; Hill 2014).

The Qur'an does not specifically mention whether women can lead men and women in the Friday prayer, conduct memorial or funeral services, visit the sick, etc. The traditions of the Prophet Muhammad also inspired some Muslim women to be leaders in prayer.[1] The hadith of Umm Waraqa especially has gained wide popularity to explore the Sunna with respect to women's role in spiritual care.[2] In addition to following the Qur'an and the Prophetic tradition, according to the majority of schools of thought, i.e., Shafi, Hanafi, and Hanbali, with the excep-

1 A detailed version of this hadith literature is as follows: The hadith of 'A'ishah and Umm Salamah (may Allah be pleased with them). 'Abdur-Raziq (5086), Ad-Daraqutni (1/404) and Al-Bayhaqi (3/131) reported from the narration of Abu Hazim Maysarah ibn Habib from Ra'itah Al-Hanafiyyah from 'A'ishah that she led women in Prayer and stood among them in an obligatory Prayer. Moreover, Ibn Abi Shaybah (2/89) reported from the chain of narrators of Ibn Abi Layla from 'Ata' that 'A'ishah used to say the Adhan, the Iqamah, and lead women in Prayer while standing among them in the same row. Al-Hakim also reported the same hadith from the chain of narrators of Layth Ibn Abi Sulaim from 'Ata', and the wording of the hadith mentioned here is Al-Hakim's. Furthermore, Ash-Shafi'i (315), Ibn Abi Shaybah (88/2) and 'Abdur-Raziq (5082) reported from two chains of narrators that report the narration of 'Ammar Ad-Dahni in which he stated that a woman from his tribe named Hujayrah narrated that Umm Salamh used to lead women in Prayer while standing among them in the same row. The wording of 'Abdur-Raziq for the same hadith is as follows: "Umm Salamah led us (women) in the 'Asr Prayer and stood among us (in the same row)." In addition, Al-Hafiz said in Ad-Dirayah (1/169), "Muhammad ibn Al-Husain reported from the narration of Ibrahim An-Nakh'i that 'A'ishah used to lead women in Prayer during the month of Ramadan while standing among them in the same row. Further, 'Abdur-Raziq reported (5083) from the narration of Ibrahim ibn Muhammad from Dawud ibn Al-Husain from 'Ikrimah from Ibn 'Abbas that the latter said, "A woman can lead women in Prayer while standing between them."

2 The hadith is reported that Umm Waraqah, the daughter of Nawfal reported, "When the Prophet (peace and blessings be upon him) proceeded for Badr I said to him, 'Messenger of Allah allow me to accompany you in the battle. I shall act as a nurse for your patients and maybe Allah will bestow martyrdom upon me.' He replied, 'stay at your home and Allah the Exalted will bestow martyrdom upon you.' She read the Quran and sought permission from the Prophet (peace and blessings be upon him) to have a mu'adhdhin in her house. He therefore permitted her to do so. She announced that her slave and slave girl would be free after her death so one night they strangled her with a sheet of cloth until she died and ran away. The next day 'Umar announced that anyone who has knowledge of them or has seen them should bring them to him. (After they were caught) 'Umar ordered that they be crucified and this was the first crucifixion at Madinah." From Umm Waraqah, the daughter of Abdullah bin al-Harith, "the Messenger of Allah (peace and blessings be upon him) used to visit her at her house. He appointed a mu'adhdhin to call Adhan for her and he commanded her to lead the inmates of her house in prayer." Abdurrahman said, "I saw that her mu'adhdhin was an old man." [Abu Dawud (Eng. Trans. #591 & 592)].

tion of the Malikis, and very recently, the Ithna Asharis from the Shi'a school of thought, women can be *imam* (leader) of a *jama'ah* (congregation), i.e. the optional *tarawih* prayers during Ramadhan – if the congregants are females only. Therefore, it was not unusual for Muslim female spiritual caregivers to lead the congregational prayers. Also, the practice of women's recitation of the Qur'an varies from culture to culture. For example, the recitation of the Qur'an by females in public, especially in front of a mixed audience, is not welcomed in an Arab or Persian context (Safi 2013). Nevertheless, unlike the leading of Friday prayers by women, some Muslim cultures accept women's recitation of the Qur'an in public. For example, despite the patriarchal constructs of the female's role in society, the South Asian culture allows females to recite the Qur'an in public.

Nevertheless, many Muslim female spiritual caregivers started to follow the new insight provided by some Muslim female scholars such as Amina Wadud, Nevin Reda El-Tahry, etc., to develop the ability to reread the Islamic tradition in a prudent and thoughtful manner. They are encouraged by these female scholars and activists who lead the congregational prayers. For example, in a mixed audience since 1995, a woman-led prayer which occurred in Johannesburg in South Africa still inspires many Muslim females who deliver either *adhan* (call for prayer), *khutbah* (a sermon) or lead the mixed audience in prayer: Shamima Sheikh (1960 – 1998) in South Africa, Amina Wadud, Lubna Nadvi, Zaytun Suleyman, Fatima Seedat, Fatima Hendricks, and Dr. Mariam Seedat in United States, Maryam Mirza, Yasmin Shadeer, Raheel Raza, Pamela Taylor, and Nevin Reda in Canada have successfully led mixed congregations in Friday or Eid prayers. In this context, the March 18, 2005 woman-led prayer in New York City was a ground breaking event. As Juliane Hammer points out:

> The imam was a woman, who also delivered the khutbah; the congregation she addressed and led in prayer was not separated by gender; and the adhan (call to prayer) was pronounced by a woman. It is in these three departures from established ritual practice that the March 18 prayer became an embodied performance of gender justice in the eyes of its organizers and participants. They symbolically challenged the exclusively male privilege of leading Muslims in ritual prayers and at the same time blurred the lines of gender segregation in ritual prayers (Hammer 2012, 15).

Following their footsteps, some Muslim female spiritual caregivers, especially those who provide spiritual care in multi-faith settings, take radical revolutionary steps by reciting the Qur'an loudly in a mixed gender audience. For example, Tahera Ahmed, one of the chaplains at Northwestern University, publicly recited the Qur'an at the National Islamic Society of North America (ISNA) conference titled "Beyond the Ceiling: Ground-breaking Voices of American Muslim

Women," where Muslim Public Affairs Council in U.S. and the White House recognized over 80 American Muslim Women in the fields of STEM (Science, Technology, Engineering and Math), business development, government, communications and entrepreneurship in April 2014. Recently, Sherin Khankan and Saliha Marie Fetteh, Muslim female imams in Denmark, also declared that along with providing spiritual care and counselling to Muslims, other aspects of the Islamic tradition such as announcing the *adhan* (call to the prayer), delivering the *khutbah* and reciting the Qur'an in public, are also an important part of what they do.

These cases, as Khoja-Moolji suggests, are "a *symbolic* or *representational* issue" for many Muslim female leaders, including Muslim female spiritual caregivers because of the scope of their impact on women's religious leadership in many areas of life, including the spiritual and religious domains "that were previously not available to them" (Khoja-Moolji 2011, 6).

Recommendations for an egalitarian Islamic spiritual care practice

Despite the geographical differences (i.e. the US context versus South African or Canadian contexts), the leadership role in prayers and reciting the Qur'an in Islamic spiritual care still constitute a significant source of power and a sacred duty that provide Muslim spiritual caregivers with unique opportunities to express and perform their religious authority and also educate clients about a range of religious and practical issues in Islamic spiritual care practice. Taking away this important role from Muslim female spiritual caregivers means losing a significant source of power and authority in Islamic spiritual care.

Therefore, at the heart of our discussion is our inquiry of power and how knowledge is built in the Islamic spiritual care profession. Furthermore, we question structural and historical arrangements that inhibit and disadvantage Muslim females more than males in the Muslim community. Such a critical approach to the Islamic spiritual care practice aims to shed light on the form and function of power and hierarchy across a range of spiritual and religious care duties to others, and then seeks to give voices to women who may feel displaced by gender disparity.

From this angle of thought, the patriarchal approach to Islamic spiritual care reduces the potential professional development of Muslim female spiritual caregivers. Although Muslim female spiritual caregivers are committed to advocating for the spiritual and emotional welfare of their clients and to advocating for justice for people, very often they find themselves marginalized because they hold a "minority" status in the Islamic spiritual care profession. Therefore, a critical theological framework of the majority of Muslim feminist and egalitarian female scholars are resources for Muslim spiritual caregivers to see the interconnectedness of gender, religion, and spirituality.

Second, the female presence in the field of Islamic spiritual care by no way challenges religious and spiritual authority of Muslim leaders. This is mainly explained with the Muslim community views of Muslim spiritual caregivers simply as facilitators of discussion of existential, relational, mental, physical, as well as religious issues and performers of rituals in various institutions. Jalalzai (2016) quotes from Mattson who acknowledges the Islamic spiritual care profession seeks to "decenter[s] the figure of the imam, and to open up new leadership opportunities for women [...]" (238). Such an attempt to deconstruct patriarchal narratives in Islamic spiritual care starts with the training of Muslim female spiritual caregivers. The availability of educational programs and demand for them mean that the Islamic spiritual care profession is the field that many Muslim women pursue because they want to help those in crisis. In addition, in the religious and spiritual leadership realm, Islamic spiritual care is the only profession that "helps to forge new paths for Muslim women [...]" (Jalalzai 2016, 177) and offers "women innovative opportunities to exercise religious knowledge and leadership" (Jalalzai 2016, 243). Perhaps, this is the main motivation of Muslim leadership and spiritual care and counselling programs at Hartford Seminary, Emmanuel College and the Bayan Claremont that open new avenues for Muslim females to pursue careers in Islamic spiritual care. However, the task to make Muslim female spiritual caregivers confident in this growing and evolving field of Islamic spiritual care is not that easy. For example, there are criticisms against the aforementioned programs, some interpret their support of the profession of female Muslim chaplaincy as saying it "challenges prevailing stances on the exclusivity of male ritual leadership, and instead reinforces underlying gender constructions and norms" (Jalalzai 2016, 244). It is indeed the reality, as Jihad Turk from Bayan Claremont points out, that Bayan's long-term goals of Islamic spiritual care education is to tackle "some of these issues [related to women and authority], and do it in a way that does not alienate the institution [from Muslim communities]...That is a long term policy [...] but part of our vision" (Jalalzai, 2016: 242).

Furthermore, many Muslim female spiritual caregivers bring ideas, principles, and tenets to the inquiry process to contribute their perspectives within Islamic spiritual care. As a perspective, Olesen quotes from Eichler (1986), stating they focus on these important aspects of feminist and egalitarian inquiry (a) "[the work] problematizes women's diverse situations as well as the gendered institutions and material and historical structures that frame those;" (b) "It refers the examination of that problematic to theoretical, policy, or action frameworks to realize social justice for women (and men) in specific contexts"; and (c) "It generates new ideas to produce knowledge about oppressive situations for women, for action or further research" (Olesen 2005, 236).

In general, the egalitarian approach in Islamic spiritual care requires addressing various inequalities in the practice, encourages the application of historical and social context to understand why the voices of females are heard less in society, and rereading the principle of modesty within the Islamic tradition. This approach has been inspired by the Qur'an, which teaches the fundamental equality of women and men regardless of their race, ethnicity, economic and political status. Therefore, contextualizing, rereading and reinterpreting the Islamic tradition in the context of Islamic spiritual care is an important endeavour of Muslim female spiritual caregivers. Such an approach challenges the Qur'an's patriarchal exegesis of conservative males by emphasizing the idea that only God knows the true meaning of the Qur'an and doubts the authenticity of the male-dominated Islamic classical tradition that very often neglects to deal with the oppression of females in Muslim societies.

Conclusion

Discussions of the role of Muslim female spiritual caregivers in Islamic spiritual care extend debates concerning the role of females as Muslim leaders in the context of the still male-dominated field of Islamic spiritual care. We witness the challenges of Muslim female spiritual caregivers and how they are ready to give up or accept some sources of authority and power in Islamic spiritual care by adjusting their own theological position. Therefore, women and gender issues should constitute one of the central categories of analysis in Islamic spiritual care. Inequality in Islamic spiritual care arises when female spiritual caregivers who choose to work in this field do not have the power to perform traditional Islamic spiritual care practices in public spaces. For example, one of the needs emerges from the controversies in the debates of females leading the Friday or holiday prayers in Islamic spiritual care in different institutional settings.

Thus, in order to prevent inequality in Islamic spiritual care practice, there is a need to open up academic and professional spaces for the voices of Muslim female spiritual caregivers. This will help to address the structural issues and forces that impact and inform Islamic spiritual care as a profession. Without addressing the issue of existing gender tensions in the Islamic spiritual care profession, Muslim female spiritual caregivers will have no access or only limited access to opportunities in the Islamic spiritual care profession.

References

Ahmed, Leila. 1992. *Women and gender in Islam: historical roots of a modern debate.* New Haven: Yale University Press.
Ali, Kecia. 2006. *Sexual ethics and Islam: Feminist reflections on Qur'ān, hHadith and jurisprudence.* Oxford, UK: Oneworld Publications.
Badran, Margot. 1999. "Towards Islamic feminisms: A look at the Middle East." In: Asma Afsaruddin (ed.) *Hermeneutics and Honor: Negotiating female "public" space in Islamic/ate societies.* Cambridge, MA: Harvard Middle Eastern Monographs. 166–167.
Bakhtiar, Laleh. 2011. "The sublime Qur'ān: The misinterpretation of chapter 4 verse 34." *European Journal of Women's Studies* 18/4: 431–439.
Barazangi, Nimat Hafez. 2006. *Woman's identity and the Qur'an: A new reading.* The University Press of Florida.
Barlas, Asma. 2002. *Believing women in Islam: Unreading patriarchal interpretations of the Qur'an.* Austin, TX: University of Texas Press.
Burt, Sandra, and Lorraine Code. 1995. *Changing Methods.* Ontario, Canada: Broad View Press.
Chaudhry, Ayesha S. 2013. *Domestic violence and The Islamic tradition: Ethics, law, and the Muslim discourse on gender.* Oxford: Oxford University Press.
Fonow Mary Margaret, and Judith A. Cook. 1991. *Beyond methodology: Feminist scholarship as lived research.* Bloomington: Indiana University Press.
Gilliat-Ray, Sophie, Mansur Ali, and Stephen Pattison. 2013. *Understanding Muslim chaplaincy.* Surrey, U.K.: Ashgate Publishing Ltd.
Hammer, Juliane. 2012. *American Muslim women, religious authority, and activism. More than a prayer.* Austin: University of Texas.
Harding, Sandra. 1991. *Whose science? Whose knowledge?* Ithaca, NY: Cornell University Press.
Isgandarova, Nazila. 2011. "The concept of effective Islamic spiritual care." *The Journal of Rotterdam Islamic and Social Sciences* 2/1: 87–117.
Isgandarova, Nazila. 2012. "Effectiveness of Islamic spiritual care: Foundations and practices of Muslim spiritual caregivers." *The Journal of Pastoral Care & Counseling* 66/3: 1–16.
Isgandarova, Nazila. 2005. "Islamic spiritual care in a health care setting." In: Augustine Meier, Thomas St. James O'Connor, and Peter L. VanKatwyk (eds.). *Spirituality and health: Multidisciplinary explorations.* Waterloo: WLU Press. 85–104.
Jalalzai, Sajida. 2016. *Translating Islamic authority: Chaplaincy and Muslim leadership education in North American protestant seminaries.* PhD thesis. Columbia Unviersity, 2016. https://academiccommons.columbia.edu/.../ac.../Jalalzai_columbia_0054D_13340.pdf (accessed August 3, 2016).
Khoja-Moolji, Shenila. 2011. *An emerging Model of Muslim leadership: Chaplaincy on university campuses.* The Pluralism Project, Harvard University.
Mann, Susan A., and Lori R. Kelley. 1997. "Standing at the crossroads of modernist thought: Collins, Smith, and the new feminist epistemologies." *Gender & society* 11: 391–408.

Mattson, Ingrid. 2005. *Can A woman be an imam? Debating form and function in Muslim women's leadership.* (http://www.onbeing.org/program/new-voice-islam/feature/can woman-be-imam-debating-form-and-function-muslim-women (accessed on May 20, 2021).
Mernissi, Fatima. 1987. *The veil and the male elite: A feminist interpretation of women's rights in Islam.* Reading, MA: Addison-Wesley Publishing.
Olesen, Virginia. 2005. "Early millennial feminist qualitative research: Challenges and contours." In: Norman K. Denzin, and Yvonna S. Lincoln (eds.) *The Sage handbook of qualitative research.* Thousand Oaks, CA: SAGE. 235–278.
Reinharz, Shulamit. 1992. *Feminist methods in social research.* New York, NY: Oxford University Press.
Richards, P. Scott, and Allen E. Bergin. 1997. *A spiritual strategy for counseling and psychotherapy.* Washington, DC: APA.
Safi, Omid. 2013. "Words of God in women's voices: Women reciting the Qur'an in public." *Religion News Service.* http://omidsafi.religionnews.com/2013/09/09/tahera/#sthash.vEmgrySf.dpuf (accessed May 20, 2021).
Shaikh, Sa'adiya. 1997. "Exegetical violence: *Nushuz* in Quranic gender ideology." *Journal for Islamic Studies* 17: 49–73.
Shaikh, Sa'adiya. 2007. "A tafsir of praxis." In: Daniel C. Maguire, and Sa'adiya Shaikh (eds.). *Violence against women in contemporary world religion.* Ohio: The Pilgrim Press.
Turk, Jihad. May 12, 2015. *Interview with Dr. Jihad Turk on Bayan Claremont and Interfaith in Islam.* Pacifica Institute. http://pacificainstitute.org/san-diego/2015/05/12/interview-with-dr-jihad-turk-on-bayan-claremont-and-interfaith-in-islam/ (accessed May 30, 2021).
VanKatwyk, Peter. 2008. "Seeing the same different: The 'living human document' in a postmodern context of Clinical Pastoral Education." In: Thomas St. James O'Connor, Colleen Lashmar, and Elizabeth Meakes (eds.) *The spiritual care giver's guide to identity.* CAPPESWONT & Waterloo Lutheran Seminary.
Wadud, Amina. 1999. *Qur'an and woman: Rereading the sacred text from a woman's perspective.* Oxford: Oxford University Press.

Anke I. Liefbroer, Stef Lauwers, Pieter Coppens, Bikram Lalbahadoersing[1]

Spiritual care in an interfaith context: Implications for Buddhist, Muslim, and Hindu spiritual care in the Netherlands

Abstract: This chapter considers the implications of an interfaith context for the way in which spiritual care takes shape. We focus on Buddhist, Islamic, and Hindu perspectives that represent relatively 'new' traditions in the field of spiritual care in the Netherlands. We describe the developments and characteristics of spiritual care in this context from each of these traditions, and discuss the implications of working with clients with a different religious or spiritual orientation. A comparison of the three perspectives shows both similarities and differences that help us to deepen our understanding of the implications of religious and spiritual diversity for spiritual care provision in the Netherlands.

Introduction

The religious and spiritual landscape in many Western societies has changed over the past decades: from a landscape in which many, or even most, people adhere to a religious—often Christian—tradition, to a situation in which 'being religious' no longer is the default-option and a secularized worldview has become dominant (Taylor 2007). In addition to processes of secularization, the landscape has become pluralized, with people with a variety of religious, spiritual and cultural backgrounds living together, including people who combine elements from various religious traditions (Berghuijs 2017; Pew Research Center 2009; Vertovec 2007; Woodhead, Partridge, and Kawanami 2016). For spiritual caregivers or chaplains—often working in secular institutions (e.g., the military, healthcare institutions) while at the same time formally ordained or authorized by a religious institution (Doolaard 2006; Swift 2013)—questions arise concerning what the specific religious ordinations entails and how this relates to spiri-

1 This chapter is written by all authors, but each author also has a specific focus: Anke I. Liefbroer is the main author of the 'Introduction' and 'Discussion' (sections 1 and 5); Stef Lauwers is the main author of 'a Buddhist perspective' (section 2); Pieter Coppens is the main author of 'an Islamic perspective' (section 3), and Bikram Lalbahadoersing is the main author of 'a Hindu perspective' (section 4).

 https://doi.org/10.1515/9783110717365-008

tual care provision to a spiritually diverse client population. In this chapter, we consider the implications of this diversified religious and spiritual landscape for the way in which spiritual care takes shape in the multicultural and multifaith society of the Netherlands.

As in other Western European countries, people from secular as well as a diversity of spiritual and religious backgrounds live in the Netherlands: around half of the Dutch population does not (or no longer) adhere to a religious tradition (51%), and others belong to a variety of Christian denominations (24% Roman-Catholic; 15% various Protestant denominations), Islam (5%) (CBS 2017), or other, smaller, religious traditions, such as Hinduism (0.6%) and Buddhism (0.4%) (CBS 2015). Here, we focus on these three latter traditions, which can be considered three relatively 'new' religious denominations represented in the field of spiritual care.

Historically, spiritual care in Dutch institutions used to be mainly provided by Protestant, Catholic, and Humanist spiritual caregivers. However, over the past decades, other spiritual caregivers were employed in state-funded institutions as well, both those affiliating with other denominations as well as those without formal affiliation. Specifically, spiritual caregivers from religious traditions previously not formally represented—e.g., Buddhist, Islamic, and Hindu spiritual caregivers—started providing spiritual care and educating spiritual caregivers to become authorized chaplains for these 'new' denominations (Doolaard 2006; Ganzevoort, Ajouaou, Van der Braak, De Jongh, and Minnema 2014; Liefbroer and Berghuijs 2019). Also, in response to processes of secularization and professionalization of spiritual care as a discipline, spiritual caregivers started working as unaffiliated (i.e., not formally authorized/ordained by a religious or Humanistic institution) spiritual caregivers.[2]

These historical developments are reflected in the way in which spiritual care provision is organized in practice, although there are differences between work settings in this regard. In healthcare settings, for instance, Protestant, Catholic, Humanist, as well as unaffiliated spiritual caregivers mainly seem to work in a territorial mode (i.e., providing care to all patients in a certain department), spiritual caregivers from 'newer' denominations (e.g., Islamic spiritual caregivers) are more likely to work in a categorical mode (i.e., providing care to patients with the same religious or spiritual orientation) (Liefbroer and Berghuijs 2019; Van Buuren and Van Dijk 2006). By contrast, within penitentiary institutions

2 Unaffiliated spiritual caregivers can be recognized by the Dutch "Stichting RING-GV", which examines spiritual caregivers' spiritual competence. Recognition by the "Stichting RING-GV" is seen by the organization of spiritual caregivers in the Netherlands (VGVZ) as equivalent to religious or Humanistic authorization.

all job positions are allocated along denominational lines and spiritual care is mainly provided in a categorical mode to clients with the same religious or spiritual orientation as the spiritual caregiver has (Ajouaou and Bernts 2015; Bernts, Ganzevoort, Leget, and Wojtkowiak 2014; Van Iersel and Eerbeek 2009; Liefbroer and Berghuijs 2019). However, as shall become clear from this chapter, in each of these settings spiritual caregivers still meet clients with a variety of spiritual or religious orientations. In this chapter, we consider the developments in each of the main spiritual care settings (healthcare, prisons, the military), since the way in which each setting organizes their spiritual care provision has consequences for the way in which spiritual caregivers position themselves in this context and for the way in which they perceive spiritual caregiving to a diverse patient population (Liefbroer and Berghuijs 2019).

Education for the Buddhist, Islamic, and Hindu spiritual caregivers recently started at Vrije Universiteit Amsterdam, containing both faith-specific (40% of the curriculum) and generic courses (60% of the curriculum). In 2014, when the curricula for these denominational spiritual care programs were being developed, several colleagues reported on specific aspects of spiritual care provision from these various traditions (Ganzevoort et al. 2014). Now, several years later, we aim to reflect on the developments that have taken place over the past years, and to further explore the implications of spiritual care provision from these three denominations for providing spiritual care in an interfaith setting, i.e., when providing spiritual care to clients from a diversity of spiritual or religious orientations. In addition, we aim to compare these three perspectives to identify similarities and differences, thereby deepening our understanding of the implications of religious and spiritual diversity for the way in which spiritual care takes shape in the Netherlands.

In the following sections, we first describe for each of the denominations—Buddhism, Islam, and Hinduism—how this form of spiritual care was developed in the Netherlands. Second, we describe the characteristics of spiritual care as seen from these denominations. The core aspects of spiritual care from each tradition are explored, as well as the roles the spiritual caregiver takes when providing spiritual care and the practices that are typical for spiritual care provision by each denomination. Third, we discuss what the implications of working from a denominational background are for providing spiritual care to clients with a different religious or spiritual orientation. Finally, in our discussion section, we compare the perspectives and look at similarities and differences between them, and discuss the implications for practicing spiritual care in an interfaith context.

A Buddhist perspective

A brief history of Buddhist spiritual care in the Netherlands

The Ministry of Justice played an important role in the establishment of Buddhist chaplaincy in the Netherlands. There had been cases of Buddhists volunteers visiting Dutch prisons prior to 2000, but what is by many people considered as the official beginning of Buddhist chaplaincy in the Netherlands was a Turkish prisoner with a Muslim background asking a prison director for a Buddhist chaplain to talk about some Buddhist books he had read (interview Meindert van de Heuvel in Van den Berg-Mulder 2010, 127). His request was initially refused, since in prisons only Roman-Catholic, Protestant and Humanist chaplains were available at that time. However, on 21 August 2000 the "Complaints Committee Krimpen aan de Ijssel Prison" told the director that a Buddhist chaplain had to be found. Eric Soyeux, a Rigpa volunteer, went to visit the Turkish prisoner and described his spiritual care provision as follows: "Soon we meditated together (...). After some time, my client invited other inmates, so gradually I had a meditation group of about seven people. I often showed a video with teachings of Sogyal Rinpoche. We regularly sang the Vajra guru mantra, which created a peaceful atmosphere. I tried to establish a meditation practice and if that succeeded I tried to follow up with regular Rigpa teachings. We did a lot of talking and I was seen as a person of trust, prisoners could share their experiences." (Hoek 2012, translated by Stef Lauwers). When Soyeux's client, the Turkish prisoner, found out that Soyeux was not paid for his visits like the Christian and Humanist chaplains he went to court again, and won (Centrale Raad voor de Strafrechttoepassing/Administration of Criminal Justice, court case number 00/1737, 8 January 2001). Since then, the Buddhist volunteer was considered a chaplain and had to be financially supported.[3] Van der Sande, in his report on the recognition of the Dutch Buddhist Union as endorsing organization for Buddhist chaplains, notes that from that date on the Ministry of Justice started corresponding with the Dutch Buddhist Union (Hogendoorn 2015, 2).

The second important step in the establishment of Buddhist chaplaincy is that in 2004 a centralized organization for chaplaincy services within the Dutch prisons became active and Buddhist chaplains were able to enter. In

3 Soyeux, in the same interview, mentioned that this decision created tension with Christian and Humanist chaplains: "Who is he? We need a degree but he, just like that, becomes a chaplain" (Hoek 2012, translated by Stef Lauwers).

2008, the Dutch Buddhist Union was, on a temporary basis, recognized as the endorsing committee for Buddhist chaplains in prisons (Bernts, Van der Velde, and Kregting, 2012a, 5). The head of the Dutch Buddhist Union was appointed head of Buddhist chaplaincy in prisons. A Buddhist Endorsement Committee was established on 3 April 2009 (Bernts, Van der Velde, and Kregting 2012a, 43). Two already active Buddhist chaplains, on the condition of earning a master's degree in religion in the near future, and three new, already academically qualified, Buddhist chaplains (including one of the authors of this article), started January 2011 as the new Buddhist chaplaincy team in prisons. Four chaplains had a background in Zen, and one in Tibetan Buddhism. For permanent recognition of the endorsing committee, a study into whether the Buddhist Union represented most Buddhist in the Netherlands was conducted. Also, the demands for chaplains with a master's degree and the establishment of a Master education trajectory for Buddhist chaplains at a Dutch University had to be met. In 2011, the Vrije Universiteit Amsterdam asked the ministry of Education, Culture and Science for a "Special facility Buddhist seminar education trajectory". This Buddhist seminary had to establish the formation of Buddhist chaplains in a joint venture of the Vrije Universiteit and the Buddhist Endorsement Organization. The request was honored in 2012 and in December 2012 the license recognizing the Dutch Buddhist Union as endorsing organization became permanent.

The third step in the history of Buddhist chaplaincy in the Netherlands is this establishment of the education trajectory at Vrije Universiteit Amsterdam. First, a curriculum committee was set up, and members of the University and the Dutch Buddhist Union were involved. A bachelor's, master's and a post-academic endorsement trajectory were gradually deployed. The bachelor's students had to take part in the Bachelor in Religion and complete 60 % general and 40 % Buddhist courses. The master's students had to register in the Master Spiritual Care Buddhist trajectory, consisting of 60 % general and 40 % Buddhist courses. Meanwhile, the curriculum committee had established a post-master program that could give extra weight to the Buddhist chaplaincy education and was imperative for endorsement. Ten courses were offered, in the first year (2014–15) in a full-time mode, and from 2015–16 in a part-time two-year program. The two-year program offered students more time for introspection and reflection and added to their maturity as Buddhist chaplains. To take part in this 60 ECT two-year post-academic program, students are required to have a Master in Religion (preferably option Spiritual Care Buddhist trajectory at Vrije Universiteit) or a comparable degree.

Currently, in Summer 2019, Buddhist chaplains not only work in prisons, but in other settings as well. Graduates of the Buddhist endorsement trajectory at the Vrije Universiteit are employed as general chaplains in psychiatric, hospital, elderly and juvenal care. Also, the Dutch army currently started vacancies for Buddhist chaplains.

Characteristics of Buddhist spiritual care

Content of Buddhist spiritual care

While the first volunteers offered spiritual care very much related to their own Buddhist tradition, from 2011 this changed. The endorsement committee stated that Buddhist chaplaincy in the Netherlands should not be related to a specific Buddhist tradition (Vrije Universiteit Amsterdam 2019). In practice, the specific background of each Buddhist chaplain can still be traced in the way he or she operates, but Buddhist chaplains at this date are making a serious effort to work client-centred and to use a variety of skills based on materials from various Buddhist and secular mindfulness traditions. The education program at Vrije Universiteit supports this diversity as much as possible, but also has to rely on available books and articles that are often American and zen-b(i)ased. In the following, we will briefly describe the content of Buddhist spiritual care based on this literature.

From the start of the education program, Bernie Glassman's "the three tenets"—"Not-Knowing", "Bearing witness", and "Doing the Actions that Arise from Not-Knowing"—proved an important concept (Glassman 1998; Nakao 2017). Students use these three tenets as a way of approaching clients. Even if a chaplain has visited a client numerous times before, by following these tenets every contact can be open and new. Joan Halifax's "Being with Dying" (2008), Andrew Bein's "The Zen of Helping" (2008) and also articles such as Mikel Monnet's "Developing a Buddhist Approach to Pastoral Care, a Peacemaker's View" (2005) are commenting on the tenets as beneficial for Buddhist (spiritual) care. The tenets are very much in line with the 'theory of presence' (Baart 2002) that is often used in Dutch spiritual care, but offer a more contemplative approach as the foundation of the first two tenets is rooted in meditation practice. In the third tenet—"Action" or "Doing what needs to be done"—the chaplain uses mindfulness and wisdom to see what particular needs the client has, and these needs are then met with "Upaya, skillful means" using the abundance of the dharma in its broadest sense. This 'toolkit' of the Buddhist chaplain is filled with beneficial stories, ritual, and meditation techniques from the various Buddhist traditions. Opinions differ concerning whether a Buddhist chaplain should be able to use materials from non-Buddhist traditions if beneficial for the client. Some claim that from a Mahayana point of view this should be possible (White 2014).

In addition to Glassman's three tenets, Jennifer Block's principles of Buddhist chaplaincy (2012) are important in the education program. Block also starts with one of the tenets, "the willingness to bear witness", and then adds:

> *"The willingness to help others discover their own truth, willingness to sit and listen to stories that have meaning and value, helping another to face life directly, welcoming paradox & ambiguity into care and trusting that these will emerge into some degree of awakening and the last principle: creating opportunities for the people to awaken to their True Nature".*

For rituals, the eight categories of Gil Fronsdal's "Rituals in Buddhism" are used. Harvey's "An introduction to Buddhist ethics" (2000) is the main manual for Buddhist ethics, and for leadership and community building students read "A thousand hands, a guidebook to caring for your Buddhist community" (Nathan and Fisher 2016) and "Waking up from war: a better way home for veterans and nations" (Bobrow 2015).

Relating to "Mindfulness", in the sense of John Kabat-Zinn's mindfulness-based stress reduction/mindfulness-based cognitive therapy (MBSR/MBCT) eight-week program, also became an important part of the Dutch chaplaincy discourse (Van Baarsen, Oldenhof, and Kruijne 2016). As MBSR/MBCT became very popular in the Netherlands over the past years, a lot of clients asking for a Buddhist chaplain have a background in mindfulness. To be able to provide spiritual care to these clients, the education program consists of three major courses on mindfulness. In the Master's program there is a Buddhist elective course "Multidisciplinary reflections on Mindfulness". In the post-academic trajectory students participate in a MBSR-trajectory which focuses on literature by Bhikkhu Analayo "Satipatthana, the direct Path to Realization" (2004) and by David McMahan "The Making of Buddhist Modernism" (2008), thereby reflecting on the Buddhist roots of the program.[4]

Roles of the Buddhist spiritual caregiver

In the general spiritual care program at Vrije Universiteit the book "Zorg voor het verhaal/ Caring for the story" (Ganzevoort and Visser 2007) is used as the basic

4 In the Netherlands MBSR is often used in general or denominational chaplaincy. As most Buddhist chaplains are trained mindfulness teachers, educated by external institutions (mostly at Radboud University Medical center), questions by candidate Buddhist chaplains were raised if this teacher training could not be included in the program at Vrije Universiteit. Until now this has not been the case.

manual. Ganzevoort and Visser (2017) describe three roles of the pastoral caregiver: the witness (representative of tradition), the helper (professional role), and the companion (or friend). In trying to find a Buddhist counterpart for these roles and to include the three major Buddhist traditions we identified: spiritual friend (kalyana mitta), bodhisattva (helper), and spiritual warrior (the chaplain as a critical mirror, the tradition as counter culture).

First, there is the role of the Buddhist chaplain as a spiritual friend. In Angutarra Nikaya, Mitta Sutta 7.35, a spiritual friend—kalyana mitta—is described as follows:

> Monks, a friend endowed with seven qualities is worth associating with. Which seven? He gives what is hard to give. He does what is hard to do. He endures what is hard to endure. He reveals his secrets to you. He keeps your secrets. When misfortunes strike, he doesn't abandon you. When you're down and out, he doesn't look down on you. A friend endowed with these seven qualities is worth associating with.

Most students recognize a lot of what a chaplain does in the description of these seven qualities. The 'keeping your secrets'-part is seen as very important. Chaplains create a safe haven and have the right and duty to keep silent about what people tell them. (Buddhist) chaplains should never reject clients and feel the obligation to use everything in their power to help.

Second, and relating to this power to help, the Buddhist chaplain is described as bodhisattva. In Mahayana tradition the bodhisattva is a being that compassionately refrains from entering Nirvana in order to help and liberate others, and will continue doing so until all living beings are saved. It is often used as a metaphor for Buddhist chaplaincy by American authors, especially if they are Zen- or Tibetan Buddhism-inspired (Fronsdal 2012; Meyeonghbeop 2016; Elliot 2012).

The third model focuses on the chaplain as a spiritual warrior. The term spiritual warrior is used in Tibetan Buddhism for the bodhisattva fighting greed, anger and delusion (Maguire 2017). This is a particularization of the bodhisattva ideal, just as Tibetan Vajrayana is also a part of Mahayana. Here the spiritual caregiver can take the role of a counterpart, e. g., against a harmful belief a client may have or, at a macro-level, against a non-beneficial system. Another possibility is to replace the metaphor of spiritual warrior by wounded warrior (Kittisaro and Thanissara 2014, 181–205).

Working with these three models, students should be aware of their personal preference while at the same time looking for what a particular client or system needs. For this mindfulness, wisdom, and compassion are necessary (Beroepsprofiel BZI).

Practices of Buddhist spiritual care

Buddhist chaplaincy is very much based on the idea of the 'client central and the tradition as supportive' (Sudholter 2018). This seems to imply a demand-driven rather than a supply-driven approach. In reality, in prison and healthcare, supply-driven group programs in meditation and mindfulness were initiated and soon became very popular. As mindful yoga is part of the MBSR courses and appears to be much appreciated by clients, it is worth mentioning that some Buddhist chaplains act as yoga instructors as well. Buddhist chaplains in the penitentiary system all have part-time jobs working in more than one prison. In addition to meditation and mindfulness group activities, individual pastoral care is provided (Sudholter 2018).

Implications for interfaith spiritual care

Buddhist chaplains in the Netherlands from the beginning have been working with clients from a variety of denominations. It is stated above that the first official client was a prisoner with a Muslim background and that a lot of clients come from secular mindfulness programs. Although the number of official Buddhists in the Netherlands is small, Buddhism is considered by many people as a secondary source of religious inspiration (Boeddhistische Unie Nederland 2018). Buddhism is often associated with relaxation, compassion and friendliness. Because of this, the Buddhist chaplain is popular also among non-Buddhists. In prisons, Buddhist chaplains are often asked by non-Buddhist clients for help with stress reduction. Meditation and mindfulness are considered by many as very helpful (Sudholter 2018). In healthcare settings, Buddhist chaplains all work as general chaplains without much problem. Their specific Buddhist knowledge is considered as an additional aspect they can use in their spiritual care practice. Apart from meditation and mindfulness, the arrow sutras from the pali canon (Sala Sutta, Sanyutta Nikaya 3.8 and Cula Malunkyovada Sutta, Majjhima Nikaya 63) are experienced to be very helpful in serving non-Buddhist clients. Translated in popular jargon these sutras state that "pain is unavoidable but suffering is optional" and that all questions about a "why" are a part of this unfruitful suffering. In some mindfulness courses this theory is already included.

In the education program at Vrije Universiteit Buddhist staff also work in an interfaith setting. Last year, an introductory lecture on Buddhist chaplaincy was given in the general spiritual care course. After the internship period, students from various denominations mentioned that 'the three tenets' explained in this course proved very helpful in approaching clients during their chaplaincy internship. Also, the seven qualities of the spiritual friend as a metaphor for what a chaplain can be, received a positive response from students from non-Buddhist traditions. A month after the lecture, a student mentioned that he had used the seven qualities in his inauguration speech as a Protestant minister. Topics as empathy fatigue and secondary trauma, part of the Buddhist program, were also found very interesting by other students. In the general master's program an introduction and seminar on Buddhist ethics is given to all chaplaincy students. Buddhist staff also take part in the supervision of all spiritual care students during their internship period.

An Islamic perspective

A brief history of Islamic spiritual care in the Netherlands

Islamic spiritual care in the Netherlands is primarily present in three domains: healthcare, penitentiary institutions, and the army. The history of Islamic spiritual care in penitentiary institutions is the oldest, with an officially embedded civil service history starting in 2008, preceded by a period of 10 years of voluntary and freelance work of Imams in prisons (Ajouaou 2014, 23–4). The history of Islamic spiritual care in the army starts in April 2009, when two Imams are officially appointed (Michalowski 2015, 46–7). The institutional embedding of Islamic spiritual care in these government organs was made possible by the establishment in 2004 of *Contactorgaan Moslims en Overheid* (CMO), an official representative of the Dutch Muslim communities towards the Dutch government (Boender 2014, 255, 264). To work as an Islamic spiritual caregiver at the Ministry of Justice or Defense an official recognition by CMO is needed. This recognition is granted on the basis of a couple of prerequisites, among which formal, like a relevant university diploma and the will to keep following education, but mostly religious prerequisites like proven religious knowledge, personal and public piety, and a proven history of decent behavior and integrity (CMO).

On Islamic spiritual care in healthcare institutions no concrete historical data are prevalent in academic studies, but it has a similar prehistory of freelance and voluntary work. It has a more institutionalized presence since 2001, when the Dutch professional organization for spiritual caregivers in healthcare (VGVZ) established an official branch for Muslim spiritual caregivers. This was the result of a VGVZ-committee on 'multicultural' spiritual care in the 1990s that explored the need for Hindu and Muslim spiritual caregivers in healthcare institutions (Karagül 1999; Van den Akker and Van Wersch 2003). In healthcare settings official recognition by CMO is not always necessary and depends on the particular demands of the institution.

On university level, the VU Master of Spiritual Care offers the only Islam-specific track in the Netherlands, thus being the main deliverer of Islamic spiritual caregivers to named institutions with recognition by CMO. Students of the Islam-track follow the general curriculum in an interfaith setting, consisting of two courses in the theory of Spiritual Care, a course in Hermeneutics, a course in Comparative Ethics, and Supervision. They thus are from the very beginning of the curriculum trained in interfaith skills. Besides these courses in an interfaith setting, they follow two courses specifically with the students of the Islam-track: *Theory of Islamic Spiritual Care* (TISC), and a master seminar in which they relate practical matters of their internship to the theory learned during the Master program.

A specific challenge for the field of Islamic spiritual care in the Netherlands, and perhaps also globally, is the relative lack of academic studies on the practice of the field and of a proper theorization of that practice. To date there is only one encompassing study in the Netherlands, that combines both a study of the practice of Islamic spiritual caregivers in Dutch penitentiary institutions as well as a theorization of the field of Islamic spiritual care in this regard (Ajouaou 2014). It thus still largely is a field that is developing itself through practice alone. This has ramifications for the way it is taught in the course *Theory of Islamic Spiritual Care* (TISC) in the VU master program: the literature prescribed is not firmly rooted in a separate Islamic discourse on spiritual care particular to the Dutch situation, comparable to existing handbooks that Christian chaplaincy traditions have managed to bring forth over the decades (Doolaard 2006; Ganzevoort and Visser 2007; Heitink 1998). The creation of such a handbook for the Islamic context therefore forms a priority for the field. The course literature currently is improvised from studies on international developments in the field, Islamic primary and secondary sources on belief, ethics and spirituality, and Dutch sources on Christian chaplaincy. In what follows, we describe the curriculum of the Islam trajectory within the master Spiritual Care at VU, and how it aims to cater for the particularities of the field. We discuss the content, role and practice of Islamic spiritual care and its implications for interfaith spiritual care based on the contents of this course.

Characteristics of Islamic spiritual care

Content of Islamic spiritual care

According to the so-called Hadith of Gabriel, a famous narration in which archangel Gabriel visits Muhammad and his Companions to teach them the core of their religion through a set of rhetorical questions to Muhammad, Islam consists of three domains: the ethical-practical domain of religious rituals, duties and prohibitions (*islām*), the domain of religious beliefs (*īmān*) and the domain of inner spiritual life (*iḥsān*) (al-Nawawī 2007 31–48). The content of Islamic spiritual care, one may argue, consists of all these three domains, and may also take its model for the 'therapeutical' relationship between caregiver and client from the pedagogical relationship between Gabriel and Muhammad in said narration. The course TISC in the VU Master, a 6ECTS-course consisting of 12 gatherings, is structured around these three domains. The three meetings in the course on the domain of religious duties and prohibitions (*islām*) focus on both Islamic rituals and ethical thought. The two meetings that deal with the domain of religious beliefs (*īmān*) focus on the question of theodicy in the work of Islamic spiritual care. The two meetings on inner spiritual life (*iḥsān*) in the course put the 'spiritual' into Spiritual Care, so to speak, and consists of an application of core themes of Islam's spiritual tradition in the practice of spiritual care. The application of this emic paradigm creates a sense of recognition among Muslim students in the curriculum. It avoids a reliance on purely etic academic concepts, and invites students to engage in the curriculum on their own terms and values, within a further thoroughly academic setting.

Roles of the Islamic spiritual caregiver

TISC starts with two meetings on the discussion of defining the field of Islamic spiritual care and legitimizing it from the perspective of Islamic tradition(s). Although traditional roles of Islamic leadership certainly contain elements of it, the term spiritual care in itself is alien to Islamic tradition. Students are challenged to find conceptual common ground with other terms and concepts of spiritual leadership in Islam, like the mosque-imam, the Mufti, the giver of guidance (*murshid*) or the inviter to religion (*da'ī*). Seminal in this discussion is understanding how the more complex institutional environment radically changes the role of the spiritual caregiver compared with the traditional mosque-imam. Following a scheme of Asim Hafiz (2015), students learn to reflect on how the practice of Islamic spiritual care is seated in four different associations of the spiritual caregiver: the vocational, the professional, the religious/communal associations, and the educative/reformative association (Hafiz 2015, 90). Because of this plurality of associations the role of normativity becomes different compared to the traditional mosque-imam, whose work is only defined by the religious/communal association. It changes from a more directive to a more hermeneutical, question-based approach. Also, the responsibilities towards non-Muslim institutions change the way religious norms may be expressed and practiced as a spiritual caregiver (Hafiz 2015; Ajouaou 2014).

In the context of rituals and ethics (*islām*), the educative/reformative association of the spiritual caregiver becomes prominent, which may be considered a novelty in Islamic tradition (Hafiz 2015, 91–2). Islamic spiritual caregivers are pioneers in many ways, and necessarily take upon them a role as educators and reformers, both within their profession, but also towards the religious communities in which they are rooted. They come across ethical dilemmas that a traditional Islamic leader would not be confronted with in the same manner, and have to contextualize Islamic rituals in new institutional contexts. This means that Islamic spiritual caregivers need to constantly and thoroughly educate themselves and others in Islamic practical ethics to be able to proactively deal with their specific cases, and that they need a good set of interfaith and interpersonal skills to be able to communicate their ethical advices to their non-Muslim institutional environment, and actively involve this environment in their ethical deliberation process. Finding the right balance between all these roles and factors is the main focus in the course. The interfaith courses on Hermeneutics and Comparative Ethics in the curriculum are a very good addition to this process of ethical deliberation in a predominantly non-Muslim environment.

Practices of Islamic spiritual care

The domain of religious duties and prohibitions (*islām*) is where arguably the practice of Islamic spiritual care becomes most visible. In our course extra attention goes to the institutional embedding of the spiritual caregiver, according to earlier mentioned scheme of Hafiz (2015). It partly focuses on rethinking the practice of rituals in Islamic spiritual care in its specific contexts (e.g., Friday prayer in prison, Islamic 'alternative' rituals in the context of mental healthcare), but most attention is drawn to the contextualization of Islamic ethics. Students learn to reflect on how assistance in ethical decision-making of their clients takes place in the complex relationship between the four different associations of the spiritual caregiver. In their task as ethical advisors, Islamic spiritual caregivers have to be sensitive not only towards the wishes of their clients, but also to the norms and values current in their religious community, to the ethical demands and professional code of their vocation as spiritual caregivers, and to the laws to which the professional institution is bound, as well as the practical implications of their ethical advice for this institution.

In the domain of religious beliefs (*īmān*) the focus is on the question of theodicy in the work of Islamic spiritual care. An important practice for the spiritual caregiver is to offer support to clients in their experiences of contingency, crisis or trauma. Such experiences may lead to a crisis in one (or more) of three assumptions of a theodicy-triangle: (1) the assumption that God is Almighty and that the world therefore is meaningful; (2) the assumption that God cares and the world is therefore benevolent; and (3) the assumption that the person him/herself is good and valuable and that inflicted evil is not a form of divine punishment (Ganzevoort and Visser 2007, 307–12; Janoff-Bulman 1992). Students become acquainted with Islamic models of theodicy and their applicability in the domain of spiritual care (Ghaly 2014; Jackson 2009). Through discussion of a couple of concrete cases in the context of healthcare, the army and prisons, students evaluate together what the guiding practice of the spiritual caregiver may be in a theodicy-related crisis of faith caused by trauma, which theodicy models have 'therapeutic' value and can offer a form of consolation, and whether the preservation of faith is a task of the caregiver.

Implications for interfaith spiritual care

One could argue that Islamic spiritual care is currently developing as a field strongly rooted in its own tradition aiming at clients of its own particular denomination, against the rising trend of interfaith spiritual care (Liefbroer and Berghuijs 2019). On a short term it seems unlikely that interfaith spiritual care will become more prominent in Islamic spiritual care: in the army and prison the primary aim remains the presence of an Imam to fulfill the religious rights of Muslims, and also in healthcare institutions tradition-specific care seems to remain highly relevant (Ajouaou 2014; Michalowski 2015). Despite a high level of intra-religious pluralism, which is a challenge in itself for the Islamic spiritual caregiver, there is thus far no clear sign of an increase of secularization or multiple religious belonging among the Muslim population of the Netherlands (Huijnk 2018). Interfaith spiritual care and the corresponding set of skills needed is however still very urgent because of the interfaith setting in which the Islamic spiritual care activities are undeniably taking place: the plurality of associations of the Islamic spiritual caregiver necessitates that he/she can work in an interfaith context, even if mainly working with Muslim clients. One could thus argue that this complex set of associations makes the work of an Islamic spiritual caregiver interfaith by definition: even if the client base still primarily consists of Muslims, one operates in an environment with many (non-)religious and spiritual orientations and constantly has to be sensitive about this and navigate one's own values and presuppositions through the challenges of such an environment.

The applicability of Islamic spiritual care in an interfaith setting further seems to have two main challenges: the challenge to make spiritually inclined Islamic traditions suitable for caregiving to non-Muslims, and intra-religious controversy about the Islamic validity of these traditions among Muslims. Concerning the first challenge, one can state that the domain of religious rituals, duties and prohibitions (*islām*) is less suitable as reservoirs for interfaith spiritual care practices compared to other denominational forms of spiritual care. The domain of religious beliefs (*īmān*) may have something to offer to non-Muslims through certain aspects of the theodicy question. Given the universality of the questions related to theodicy and the concept of 'shattered assumptions', one may argue that this is a typical topic that could also be tackled in the interfaith curriculum of the master, and a topic in which the Islamic spiritual caregiver can also be of high relevance to non-Muslim clients. In conversational practice related to these themes, the Islamic spiritual caregiver may offer comfort and solace to a non-Muslim client by operationalizing Islamic perspectives on theodicy that can be universalized.

The domain of inner spiritual life (*iḥsān*) has the most potential in this regard, and may very well be 'universalized' without losing its rootedness in the Islamic tradition. This needs further exploration, both in academia and in practice. Islam's discursive tradition has a very rich body of wisdom literature, analyzing humanity's inner spiritual life and offering suggestions for 'the purification of the soul' (*tazkiyyat al-nafs*) with a centuries-long praxis, mostly associated with the Sufi tradition. The language of this literature is clearly embedded in Islamic tradition and practice, but also universal in its appeal: the writings of Rumi for example are a best seller in the USA, and also the works of Farid al-Din Attar have found their way to a much larger non-Muslim audience. For Islamic spiritual caregivers working in an interfaith setting, this would be a very suitable repertoire to make a significant part of Islam's discursive tradition relevant for non-Muslims as well.

From the 19th century onwards however, this spiritual tradition has become increasingly problematized within Islamic tradition, due to the rise of Islamic reformist movements with anti-mystical inclinations (Jackson 2012, 12–27). A major challenge for theorists of Islamic spiritual care is to 'translate' this rich discursive tradition into a common language that is acceptable for a large segment of Muslims, Sufi and non-Sufi, in the first place: secondly, to make the relevant aspects of Sufism for spiritual care acceptable for a non-Muslim audience as well. Research on to which extent this is already happening in the practice of Islamic spiritual care is an important priority for the field.

Within the context of our education program, the final three meetings of the course TISC are a first step in that endeavor of 'translating' Islam's controversial mystical tradition to a larger audience. The last part of the seminal work of Ganzevoort and Visser (2007) consists of chapters that deal with some basic emotions and spiritually transitional experiences relevant to chaplaincy work, substantiated with Christian theological perspectives. Students are challenged to analyze these Christian theological perspectives for compatibility with Islamic teachings, and to present their own vision on these overarching themes from their perspective as Islamic spiritual caregivers. They thus present their vision on topics such as anger and violence, anxiety and desire, guilt and shame, loss, trauma and sadness, substantiated with their personal explorations of Islamic theology and its spiritual tradition. Through this approach they help create an independent Islamic discourse on these matters, meanwhile also becoming familiar with Christian perspectives on these grand life themes which significantly contributes to their interfaith skills. Given the universality of these experiences of contingency and related emotions, this may very well be operationalized in an interfaith setting. This approach offers our students a conceptual common ground when offering care to non-Muslims from different persuasions in their future profession as Islamic spiritual caregivers.

A Hindu perspective

A brief history of Hindu spiritual care in the Netherlands

Hindu spiritual care in the Netherlands has first developed within hospitals and penitentiary institutions and later also within the context of defense.[5] It started when Christian chaplains felt that they were unable to provide spiritual care to Hindu clients as they did for Christian clients, because they lacked knowledge of the Hindu tradition and had no religious authority. So, Hindu priests (pandits) were attracted from their own network or well-known Hindu organizations and were asked to provide spiritual care to these Hindus. These pandits were trained

5 This article is based on an earlier publication by Bikram Lalbahadoersing in *Tijdschrift Geestelijke Verzorging* (2015, issue 78), titled 'Een filosofisch kader voor hindoe geestelijke verzorging' ['A philosophical framework for Hindu spiritual caregiving'].

in the work of mental care in hospitals or in penitentiary institutions and appointed on a freelance basis. Since this type of spiritual care provision happened on an individual basis and there was no consultation between the different priests (who were working in different hospitals and prisons), every Hindu priest applied his/her own approach (Van Dijk 1998, 40 – 52; Lalbahadoersing 2015, 14; Rambaran 2015, 10).

In practice, this meant that the pandit, traditionally trained to conduct the rituals on occasions like marriage, birth of a child, or death of a person, was able to continue his religious work in the institutions in an adapted way. The adjustments mainly concerned that there was no open fire available in the penitentiary institutions or hospitals for sacrifice rituals and the various ingredients for sacrifices were often not available. Furthermore, since pandits started following spiritual care courses on conversation techniques and counseling, the provision of Hindu pastoral counseling was initiated. After the recognition of the Hindu Council of the Netherlands (HRN) as a sending agency for Hindu spiritual caregivers in penitentiary institutions in June 2009 (Bernts, Van der Velde, and Kregting 2012b, 5), the Hindu Council of the Netherlands began a more structured process of professionalizing Hindu spiritual care.

The start of Hindu spiritual care in defense has a clearer mark. In 2004, the Hindu Council of the Netherlands was recognized by the Ministry of Defense as a sending institution (Rambaran 2015, 10). One of the most prominent activities of Hindu spiritual care in defense is yoga (Snel 2018; Keultjes 2018; Bijl 2019). This started as early as 2004 when a first yoga workshop was organized by the Hindu Spiritual Care Department. There was a lot of interest and many workshops were offered in the following period. Due to the high demand for yoga, several yoga teachers were trained in 2016 and there is a network of defense personnel who practice and teach yoga.

In the meantime, there have hardly been any scientific studies or publications on Hindu spiritual care in the Netherlands, which in part explains the variety of individual approaches in this new field. Since May 2019, a professor for Hindu studies has been appointed at the Vrije Universiteit Amsterdam, which will stimulate academic reflection on the theory and practice of Hindu spiritual care.

Characteristic of Hindu spiritual care

Content of Hindu spiritual care

In 2010 a Head of Hindu chaplaincy was appointed at the Ministry of Justice. One of his tasks was to develop a method that Hindu chaplains should use in their work with prisoners. As a first step, the team of Hindu spiritual caregivers in the prisons took the initiative to formulate several principles for their own field of work, so that there was a framework from which Hindu spiritual caregivers could provide spiritual care (Lalbahadoersing 2015, 16). For this exercise, they first looked at the common cultural elements that the Hindu community in Suriname—from which most Hindus originate in the Netherlands—had embraced, such as the Hindi language, public celebrations of religious festivals, solidarity with their own temples and marrying within one's own community.

However, there were also differences between the Surinamese tradition and the contemporary Dutch context. A great deal of knowledge about Hinduism became available in the Dutch or English language, as a result of which highly educated laymen were given access to information that was previously only accessible to those familiar with the Hindi and Sanskrit languages. Consequently, there was an increase of interest among laymen in the fundamental philosophical concepts of the Hindu tradition. Hindu chaplains therefore soon realized that the development of Hindu spiritual care required a framework containing the four philosophical concepts that form the basis of Hindu life: way of life, growth of consciousness, solidarity, and karma (Rambaran 2015, 106).

The first principle for Hindu spiritual care is that the spiritual caregiver pays specific attention to the entire way of life of the client or conversation partner (Rambaran 2015, 106). Hinduism as a religion has various forms, as there are Hindus who believe in a personal God, while there are also Hindus who hold an impersonal image of God. Since Hinduism has no central authority, Hindus have traditionally had much freedom to make personal choices, and there is a lot of diversity amongst Hindus. This is also translated in the rules of life Hindus follow. For example, it may be that one Hindu only wants to eat vegetarian food one day a week, while another wants a vegetarian diet every day, or only during religious festivals. This diversity does not mean that people do not commit to these rules: it puts heavy pressure on a Hindu's conscience if he/she is unable to comply with the 'self-chosen religious rules'. That is why Hinduism is called a "way of live".

Secondly, the Hindu spiritual caregiver strives—through a variety of religious and spiritual practices—to increase the awareness of the individual (Rambaran 2015, 107). By broadening one's consciousness, people may experience a deeper connection to fellow human beings, feel more inspired by the environment, and become better in self-reflection. Increasing moral awareness, attention to norms and values, and the development of responsibility for one's own actions starts with attention to the quality of consciousness. Another characteristic of an expanded consciousness is that one can experience reality on a different level, namely on the level of spiritual experiences. The Vedas, source scriptures from the Hindu tradition, speak of "Ekam sad vipra bahudha vadanti", which means that there is one ultimate spiritual Truth about which "rishis" (seers) speak in different terms. This principle enables Hindus to open themselves to other traditions and philosophies of life.

A third characteristic of Hindu spiritual care is that it strives to strengthen the client's connection with his/her environment on three different levels (Rambaran 2015, 108). Hindu texts set out a holistic approach to people and society. At the micro level, the individual tries to attain higher forms of consciousness, enabling him/her to get to know his deeper being, the Atman. At the meso level, the individual develops within a social context, where he/she learns to give space to the needs and concerns of the community in addition to the pursuit of personal happiness. At the macro level, the aim is to bring the relationship of the individual human (micro level) within a social context (meso level) into relation with the cosmos and the Supreme; the development of people and society must be in harmony with the natural environment.

Fourthly, the principle of karma plays an important role within Hindu spiritual care (Rambaran 2015, 132). In the Hindu tradition, it is assumed that there is no randomness in the universe, and the principle of karma implies that there is a causal relationship between the actions someone performs and the consequences these actions have. When the actions and consequences are closely linked, karma is often testable with everyday practice (e.g., working on a job and getting paid; refusing to complete a job and getting fired). However, sometimes the causes of consequences cannot be traced so easily by our consciousness. Hindus can then rely on testimonies from the great teachers or mystics of tradition, such as seers and saints, as it is said that they can interpret such remote links because of their expanded awareness. Although it is not up to the spiritual caregiver to explain what has caused something to happen, he/she can assist a client on his/her journey to the growth of consciousness and the ultimate realization of the eternal soul.

Roles of the Hindu spiritual caregiver

The start of Hindu spiritual care in the Netherlands meant a double translation of an age-old tradition into a modern context. Firstly, Hinduism is an ancient belief tradition that has evolved on the Indian subcontinent. Because of this, historical characteristics of Indian society are closely intertwined with the structures and customs in Hinduism. Typical is the large family system, in which grandparents, together with the children and grandchildren, form a large household. They cook together, salaries go into a joint pot and the religious rituals are also performed within the family collective. Another characteristic of the Hindu tradition is the guru. When people want to develop spiritually, they look for a guru to teach them how to do so. In the past, a student of a guru went to live with the guru and formed a temporary family with the guru and other fellow students. The religious expert or academic scholar in the tradition is the third type of spiritual counselor, who focuses on transferring information. These three separated roles—that of the wise elder, the guru, and the expert—are the three traditional forms of spiritual guidance (Lalbahadoersing 2015, 15).

The second translation of the age-old tradition into a modern context concerns the translation of Hindu-Suriname aspects of the Hindu tradition to the Dutch context. The Hindu tradition as practiced by most of the Hindus in the Netherlands does not directly originate from India, but from Suriname (South America). In 1863, slavery was abolished in the Kingdom of the Netherlands. However, to continue the labor on the sugar cane plantations, people from (amongst others) India were brought to Suriname. By the time Suriname became independent (1975), about half of the Hindu population moved to the Netherlands (Choenni 2003, 56). In the hundred years in which the Hindu community lived in Suriname, the appearance and experience of the Hindu religion underwent a radical change into a more homogeneous Hindu community (Bakker 1999, 263). This contrasts with the enormous diversity that is found in the mother country of India. Furthermore, there was great emphasis on rituals, and the magical practices surrounding healing and incantations were given a more prominent place in the cultural experience. Some attribute this to the village religion that the workers had brought with them (Choenni 2003, 106; Rambaran 2015, 16). A final relevant change concerned life as a large minority in a multi-religious and multi-racial society. This has had a strong conservative influence on the identity experience of Hindus. The Hindu language, the public celebrations of heyday, the solidarity with one's own temples and marrying within one's own community, therefore became the collective core values for the community (Choenni 2003, 106).

A new type of authority bearer arose in this new situation, namely that of the Hindu priest or pandit (Bakker 2005, 19–20; Schouten 2005, 37–38; Van Dijk 1998, 33–34). Due to a lack of qualified people (hardly any clergy were imported to Suriname), the different religious needs of believers were all addressed by one and the same person. This made the pandit fulfill the roles of the guru, the scholar, and the wise elder as well as the ritualist, the magician and the cultural foreman. The Christian example of the pastor and priest may also have contributed to the contraction of the functions to a person. Meanwhile, the fulfillment and performance of this new function had a strong ritualistic approach, because most pandits at that time mainly had knowledge on performance of rituals. This meant that spiritual practices as well as knowledge of Hindu scriptures became strongly ritualized, which until now remains the common practice of Hindu priests, as their services are mostly required at rites de passage and other special moments. However, for Hindu spiritual caregivers this ritualistic approach poses a challenge, since many rituals consist of fire offerings that are usually not permitted in the official buildings in which Hindu chaplains work (e.g., in hospitals, prisons and military buildings). Therefore, Hindu spiritual caregivers started looking for alternative concepts in their own tradition by going back to the core of the different religious functions in order to form a new conceptual frame for the role of Hindu chaplain (Lalbahadoersing 2015, 16).

Practices of Hindu spiritual care

Hindu spiritual caregivers, working in the prison system, have been working for several years with the above-mentioned philosophical framework of four basic principles, giving meaning to activities such as meditation, mantra recitation, religious celebrations and yoga. Prisoners often say that they feel different after a yoga class; they are more relaxed and better able to sleep. "My mind refreshes after I have done yoga," one prisoner commented (Rambaran 2015, 193). Another prisoner said that after a long period of yoga he was able to sleep tight again. Another prisoner, who had practiced yoga for the first time, called his wife to tell her that he had experienced something special and that he wanted to share it with friends and family. He also encouraged his wife to practice yoga (Rambaran 2015, 195).

Ultimately, the aim is for the Hindu prisoner to adopt a way of life that triggers a growth of consciousness, because of which he/she can experience a closer connection to others and become more aware of the consequences of his/her actions. This objective is for instance reflected in the concrete activity of restoring family relationships—relationships that are important to Hindus because religion is primarily practiced in the family, and because religious values and norms are transmitted and confirmed in the same family context (Jaggan 2016).

In addition to these practices, Hindu spiritual caregivers also provide individual pastoral counseling, for instance in healthcare settings in accordance with the practices of the other chaplains, like Christian and Humanist. In doing so, patients' expectation of the spiritual caregiver in a healthcare institution sometimes come very close to that of the traditional healer, who, with the help of prayer, assists those in need (Lalbahadoersing 2015, 16). If the patient feels the need to perform a ritual, the Hindu chaplain can provide a (simple) ritual. For extensive rituals, the patient is expected to call in his own family priest and do the rituals at home.

Implications for interfaith spiritual care

In the characteristics of Hindu chaplaincy as described above, spiritual care provision is commonly assumed to take place in interaction between a Hindu spiritual caregiver and a Hindu client. However, for instance in healthcare settings, Hindu spiritual caregivers often feel the need to adhere to the format of working in a territorial manner—for all clients regardless of one's religious or spiritual orientation, in accordance with the format that is commonly used by Protestant, Catholic and Humanist chaplains. For a Hindu spiritual caregiver such interfaith spiritual care seems possible, as Hindu spiritual caregivers can provide spiritual help to anyone who asks for it. However, it should be a conscious choice by the client asking for this, and he or she should be open for Hindu spiritual care. When this is the case, the spiritual caregiver can offer any kind of spiritual care.

One of the consequences of the territorial working manner is that a 'light version' of the tradition has developed for the 'average Westerner', or non-Hindu client, and another practice has developed for Hindu believers. For example, non-Hindu clients mainly expect pastoral conversation, yoga and meditation from Hindu spiritual caregivers. The Hindu believers, on the other hand, seek more religious substantive guidance in which simple rituals play a role. In the latter case, a worldview with a clear place for the divine aspects of the Hindu tradition is presupposed, and needs to be present and shared with both the spiritual caregiver and the client.

Discussion

In the previous sections, we have described how Buddhist, Muslim, and Hindu spiritual care takes shape in the multifaith and multicultural context of the Netherlands. As each of these 'new' spiritual care denominations are rooted in a non-Western context, the descriptions show how each denomination is challenged to 'translate' and recontextualize their faith-specific characteristics to the spiritual care setting of the Netherlands. We will compare the three perspectives in order to identify their similarities and differences, and discuss the implications for practicing spiritual care in an interfaith context.

Spiritual care from Buddhist, Muslim, and Hindu denominations seem to have developed in a similar vein. For all three denominations, official recognition and employment as Buddhist, Islamic, or Hindu spiritual caregiver was preceded by a period of ad-hoc, voluntary or freelance work, especially within penitentiary institutions and (sometimes) in healthcare settings. Subsequently, for each denomination an official representative council or organization was established that could authorize/ordain spiritual caregivers as representatives of that tradition. Such authorization required spiritual caregivers—in addition to other requirements—to complete a relevant bachelor's or master's degree, such as one of the faith-specific trajectories that were accordingly provided at Vrije Universiteit Amsterdam. Currently, spiritual caregivers authorized by Buddhist, Muslim, and Hindu denominations are (being) employed in penitentiary institutions, healthcare settings, and the army.

The specific characteristics of each denomination, however, seem to contain both similarities and differences. The faith-specific content differs between the traditions, with Buddhists focusing on concepts such as 'not-knowing', 'bearing witness', and 'doing the actions that arise from not-knowing' (Glassman 1998), Muslims focusing on three domains of religious rituals, duties and prohibitions (*islām*), religious beliefs (*īmān*) and the inner spiritual life (*iḥsān*) (al-Nawawī 2007, 31–48), and Hindus emphasizing the concepts of 'way of life', 'growth of consciousness', solidarity, and karma in their spiritual care practice (Rambaran 2015).

Meanwhile, when focusing on the specific roles and practices of spiritual caregivers from these three traditions, we do see several parallels. In line with the roles identified among Christian spiritual caregivers as 'companion', 'counselor', and 'spiritual guide' (Ganzevoort and Visser 2007; Liefbroer, Ganzevoort, and Olsman 2019), from a Buddhist perspective the spiritual caregiver may represent the roles of the 'spiritual friend' (kalyana mitta), the 'helper' (bodhisattva), and the 'spiritual warrior'. Similarly, from an Islamic perspective the spiritual caregiver is associated with his/her vocational, professional, religious/communal role, and from a Hindu perspective the spiritual caregiver may function in the roles of the wise elder, the expert/scholar, and (as confessional caregiver) in the role of the guru, the ritualist, the magician and the cultural foreman. From a Muslim perspective the role of the spiritual caregiver as educator/reformer is added to these, and is seen in relation to the context in which spiritual caregivers work as well as in relation to their religious community.

The practices also show some parallels, as from all three perspectives the ritual dimension of spiritual care practices is emphasized. From a Buddhist and Hindu perspective this is mostly seen in relation to (group) practices such as meditation and yoga, mindfulness (Buddhism), mantra recitation and religious celebrations (Hinduism). From an Islamic perspective ritual practices such as Friday prayers form an important part of the spiritual care practice. Furthermore, for all three perspectives individual spiritual care or counseling is part of spiritual care provision. In contrast to the Buddhist and Hindu perspectives, the practice of ethical decision-making is mentioned from an Islamic perspective.

Finally, there are differences in terms of interfaith practices for each of the perspectives. From a Buddhist perspective it is emphasized that Buddhist chaplaincy originated in an interfaith setting, and that various practices (e.g., meditation, mindfulness, arrow sutras) can be helpful in spiritual care provision to non-Buddhist clients. By contrast, from an Islamic and Hindu perspective the character of providing spiritual care to adherents of the same faith tradition is primarily focused on, although from these perspectives also possibilities for interfaith spiritual care provision are noted. From an Islamic perspective, the domain of religious rituals, duties and prohibitions (*islām*) seems difficult to apply to spiritual care encounters with non-Muslim clients, but the domains of religious beliefs (*īmān*) and of inner spiritual life (*iḥsān*) may prove fruitful for spiritual care provision to non-Muslims. For Hinduism, a difference is made between a ‘light version’ of Hindu spiritual caregiving for non-Hindu clients (e.g., providing yoga, meditation, pastoral counseling), and another practice for Hindu clients containing tradition-specific content and rituals.

Conclusion

In this chapter we have considered the implications of the multicultural and multifaith society of the Netherlands for the way in which spiritual care takes shape, with a focus on Buddhist, Islamic, and Hindu perspectives. These relatively new denominations in the field of spiritual care have followed similar trajectories in gaining recognition as formal representatives of those traditions in addition to their Christian, Humanist and unaffiliated colleagues. Although the faith-specific content of each tradition differs, the roles and practices of spiritual care provision show several parallels in the way in which spiritual care from each of these traditions is performed. From a Buddhist perspective providing interfaith spiritual care seemed to have been common practice from its origin, whereas from an Islamic and Hindu perspective spiritual caregiving to adherents of the same faith tradition is primarily focused on, although from these perspectives also possibilities for interfaith spiritual care provision are identified. Considering these various perspectives is one of the steps needed for deepening our understanding of the implications of religious and spiritual diversity for the way in which spiritual care takes shape in the Netherlands.

References

Ajouaou, Mohamed. 2014. *Imam behind bars: A case study of Islamic spiritual care in Dutch prisons towards the development of a professional profile.* USA: CreateSpace Independent Publishing Platform.

Ajouaou, Mohamed, and Ton Bernts. 2015. "The effects of religious diversity on spiritual care: Reflections from the Dutch correction facilities." In: Irene Becci, and Olivier Roy (eds.) *Religious diversity in European prisons: Challenges and implications for rehabilitation.* Cham: Springer. 31–45.

al-Nawawī, Yahya. 2007. *Das Buch Der vierzig Hadithe Kitāb al-Arbaʿīn mit dem Kommentar von Ibn Daqīq al-ʿĪd.* Translated by Marco Schöller. Frankfurt: Verlag der Weltreligionen.

Analayo. 2004. *Satipatthana, the direct path to realization.* Cambridge: Windhorse Publications.

Author unknown. Year unknown. *Beroepsprofiel boeddhistisch chaplain [Professional profile Buddhist chaplain].* Unpublished document, via personal correspondence.

Baart, Andries J. 2002. *The presence approach: An introductory sketch of a practice.* Utrecht: Actioma / Catholic Theological University in Utrecht.

Bakker, Freek L. 1999. *Hindoes in een creoolse wereld [Hindoes in a creole world].* Zoetermeer: Boekencentrum B.V.

Bakker, Freek L. 2005. "De pandit en de dominee." [The pandit and the priest.] In: Reender Kranenborg (ed.) *Voorgangers in Nederland. Onderzoek naar de positie van de pandit, de imam, de predikant, de rabbijn en de charismatisch leider in de religies van Nederland [Ministers in the Netherlands. A study investigating the position of the pandit, imam, priest, rabbi, and the charismatic leader in religions in the Netherlands].* Zoetermeer: Meinema.

Bein, Andrew. 2008. *The zen of helping, spiritual principles for a mindful and openhearted practice.* Hoboken, NJ: John Wiley and Sons.

Berghuijs, Joantine. 2017. "Multiple religious belonging in the Netherlands: An empirical approach to hybrid religiosity." *Open Theology* 3/1: 19–37. DOI: 10.1515/opth-2017–0003

Bernts, Ton, R. Ruard Ganzevoort, Carlo Leget, and Joanne Wojtkowiak. 2014. *Omvang en verdeling van de geestelijke verzorging in de krijgsmacht vanaf 2016 [Size and distribution of spiritual care in the armed forces from 2016].* Nijmegen: Radboud Universiteit, Universiteit voor Humanistiek en Vrije Universiteit.

Bernts, Ton, Paul van der Velde, and Joris Kregting. 2012a. *Evaluatie Boeddhistische Unie Nederland. Rapport nr. 626 [Evaluation Dutch Buddhist Union. Rapport nr. 626].* https://www.ru.nl/kaski/@839066/pagina/ (accessed May 15, 2019).

Bernts, Ton, Paul van der Velde, and Joris Kregting. 2012b. *Evaluatie Hindoe Raad Nederland. Rapport nr. 623 [Evaluation Dutch Hindu Council. Rapport nr. 623].* https://www.ru.nl/kaski/@839066/pagina/ (accessed May 15, 2019).

Bijl, Natasja. 2019. *Werken bij defensie én yogales geven? Hoe combineer je dat? [Employed at the military and teaching yoga? How do you combine this?].* https://yoga-international.nu/reportage/preview-werken-bij-defensie-en-yogales-geven (accessed May 15, 2019).

Block, Jennifer. 2013. *Towards a definition of Buddhist Chaplaincy.* http://www.sati.org/wp-content/uploads/2013/05/Buddhist-Chaplaincy-definition-Jennifer-Block.pdf (accessed May 15, 2019).

Bobrow, Joseph. 2015. *Waking up from war: A better way home for veterans and nations*, Durham, NC: Pitchstone Publishing.

Boeddhistische Unie Nederland. 2018. *Inventarisatie [Inventarisation].* https://boeddhisme.nl/wat-is-boeddhisme/inventarisatie/ (accessed May 15, 2019).

Boender, Welmoet. 2014. "Polderen in de 'participatiesamenleving': De kantelende positie van het Contactorgaan Moslims en Overheid." [A society of 'participation': The changing position of the organization CMO (Contact organization Muslims and Government)]. In: Peter van Dam, James Kennedy, and Friso Wielinga (eds.) *Achter de zuilen: Op zoek naar religie in naoorlogs Nederland [Behind the pillars: Looking for religion in post-war Netherlands].* Amsterdam: Amsterdam University Press. 255–77.

CBS. 2015. *Religieuze betrokkenheid van bevolkingsgroepen, 2010–2014 [Religious affiliation of the population, 2010–2014].* Centraal Bureau voor de Statistiek: Den Haag.

CBS. 2017. *Religieuze betrokkenheid [Religious affiliation].* https://statline.cbs.nl/Statweb/publication/?DM=SLNL&PA=82904ned&D1=0-7&D2=0&D3=a&VW=T (accessed April 24, 2019).

Choenni, Chan E. S. 2003. *Hindostanen, van Brits-Indische emigranten via Suriname tot burgers van Nederland* [Hindostanis, from British Indian emigrants through Suriname to Dutch citizens]. Zoetermeer: Sampreshan.

CMO. Year unknown. *Richtlijnen en zendingsvoorwaarden islamitische zendingsorganisatie Contactorgaan Moslims en Overheid [Guidelines and conditions for authorization by Islamic organization CMO (Contact organization Muslims and Government)].* Unpublished document, requested from CMO.

Doolaard, Jaap. 2006. *Nieuw handboek geestelijke verzorging [New handbook of spirtiual caregiving].* Kampen: Kok.

Elliot, Fay Octavia. 2012. *Bodhisattva Chaplain.* https://shambhalatimes.org/2012/06/08/bodhisattva-chaplain/ (accessed May 15, 2019).

Fronsdal, Gil. Year unknown. *Rituals in Buddhism.* https://www.insightmeditationcenter.org/books-articles/articles/rituals-in-buddhism/_(accessed May 15, 2019).

Fronsdal, Gil. 2012. *Compassion and the bodhisattva vows.* http://buddhistchaplains.org/cmsms/index.php?page=compassion-and-the-bodhisattva-vows_(accessed May 15, 2019).

Ganzevoort, R. Ruard., Mohamed Ajouaou, André Van der Braak, Erik de Jongh, and Lourens Minnema. 2014. "Teaching spiritual care in an interfaith context." *Journal for the Academic Study of Religion,* 27/2: 178–197. DOI: 10.1558/jasr.v27i2.178

Ganzevoort, R. Ruard., and Jan Visser. 2007. *Zorg voor het verhaal: Achtergrond, methode en inhoud van pastorale begeleiding [To care for the story: Background, method and content of pastoral counseling].* Zoetermeer: Meinema.

Ghaly, Mohammed. 2014. "Muslim theologians on evil: God's omnipotence or justice, God's omnipotence and justice." In: Mouhanad Khourchide, Milad Karimi, and Klaus Von Stosch (eds.) *Theologie der Barmherzigkeit? Zeitgemässe Fragen und Antworten des Kalam.* Münster: Waxmann Verlag. 129–54.

Glassman, Bernie. 1998. *Bearing witness: A Zen master's lessons in making peace.* New York, NY: Bell Tower.

Hafiz, Asim. 2015. "Muslim chaplaincy in the UK: The chaplaincy approach as a way to a modern imamate." *Religion, State & Society* 43/1: 85–99.

Halifax, Joan. 2008. *Being with dying.* Boston, MA: Shambala Publications.

Heitink, Gerben. 1998. *Pastorale zorg: theologie, differentiatie, praktijk [Pastoral care: Theology, differentiation, practice].* Kampen: Kok.

Hoek, Joop. 2012. "Boeddha in de bajes, deel 2. Eric Soyeux: Wij hebben gestudeerd en hij is zo maar geestelijk verzorger geworden." [Buddha in the prison, part 2. Eric Soyeux: We have studied and he only became spiritual caregiver]. *Boeddhistisch dagblad.* https://boeddhistischdagblad.nl/achtergronden/1195-eric-soyeux-wij-hebben-gestudeerd-en-hij-is-zomaar-geestelijk-verzorger/ (accessed May 15, 2019).

Hogendoorn, Rob. 2015. *Bestaat hulpverlening aan gedetineerde boeddhisten pas sinds 2004? [Does caregiving to Buddhist prisoners only exist from 2004?].* https://openboeddhisme.nl/nl/factcheck/bestaat-hulpverlening-aan-gedetineerde-boeddhisten-pas-sinds-2004/ (accessed May 15, 2019).

Huijnk, Willem. 2018. *De religieuze beleving van moslims in Nederland: Diversiteit en verandering in beeld [The religious experience of Muslims in the Netherlands: Picturing diversity and change].* Den Haag: SCP.

Jackson, Sherman. 2009. *Islam and the problem of black suffering.* Oxford: Oxford University Press.

Jackson, Sherman. 2012. *Sufism for non-Sufis? Ibn ʿAṭāʾ Allāh al-Sakandarī's Tāj al-ʿArūs.* Oxford: Oxford University Press.

Jaggan, Soerish. 2016. *Verboden contact [Contact forbidding].* Master thesis VU Amsterdam. http://www.ubvu.vu.nl/pub/fulltext/scripties/10_2525581_0.pdf (accessed May 15, 2019).

Janoff-Bulman, Ronnie. 1992. *Shattered assumptions: Towards a new psychology of trauma.* New York, NY: Free Press.

Karagül, Arslan. 1999. *Geestelijke verzorging in de gezondheidssector in multi-cultureel perspectief. Verslag van het project 'Multi-culturele geestelijke verzorging in zorginstellingen' [Spiritual care in healthcare in multicultural perspective. Report of the project 'Multicultural spiritual care in healthcare'].* Utrecht: Utrechts Medisch Centrum.

Keultjes, Hanneke. 2018. "Al 90 yogadocenten actief bij Defensie." [Already 90 yoga teachers at the military]. *Algemeen Dagblad.* https://www.ad.nl/binnenland/al-90-yogadocenten-actief-bij-defensie~ab5355a4/ (accessed May 15, 2019).

Kittisaro and Thanissara. 2014. *Listening to the heart, a contemplative journey to engaged Buddhism.* Berkeley: North Atlantic Books.

Lalbahadoersing, Bikram. 2015. "Een filosofisch kader voor hindoe geestelijke verzorging." [A philosophical framework for Hindu spiritual care]. *Tijdschrift Geestelijke Verzorging* 18/78: 14–18.

Liefbroer, Anke. I., and Joantine Berghuijs. 2019. "Spiritual care for everyone? An analysis of personal and organizational differences in perceptions of religious diversity among spiritual caregivers." *Journal of Health Care Chaplaincy* 25/3: 110–129. DOI: 10.1080/08854726.2018.1556549

Liefbroer, Anke. I., R. Ruard Ganzevoort, and Erik Olsman. 2019. "Addressing the spiritual domain in a plural society: What is the best mode of integrating spiritual care into healthcare?" *Mental Health, Religion & Culture* 22/3: 244–260. DOI: 10.1080/13674676.2019.1590806

Maguire, Jessica. 2017. *Spiritual warrior.* http://cominghometoyourbodyretreats.com/home/2017/9/22/becoming-a-spiritual-warrior (accessed May 15, 2019).

McMahan, David L. 2008. *The making of Buddhist modernism.* Oxford: Oxford University Press.

Meyeonghbeop. 2016. *Chaplaincy on the Bodhisattva path.* https://bulletin.hds.harvard.edu/articles/winterspring2016/chaplaincy-bodhisattva-path (accessed May 15, 2019).

Michalowski, Ines. 2015. "What is at stake when Muslims join the ranks? An international comparison of military chaplaincy." *Religion, State and Society* 43/1: 41–58. DOI: 10.1080/09637494.2015.1021189

Monnet, Michael. 2005. "Developing a Buddhist approach to pastoral care: A peacemaker's view." *Journal of Pastoral Care and Counseling* 59/1–2: 57–61. DOI: 10.1177/154230500505900106

Nakao, Egyoku. 2017. *The three tenets.* https://zenpeacemakers.org/the-three-tenets/ (accessed May 15, 2019).

Pew Research Center. 2009. *Many Americans mix multiple faiths.* http://www.pewforum.org/2009/12/09/many-americans-mix-multiple-faiths/ (accessed May 15, 2019).

Rambaran, Haridat, Bikram Lalbahadoersing, Attry Ramdhani, and Sieta Motiram Sharma. 2015. *Handboek geestelijke zorgverlening aan Hindoes [Handbook for spiritual caregiving to Hindus].* Almere: Parthenon.

Schouten, Jan Peter. 2005. "De pandit als behoeder van de traditie." [The pandit as the tradition's guardian]. In: Reender Kranenborg (ed.) *Voorgangers in Nederland. Onderzoek naar de positie van de pandit, de imam, de predikant, de rabbijn en de charismatisch leider in de religies van Nederland [Ministers in the Netherlands. A study investigating the position of the pandit, imam, priest, rabbi, and the charismatic leader in religions in the Netherlands].* Zoetermeer: Meinema. 37–52.

Snel, Charlotte. 2018. "Yoga bij Defensie bezig aan opmars." [Yoga at the military is emerging]. *Defensiekrant* 17/5. https://magazines.defensie.nl/defensiekrant/2018/17/05_yoga_17 (accessed May 15, 2019).

Sudholter, Judith. 2018. *Dit doet een boeddhistisch geestelijk verzorger [Practices of a Buddhist spiritual caregiver].* https://bodhitv.nl/2018/10/03/dit-doet-een-boeddhistisch-geestelijk-verzorger/ (accessed May 15, 2019).

Swift, Chris. 2013. "A state health service and funded religious care." *Health Care Analysis* 21/3: 248–258. DOI: 10.1007/s10728–013–0252–5

Taylor, Charles. 2007. *A secular age*. Cambridge, Mass: Belknap Press of Harvard University Press.

Van Baarsen, Arend, Willeke Oldenhof, and Florus Kruijne. 2016. "Mindfulness past bij geestelijke verzorging." [Mindfulness fits spiritual caregiving]. *Tijdschrift Geestelijke Verzorging* 19/82: 36 – 45.

Van Buuren, Ari, and Alphons van Dijk. 2006. "Identiteit en interculturalisatie." [Identity and interculturalism]. In: Jaap Doolaard (ed.) *Nieuw handboek geestelijke verzorging [New handbook of spiritual caregiving]*. Kampen: Kok. 171 – 191.

Van den Akker, Piet, and Sandra van Wersch. 2003. *Naar meer pluriformiteit in de geestelijke verzorging in zorginstellingen [Towards more pluralism in spiritual care in healthcare.]* Tilburg: IVA.

Van den Berg-Mulder, Emma A. 2010. *ZENding, een onderzoek naar boeddhistisch geestelijke verzorging in Nederland en de rol van ambtelijke binding daarin [A study investigating Buddhist spiritual care in the Netherlands and the role of authorization/ordination]*. Master thesis RU Groningen. http://ggw.studenttheses.ub.rug.nl/174/1/1011-GV%20%20MULDER%20EA.%20%20Ma-scriptie.pdf (accessed May 15, 2019).

Van Dijk, Alphons. 1998. *De hindoe pandit als geestelijk verzorger in Nederlandse zorginstellingen. Achtergronden, ontwikkelingen en profielen [The Hindu pandit as spiritual caregiver in Dutch healthcare. Background, developments, and profiles]*. Best: Damon.

Van Iersel, Fred, and Jan Eerbeek (eds.) 2009. "Positie en werkwijze van het justitiepastoraat in de inrichtingen." [Position and working mode of pastoral services in prisons]. In: *Handboek justitiepastoraat. Context, theologie en praktijk van het Protestants en Rooms-Katholiek justitiepastoraat [Handbook for pastoral services in prisons. Context, theology and practices of Protestant and Roman-Catholic chaplains]*. Eindhoven: Damon. 101 – 112.

Vertovec, Steven. 2007. "Super-diversity and its implications." *Ethnic and Racial Studies* 30/6: 1024 – 1054. DOI: 10.1080/01419870701599465

Vrije Universiteit Amsterdam. 2019. *Postacademische ambtsopleiding boeddhistische geestelijke verzorger [Post-academic education for Buddhist spiritual caregivers]*. https://www.godgeleerdheid.vu.nl/nl/opleidingen/postacademische-opleidingen/postacademische-ambtsopleiding-boeddhistisch-geestelijk-verzorger/index.aspx (accessed May 15, 2019).

White, Pamela G. 2014. *Bedside Bodhisattva, a Buddhist chaplain for all faiths*. https://tricycle.org/magazine/bedside-bodhisattva (accessed May 15, 2019).

Woodhead, Linda, Christopher. H. Partridge, and Hiroko Kawanami (eds.) 2016. *Religions in the modern world: Traditions and transformations*. New York, NY: Routledge.

Cecilia Melder

Existential public health and existential care in secular and interfaith contexts

Abstract: The existential dimension, sometimes referred to as the religious or spiritual dimension, is essential for health and health-related quality of life (HQoL). Research has established a significant link between the existential health dimension and various conditions and diagnoses. The lack of an established definition of the existential dimension constitutes a challenge. Therefore, the starting point in this article is operationalisation. The World Health Organization (WHO) developed a transcultural survey for measuring health-related quality of life, including a model for spiritual, religious, and personal beliefs (WHOQOL-SRPB). This article first presents existential aspects relevant to HQoL and then a model for systematic existential health interventions with the SRPB aspects. Finally, it presents the Social Determinants of Health (SDH) model with the addition of the existential health dimension.

Introduction

In secular societies – even multicultural and multifaith ones – systematic public healthcare that addresses existential health is still lacking. Recent years have, however, seen the emergence of a field of theory and research that recognises and includes this existential dimension of health. This has consequences for the supporting environments and public institutional healthcare that can provide models, systematic methods, and interventions that address existential health issues. In this chapter, health is identified as an inter-combined continuum in which feeling well and feeling bad, being healthy and being sick are points along this continuum. In reality, health and HQoL cannot be separated, but systematisation can clarify the complexity of these concepts. Accordingly, in this chapter, health is understood as the objective evaluation of a person's physical, mental, social, and existential conditions in combination with her subjective HQoL.

In 2020 Professor Dr Niels-Christian Hvidt and Dr Peter la Cour, (Danish researchers in the field of Psychology of Religion) presented a conceptual model to frame meaning-making and existential health for secular cultures: "[The] model combines the three existential domains (secular, spiritual and religious) with the three psychological dimensions of meaning-making (knowing, doing and

 https://doi.org/10.1515/9783110717365-009

being)" (1297). This view is in line with the perspective in this chapter, which adopts Melder's (2011) stance. Melder views existential health as an existential meaning-making system encompassing the – more or less processed – combined processes of basic thoughts, actions and emotions when one life encounters different situations in relation to himself, his environment and/or a transcendent or immense overwhelming force (Melder 2011). With the clarification that the power does not have to be spiritual or religious, existential health can, for example, be related to the power of a political or ideological attitude.

Existential health is thereby defined as a person's resources (cognitive, emotional and in practice) in relation to a person's meaning (secular, spiritual or religious) on all levels (micro, mezzo and macro). The extent to which the existential health determinant can constitute a resource is related to the degree of integration among all these parameters. A more comprehensive integration increases the chances of feeling good enough for daily life and makes life challenges more manageable.

Background

Cultural development

Since World War II, there has been a cultural development in many countries characterised by increasing self-expression values and declining traditional religious values (World Value Survey Association 2021). This cultural shift has given people autonomy and individual freedom to choose how to live their lives free from earlier priorities of conformity to group norms (Inglehart 2018). Globalisation, along with this development, enhances the existential influences. We live in a time with numerous images and theories on how we can interpret life. This is especially true in so called secular countries. In interviews with Swedish adolescents, we found that understanding one's life from the perspective of a larger context (where issues encompassing the holy and profane and sorrow and joy are viewed in relation to the existence of God) have been replaced by personal beliefs that are associated with a "belief in oneself" and a "belief in [that] you will succeed" (Melder, Jyrell and Söderqvist 2016).

A worldwide decline in religiosity

Sweden is arguably an "extremely secular society" (Hagevi 2017, 499). The Nordic countries have long been the world's most secularised countries following the WVS secularisation[1] factor: Religiosity versus individual choice norms (Inglehart 2021). According to the latest WVS (waves 6 and 7) data, 50 % of the population in the Nordic countries believe in God, and 8 % have confidence in churches/religious institutions (Inglehart 2021). In the book *Religion's Sudden Decline: What's Causing it, and What Comes Next?*, Ronald F. Inglehart, founder and former director of the World Values Survey Institute, presented recent data and changes (2021). Based on WVS's extensive data covering 90 % of the world's population, he found a substantial decline in most of the world among people who believe (Inglehart 2021). When comparing 48 countries covering 60 % of the world's population over time, Inglehart found that from 2007 to 2020, 42 countries had become less religious, and six countries had become more religious, in one of the countries there was no changed (2021).

Countries around the world are now experiencing a rapidly increasing secularisation. According to WVS's latest survey, 10 % in the Baltics and 11 % in Protestant Europe answered that "Religion is very important in my life". In Catholic Europe, 21 % of the population and 35 % in the Orthodox cultural zone answered affirmatively. In Muslim-majority countries (Inglehart 2021), however, this number was 79 %.

The Nordic countries urgently need to intensify research and clinical application in existential public health. This knowledge will be crucial when other countries also will face the challenge of supporting the health promotive existential dimension in a secular context.

Existential challenges in our time

Throughout history, life has always brought challenges for individuals, groups, and entire communities. Lately there have been major events and developments (e. g., climate change, the Covid-19 pandemic, and war in Europe) that can affect existential stability. Existential challenges in the community and for individuals can impact basic approaches to life issues, health and HQoL (Saxena, O'Connell and Underwood 2002). These existential challenges affect a central dimension of

1 Only a few changes from WVS with relevance to health are presented here. A more comprehensive section on secularisation can be found later in this chapter.

being human: the existential dimension. While such values were granted to earlier generations, people today live in an era where they need to struggle constantly to find answers to questions of the purpose and meaning of life, hope and hopelessness, life and death, the existence of God, and bodily limitations. DeMarinis describes this unhealthy lack of meaning-creating structures as a threat of epidemic proportions (2006).

The complexity of health today

The Covid-19 pandemic shows the complexity of health and quality of life. The focus initially was on the harmful effects of the virus on physical health but soon began to include and highlight increased awareness of the impact on individual mental health, such as worry and anxiety, as well as social health issues such as unemployment and physical distancing. The effects on existential health should not be underestimated. A web survey of children (4 – 12 years; $N = 717$) and adolescents (13 – 18 years; $N = 330$) conducted in the spring of 2020 emphasises that even young people are affected by the pandemic (Sarkadi et al. 2021). Anna Sarkadi, professor of social medicine at Uppsala University, and her colleagues found that 63 % of children and 56 % of adolescents reported worrying about diseases or death, and 13 % of children and 17 % of adolescents reported other existential worries (Sarkadi et al. 2021). This was in a time when social restrictions were in effect, and we know that, in diverse cultures and societies, social support is crucial when life is complicated (Brooks et al. 2020). Challenges to an individual's most profound meaning-making structure regarding the purposes of life and possible futures are affected by how they are met institutionally. And for every challenge on the public level, there is a potential challenge on the personal level as well.

New opportunities

Due to the reported de facto and expected increase of existential and mental ill-health exemplified by this virus, there are consequences for healthcare that we must deal with as a society in ways that are efficient and sustainable. When a group of eminent scientists published a position paper in the *The Lancet. Psychiatry*, they called for action (Holmes, et al. 2020). In the article, Professor Emily Holmes and her colleagues present several necessary research priorities to counteract mental illness due to Covid-19; all are multidisciplinary (2020). Hopefully, the existential dimension will be included when they and outers emphasize that integration of many different disciplines and sectors is required to meet the challenge (Holmes, et al. 2020)

In A developed and systematic institutional approach to meeting existential health issues is particularly important for balance in a context where more people lack a functional existential meaning-making structure and society as a whole is becoming more divided and secularised (DeMarinis 2008; Sorgenfrei and Thurfjell 2021; Hagevi 2020).

Religious communities have an important task in supporting HQoL by providing a supportive environment through interpersonal relations and counselling. Good existential care is needed to meet increasing existential and mental ill-health, particularly for individuals in institutions such as hospitals and other care facilities where people might be more vulnerable than in other settings.

Key concepts of existential public health in practice

In the following section, key concepts used in both public health sciences and religious practice are discussed and defined for use in this text. These concepts are helpful in nuancing and systematising health-promoting initiatives, especially in planning and implementation activities that are instigated in support of existential health.

Health and public health

Each health dimension: physical, mental, social, and existential dimention, includes a various aspect. For example, the physical dimension includes mobility, muscle mass and fitness, and strength, among others. The psychical dimension contains aspects such as self-confidence, the ability to concentrate and mood. The social dimension consists of close relationships with social support and intimacy on the one hand and the wider social context with accessibility to society and the environment on the other. The difference between health and public health is that health is individual while public health is collective. As individuals, we are healthy, or we suffer from ill-health. When we refer to diseases that affect 1% of the potential population or more and lead to grave consequences for individuals and society, we are talking about public diseases (Janlert 2000). Our physical health is individual – for example, our fitness. More than 1% of the population benefit from physical activity, and thereby authorities and organisations gave physical health a place as a goal of various public health initiatives.

Health in an existential tradition

A task for religious communities is to support someone's opportunities to feel as well as possible in relation to individual conditions. In the Hebrew Bible, health is a holistic perspective that encompasses the whole person's physical, psychological, and existential well-being (Sakenfeld 2006).

The Hellenistic view of man as a unit was replaced during the first century by a more hierarchical view, where the existential part of human nature was regarded as superior to the psychological part, which was seen in turn as superior to a person's physical body (Okkenhaug 2004). From that time on, the body has been designated as subordinate to a human's mental and, above all, existential dimension. Only since the 18th century and the time of Enlightenment has the body has accorded a higher position (Medin and Alexanderson 2001).

How human health is viewed varies across time, countries and continents, between different researchers and practitioners. This article assumes a pragmatic religious, psychological view that shies away from reductionism and exclusive 'truth claims' and instead reports results that encourage further studies and in-depth knowledge (Geels and Wikström 2017). Aspects of the existential health dimension are, for example, personal faith, the meaning of life and inner peace (Melder 2014a).

Existential health and public health

What the term existential health means is a matter of ongoing discussion, and there is no definition that is widely accepted. We do know that existential health affects us in ways that can be measured and analysed – for example, in blood pressure. What the existential health dimension is based on is also difficult to define clearly, and thus any definition will be incomplete. Just like physical public health, existential public health means that not only the individual is affected but the population as well. Existential health can vary from person to person and from situation to situation. Based on the population studies conducted since the 1960s, we know that existential health affects a much larger part of the population than 1% and that shortcomings in this area can have profound consequences (Harrington 2005; Lynch 1977). Thus, the concept of existential public health falls within the framework of the public health concept.

Existential care

Existential care refers to activities that help people develop, strengthen, and maintain existential health. Existential care is not limited to faith communities, individual conversations, or counselling. By promoting existential health either as a separate intervention or as a complement to regular treatment, the efforts can support someone from a holistic perspective. Communities can make an essential contribution to health on the individual and public level with systematic efforts grounded in scientific knowledge and proven experience (Kostenius and Melder 2019). In several different faith communities, the task already is to promote existential health. Based on their preconditions, a fundamental purpose is to support people to feel as good as possible. Not only for the individual's own sake, not just for the faith community's sake, but for the sake of all that is created and for the Creator.

Health-related quality of life

Quality of Life has become a problematic concept that includes a wide range of perspectives, from PROM (patient-reported outcome measures), happiness research, and media perceptions related to consumerism (Marliani and Ramdani 2019; Brülde and Fors 2013). Quality of Life in this text is limited to Health-Related Quality of Life, focusing on the individual's self-reported health in relation to the physical, mental, social, and existential health dimensions.

Intervention

Interventions are activities intending to influence people to change. These can be efforts made in different contexts with the purpose of making people do, think and/or feel things. If we go to a doctor, a physiotherapist or a psychologist, our goal is to feel better, and even faith communities make an effort to have a good influence on their members. A health intervention is a systematic effort to influence a person or group in a way that is intended to be beneficial for health (Forsman 2014).

An existential health intervention is a systematic effort to influence a person or a group in a way that is intended to be beneficial to their existential health. Interventions can be promotions or preventions. Promotions are designed to strengthen health, whereas prevention aims to reduce ill-health (Forsman 2014). We could say that the focus in promotion is on what is healthy, but in prevention, the focus is on the unhealthy, the harmful and the sick. The purpose of prevention is to reduce ill-health, a pathogenic approach. Interventions are not black or white; the prevention of ill-health requires focusing on and strengthening the healthy parts, a salutogenic approach. In existential health interventions, promotions can focus on developing a person's existential meaning-making system through readings, group counselling and training. Promotions can, for example, include existential care in times of crises, life changes and religious anxiety.

Survey of the field

The following section outlines a brief introduction to the theoretical development of a concept of health that includes existential aspects and shows why this is important in secularised societies.

Health from a holistic perspective

Some insights from early science

In the early days, the dimension was first called religious health and then spiritual health. Today existential health is becoming more frequent, especially in northern Europe. It was identified as being the next frontier more than a decade ago when Professor John-Paul Vader
in *European Journal of Public Healths* Editorial highlighted the importance of focusing on its effects on ill-health (2006). Accordingly:

> [U]nless and until we do seriously address the question [the spiritual dimension] – however difficult and uncomfortable it may be – substantial and sustainable improvements in physical, social, and mental health, and reductions in the health gradient within and between societies may well continue to elude us. Vader 2006, 457

Meta-analyses show a preferably positive relationship between a variety of existential aspects and HQoL, but a major challenge is to define the existential dimension and then find credible ways to include the dimension in general health perspectives (Oman and Syme 2018; Shattuck and Muehlenbein 2020). In other words, to develop theories for understanding the conditions of existential health and methods for research in the field. Despite the difficulties Vader envisioned, however, he also argued that it must be possible to explore this existential dimension (Vader 2006). This is especially true in countries that are both highly secularised and multiculturally populated.

Some insights from the biblical terms

Today, more or less all forms of caregiving have emerged from a code attributed to Hippocrates (400 BCE), which comes down to: "To cure sometimes, to relieve often, to comfort always" (Shaw 2009, 955). The idea of the caregiver's obligation to comfort can be found in several documents from that time. The concept of a holistic perspective on humanity is present over time, from the ancient tradition in the Abrahamic religions to public health policies in the modern era (Genesis 2:7; WHO 1948). Given that this holistic view is fundamental and that the distinction between soul and spirit may be unclear, it is important to account for the significance of the different concepts.

Already in the Hebrew Bible, it is emphasised that the human being is created as a whole, with a body that has its physical needs and shortcomings. The body can be measured and weighed. We can even get detailed information today about large areas of the body that we cannot touch through screening and examinations. The Hebrew text uses the word *baśar,* which means 'flesh', corresponding to the Greek *sōma*, *sarx* and *skenos* in the New Testament (Sakenfeld 2006).

Even in these texts, however, the human being is more than a body. Her mental and psychological processes, as well as her cognitive abilities, are called *nephesh* in the Hebrew Bible. The Greek term in the New Testament is *psyche* (Sakenfeld 2006). In Swedish Bible translations, this concept has been translated either by 'I' or 'soul'. The third dimension of the human is called *ruach* and refers to the force of life, the holy power that, according to tradition, the Divine breathes into the person through the nose in the book of Genesis (Chipman 2001; Genesis 2:7). This corresponds to the Greek word *pneuma*, which refers to wind, breath, and life-giving power (Browning 2009).

Given the above, a human being is comprised of physical, mental, and existential dimensions. Accordingly, care for the soul/mental care is provided by the psychological and psychiatric profession. Care of the spirit, the existential dimension, is provided on the other hand by caregivers trained in meaning-making counselling, such as religious spiritual and secular caregivers (Melder 2020).

Some insights on the caregivers title

The discussion on the proper terms for existential caregivers continues; chaplain, shepherd or minister are used. An epistemological and historical reflection may contribute to what such a person could be called in a pluralistic context.

Chaplain

In a Christian context, a *chaplain* refers to a priest or a pastor responsible for people in a specific area such as a hospital or a prison. Today, this title can also include representatives of other religious and non-religious communities. The concept of *chaplain* originates in the story of St Martin of Tours. Martin was born in 316 CE in what is currently Hungary and moved to Italy to study; he became, unwillingly, a soldier at a young age (Carey et al. 2016; Schaff 1957). It is said that he was a humble and loving person (Schaff 1957). One very cold night, Martin came across a homeless war victim clothed only in rags (Carey et al. 2016). Martin did not have any spare clothes, so he took his cloak (Lat. *cappa*) and cut it into two small cloaks (Lat. *capella*): one for himself and one for the other man (Northrup 1990). That night Martin, who still was a Christian catechumen, dreamed that Jesus was wearing the cloak he had given the man (Shefferd 1957). Martin then chose to be baptised and devoted his life to the Christian church, saying: "I am Christ's soldier; I am not allowed to fight" (according to Northrup 1990). Martin then established his own monastery in Tours, the first in France and destroyed non-Christian temples (Shefferd, 1957). Martin died in 397 or 400 CE, was canonised as St Martin of Tours, and his story lived on in the French military tradition. The priest responsible for the legendary cloak was called the *cappellanus* and was carried it as a banner at the forefront of French military battles (Northrup 1990). The term *chapel* itself also originates from this tradition, from the places where the cloak was kept (Northrup 1990). It is logical, based on this background, that what began as a Christian care provider in the military, over time, became an organisational model in the Christian hemisphere. A study of the organised existential care at Swedish hospitals points out the asymmetrical power in the organisation with Christianity as the ruling religion. (Willander et al. 2019). Willander and her colleagues state the need to change this organisation to meet the increased need for religious pluralism (2019). Since *Chaplaincy* is a highly profiled Christian concept, and it is questionable if that title should be forced on all existential caregivers independent of what meaning-making system they represent.

Therapist or Minister

Terms for the existential caregiver can be therapist or minister. The term therapist is usually used for the psycho-social caregiver, but the existential caregiver can also be called a therapist or minister. Minister is used today in Christian contexts for a pastor or priest. In classic Greek, it was a non-religious term that could be used for both men and women (Rapinchuk 2012; Fisher 2016). The Greek word, θεράπων, *therapón*, which denoted a person who promptly helped, served, and healed people, especially in legal matters. According to Thomas Oden, *therapist* and *minister* are intertwined with to be a servant, from the word *Servius* (1992).

Shepherd

Shepherd is another title for a religious leader responsible for specific areas and can be found in diverse cultural and religious contexts. In the Hebrew Bible, the shepherd is usually the symbol of a good, caring leader who protects and leads the flock (Ugwu and Okwor 2013). Already in Genesis, herding sheep is performed by persons like Abel (the son of Eve and Adam), and Rachel (who married the grandson of Sarah and Abraham, Jacob later Israel) (Genesis 4:2; Genesis 29: 6, 9). The good shepherd is a symbol of the good leader found in the Muslim, Jewish and Christian traditions (Broied 2016). The symbol is also present in the Buddhist tradition and has been adopted in non-religious organisations with descriptions like "leadership, representing the shepherd, who follows behind his people, guiding others from a position of ultimate modesty, wisdom, and compassion" (van Norren and Beehner 2021, 41).

This article adopts the term *existential* for meaning-making matters and *existential care* for the support given to existential issues. To be inclusive of the variety of religious, spiritual, and secular traditions and meaning-making systems, the person who mediates the existential care is called the *existential caregiver* in this article. This term is suggested for further discussion about the title; therapist, minister, and shepherd can be respectful alternatives.

Research and existential public health

Religious participation

Today, a large amount of meta-analysis indicates a positive correlation between the existential dimension and a variety of physiological and mental health conditions. This correlation had already been noted in extensive population studies in the 1960s. Initially, it was discovered that social togetherness was crucial for our health. It was established that loneliness can lead to premature death, especially as a result of heart problems, which came to be called suffering and dying of a broken heart due to loneliness (Lynch, Katz, and Schmidt 1983). Several of these studies also found that involvement in religious associations was particularly beneficial for health (Harrington 2005). Even when other factors such as the use of nicotine, alcohol, drugs, education, and finances were taken into account, the difference remained when one could assume that religiously engaged people were healthier (Hummer et al. 2009).

From the late 1960s on, research on spirituality and religiosity in relation to health intensified (Weaver et al. 2006; Addiss 2018).

Religious practices

In addition to studying religion in reference to the human need for social context, research has emphasised the tradition of contemplation and meditation found in all world religions. A variety of other theories have also tried to explain the link, such as theories about how religiosity could have a placebo effect: if one thinks that something can have an effect, in many instances, this also affects you physiologically (Harrington 2005). The number of studies and scientific articles concerning health related to spirituality, religion and existential aspects increased by 700 % during the last three decades of the 20th century (Jager Meezenbroek et al. 2012; Weaver et al 2006). Koenig and his colleagues have, for example, collected over three thousand studies on how religious and spiritual aspects affect health and various disease states (Koenig, King, and Carson 2012). Initially, the studies were based on North American contexts, but over time studies have been conducted worldwide with similar results in various religious and cultural contexts. The studies highlight, for example, the relationship between the existential dimension of health and physical, mental and social health; the relationship between the existing health dimension and results of health promotion efforts and treatment of ill health; the connection between the existential health dimension and the health of young people, older people, of men and women (Moehling et al. 2021; Campbell, Yoon, and Johnstone 2010; Bauereiß et al. 2018; Skevington et al. 2018; Melder et al. 2016; Dew et al. 2008; SALVe 2014).

Today, studies on the existential health dimension are being conducted worldwide, which highlights the need for interventions (Gerhardt-Strachan 2022; Zarei 2021). There is a great need for a transcultural, non-normative perspective and associated measuring instruments that do not focus on religiosity or any particular cultural context. This is important not least in the Scandinavian cultural context, which is described as highly secular (Inglehart 2021).

Psychiatric organisations and existential public health

Based on the extent of studies that show the importance of the existential dimension of health, a variety of organisations and associations have emphasised the importance of including the existential dimension in their concept of health. For example, the World Psychiatric Association (WPA) and the Royal College of Psychiatrists in the United Kingdom have both officially stated that this dimension should be included in the assessment and treatment of mental illness (Moreira-Almeida, et al. 2016; Cook 2011). The American Psychiatric Associations diagnostics manual for mental illness (DSM-5), also pays attention to the importance of this existential dimension and introduced a special guide for cultural interviews that, among other things, aims to map the existential dimension in relation to a person's health status (Association, American Psychiatric 2013; Lewis-Fernández et al. 2016). The existential dimension is thus increasingly becoming an integral part of the concept of health.

Secularism and health

Secularisation is a highly polarised concept

Early on, the Swedish professor of sociology, Thorleif Pettersson, became interested in the phenomenon of secularization and began working with WVS. According to Pettersson (2006), secularism has no clear interpretation because it denotes relatively complex phenomena related to a variety of theories and models. Secularism is thus more of a paradigm, with a combination of different movements than a single theory (Pettersson 2016). Research emphasises that secularisation includes two partially opposing trends where people become more interested in the existential dimension of life while being less involved in traditional ways of expressing that existential dimension (Pettersson 2006). On the macro-level, secularity can be described as a system where religious power and dogmas are separated from political, legal, and administrative power (Lövheim, et a. 2017). On the micro-level, the traditional religious communities are being separated from religiosity in private life and the individual personal beliefs (Lövheim & Lied 2018). Central parts of secularisation that can affect existential health were established by Professor Larry Shiner. His theory focuses on three processes: the desacralization of the world; differentiation within and between a person, society, and religion; the transposition of religious beliefs and institutions from being grounded in divine power to human creation and responsibility (Shiner 1967). This process emerges and develops on different societal levels – the macro-, mezzo-, and micro-level. Dobbelaere (2002) uses the alternative terms of societal, organisational, and individual secularisation. Secularisation on the individual level denotes the dividing of the meaning-making system; the religious meaning-making system is separated into a distinct compartment and thus takes the form of an optional "religious menu" (Dobbelaere 2002).

Privatisation of belief systems

The change we today see in countries like Sweden is the subject of debate, but there is a broad consensus that religion has lost its influence on public life. This has led, among other things, to the privatisation of religion, where religion is still perceived as relevant to private and personal issues but not to public and political life (Pettersson, 2006, 232–233). A secularisation trend can also be observed in the Nordic[2] countries and internationally, for example, in the World Values Survey (WVS) (Inglehart and Welzel 2010; WVS 2010). In the WVS, changes in attitudes, values and beliefs, international comparisons show that at several important points the Scandinavian[3] countries deviate significantly from other international values on certain metrics. For example, Scandinavia is extreme in its combination of 'self-expression value' and 'secular-rational value'. The 'self-expression value' dimension includes issues of self-realisation and quality of life in relation to physical and financial security, the acceptance of homosexuality, and trust in others. The 'secular-rational value' has questions about national

2 Finland, Iceland, Denmark, Norway, and Sweden.
3 Denmark, Norway, and Sweden.

pride, respect for authorities, how important God is, how important it is for children to learn obedience and religious belief, and attitudes on the issue of abortion. Based on these results, Sweden can be seen as the world's most secularised country (Inglehart and Welzel 2010).

A secular contexts influence on health

At the same time, other research holds that while Sweden is one of Europe's most secularised countries today, it is also at the same time one of Europe's most multireligious countries (Sorgenfrei and Thurfjell 2021). This means that, rather than providing a unified existential environment, Sweden can instead be described as an existential environment based on private religiosity and individualistic multi-fragmentation (DeMarinis 2006).

DeMarinis has linked the secular context to its influence on health and claims that this context can lead to psychological dysfunction for individuals who are unable to create meaning in life, as it affects the ability to make life choices (DeMarinis 2003). DeMarinis found that a lack of functioning meaning-making structures poses a severe threat to individual health and wellness. If no action is taken for people who lack functioning meaning-making structures, a more or less complete existential dysfunction can arise, which can lead in turn to mental dysfunction and mental illness (DeMarinis 2006).

Existential public health

From demons to science

A brief historical and cultural reflection is needed to better understand the complexity of the existential dimension in health policies and organisations. In medieval times, demons were thought to cause disease, and the Black Death (1347–1713 CE) killed a quarter of the whole European population (Koening, King, and Carsson 2012). At the end of the 18th century, a scientific paradigm emerged; the time of the Enlightenment started with a desire to acquire knowledge through science instead of just referring to a divine power (Koening, King, and Carsson 2012). The split between the church and medicine that had started some hundred years earlier now deepened between religion with its difficulties in defining and measuring on the one hand and science, which emphasises empirical findings (Koening, King, and Carsson 2012), on the other.

Public health emerges

This paradigm shift does not mean that the existential dimension vanished from ordinary people's or professionals' understanding of well-being and health. Public health was first included in the official dictionary for the Swedish language in 1926 and defined as physical and spiritual health (Svenska Akademin 1926). Given arguments for the importance of existential aspects of health, the following section gives an introduction as to how this dimension has been incorporated into general concepts and policies on health. With that as its starting point, it presents how such general concepts can be modelled into valuable methods for existential health interventions.

The WHO and the concept of existential health

The existential dimensions relevance for WHO

The existential dimension has become relevant for organisations like WHO and is diversely present in public health policies found in different parts of the world. The basis of WHO's health definition is twofold and is partly based on the professional assessment of the individual's anamneses and partly on the personal assessment of one's own perceived health condition. A lot has been written about WHO's history and the history of the existential dimension in that history. It is once again clear that the interpretation of what this dimension refers, to leads to different interpretations of this history.

The inclusion of an existential dimension, by WHO mostly referred to as spiritual health[4], has been discussed since the organisation's establishment and is ongoing (Larson 1996; Solhi et al. 2019). This dimension has a long history in the UN tradition starting even before their specialized Agency WHO was formed in 1948. It was included in the first Declaration of the Rights of the Child, ratified in 1924 by the League of Nations, the predecessor of the United Nations (UN). It was considered crucial for normal development that children be guaranteed this opportunity for existential development: "The child must be given the means requisite for its normal development, both materially and spiritually" (UN 1924). This declaration has been updated and rewritten; the existential dimension is still related to the development and now also to the child's existential

---

4 The WHO's concept *Spiritual Health* will therefore be used synonymously with the existential health dimension in the description below.

well-being (UN 1989). The declaration became Swedish law on 1 January 2020 (Dotevall 2020).

The existential dimension in WHO documents

Rodrigo Toniol is a professor in social anthropology at the Federal University of Rio de Janeiro. In his *Minutes of the Spirit: The World Health Organisation and Its Forms of Instituting Spirituality* from 2019, Toniol describe how the category of spirituality was presented in nearly 1 500 official documents (physical and digital) from the UN and WHO between 1948 and 2017 (2019). Different categories could be concluded from the material; for example, spirituality is seen as a mental health dimension, a protective health factor and a vector of quality of life. But what he chooses to highlight is that "[S]pirituality is a historically situated concept which is marked by the configurations of the power characteristic of western modernity" (Toniol 2019, 5431). In his analysis, Toniol describes the development of spirituality within WHO via two axes: *the spirituality of Others* and *the spirituality of All* (2019). Spirituality has been present in WHO since its foundation, and the intensity and interpretation of the concept have shifted over time (Toniol 2019).

The relationship between WHO and faith-based actors has been studied by Simon Peng-Keller and Fabian Winiger at the department for Spiritual Care at the Faculty of Theology at the University of Zurich. Through analyses of archive material and 18 interviews with key informants, Winiger and Peng-Keller identified three phases of the relation between WHO and religious actors: 1970s–1980s: cross-pollination and institutionalisation; 1990s–early 2000s: cooling-off and crisis; and early 2000s–present: renewed interest and rapprochement (Winiger and Peng-Keller 2021).

According to Winiger and Peng- Leller, the WHO did not have that much interaction with religious actors before the 1970s (2021). During this time, the WHO was framed by the language of human rights, and there were also conflicts between religious values and health values, like population control (Winiger and Peng-Keller, 2021). This was also a time when WHO, along with the rest of the industrialised world, overestimated the curative ability that the biotech scientific thought it would bring. This approach led to "a consequence of this prevailing 'Western model' of health care, the world faced an ever-growing disparity in terms of access to health services and health status between countries and also within countries" (Jakob and Weyel 2020, 5).

Exclusive existential health

In promoting the existential dimension into WHOs policies and programs, new member countries and religious organisations have played a crucial role. From 1960 to early 1970, WHO started to redirect its efforts to find more sufficient and cost-effective ways to reduce the burden of diseases. From the early 1970s on, WHO shifted to inter-sectoral and community-driven health policies away from their earlier high-tech biomedicine approach (Hanrieder 2017). This led to a more open approach to community-based efforts and religious actors (Winiger and Peng-Keller 2021). At the same time, the power distribution among the member countries in WHO was partially altered (Toniol 2019). The political movement following post-colonialisation emphasised new dynamics within the organisation and new members demanded a more holistic non-Western approach to health (Toniol 2019). Including traditional and cultural medicine along with spirituality led to increased use of the concept of spirituality in WHO documents (Toniol 2019). During this time, more and more member states pointed out the lack of a spiritual dimension in the work WHO carried out (Toniol 2019). In 1978, the delegate from Libya and India, addressed the executive board of WHO, proposing that the health definition include the spiritual dimension (Winiger and Peng-Keller 2021; Hanrieder 2017). The Indian delegate Mr Desh Bandu Bisht predicted that all delegates might not recognise the term spiritual; he was the one introducing that this dimension, instead, should be called "Factor X" (Hanrieder 2017). Winiger and Peng-Keller point out that it was during this time that WHO was challenged to stop the spread of malaria and other infections, which forced them to alter their strategy (2021). This led to collaboration with the Christian Medical Commission (CMC), founded in 1968 in the World Council of Churches (WCC), and the Lutheran World Foundation (Winiger and Peng-Keller 2021).

The CMC had developed community-based care and incorporated spirituality into their medical work (Winiger and Peng-Keller 2021: Toniol 2019). Its works focused on primary health care (PHC) and inter-religious dialogue and worked with traditional medicine, including traditional care for the spirit (Toniol 2019). The CMC's position impacted WHO's viewpoint on spirituality: "In short, traditional medicine is the medicine of the Others who, by way of their specific cultural conditions, would conceive the spiritual dimension as the unavoidable face of their healing process (Toniol 2019, 5438). In 1978, an institutional partnership between WHO and the CMC led to WHO officially incorporating the CMC's model for primary health care into their document, thereby legitimising the idea of spirituality linked to culture and specific needs of non-Western peoples (Toniol 2019). Joining forces, CMS and WHO worked together on 'Health for All by the Year 2000' (Winiger and Peng-Keller 2021).

Winiger and Peng-Keller call this first phase 'cross-pollination' and institutionalisation due to the close and fruitful collaborations between WHO and the traditional medicine that the new member countries and the CMC contributed (Toniol 2019; Winiger and Peng-Keller 2021). The axis Toniol refers to as *the spirituality of Others* became manifest when traditional medicine was included in WHO's official statement in 1978 through the Alma-Ata declaration (2019). Traditional medicine is described by its attachment to cultures distant in time and locations from the West, with emphasis on primary health care and a holistic approach to health, including the existential dimension (Toniol 2019).

Generic existential health

The existential practice in traditional medicine and the increased body of science confirms a variety of existential qualities that have a beneficial impact on health not just for people from a particular tradition but people in general. Toniol exemplifies the changes in the axes in two WHO documents on the medical effects of yoga (2019). The first document from 2002 describes yoga as a traditional medicine in Asia, a spiritual evolution that can provide relief from disease (Tonil 2019). In a second document dated seven years later, yoga is no longer described as a traditional medicine just for some. Yoga was presented in 2009 as scientifically validated for tackling common risk factors, preventing lifestyle-related diseases, and promoting existential, mental, and physical health (Tononil 2019).

Spirituality was considered by some to be a generic dimension of health, and there have been attempts to include the existential dimension in WHO's definition. In 1983, Bisht's proposal made in 1978 was followed up by Dr Samuel Hynt, Swaziland's delegate, who addressed the existential dimension concerning the 'Health for All' strategy (Hanrider, 2017; Toniol 2019). Hynt's proposal was discussed at WHO's 36th General Assembly, where a representative from the CMC was present and played an active role in the collaboration (Toniol 2019). Winiger and Peng-Keller characterise the time between 1990s–the early 2000s as a cooling off and crisis period due to the lack of possibilities for religious actors to co-operate with WHO (2021). But the existential progress was by no means in cooling off and crisis phase. According to Toniol, spirituality became used more frequently in WHO documents after the legitimation of traditional medicine (2019). This is a time when the extended work was initiated to adapt WHO work to the new millennium, and the axis of the spirituality of All is beginning to take shape (Toniol 2019), see below: “5.5 Supportive Environments in ‘Health for All’ Strategies”.

The existential dimension included in WHO’s health definition

The inclusion of the existential dimension into the definition of health was discussed again in 1998, now at the WHO 101 Executive Board (WHO 1998). A proposal from the WHO Regional Office for the Eastern Mediterranean, which included members from Islamic countries, led to a discussion by the WHO’s executive board to supplement the definition of health adopted in 1948 with the existential dimension (Nagase 2012). But difficulties regarding consensus on the definition of this dimension led to retaining the original description of health related to physical, mental, and social well-being (WHO 1998; WHO 1948; Nagase 2012). Instead of including the existential dimension in the definition, WHO encouraged member countries to include this dimension in culturally appropriate ways depending on the individual cultural setting in resolution WHA37.13: “Understanding the spiritual dimension to imply a phenomenon that is not material in nature but belongs to the realm of ideas, beliefs, values and ethics that have arisen in the minds and conscience of human beings, particularly ennobling ideas” (WHO 1985, 5 f.). Even so, the significance of the existential dimension of health is clearly stated in WHO official documents. Countries have taken their own initiatives in including existential health in their respective health definitions. For example, Thailand has defined health as a dynamic state of physical, mental, social, and spiritual well-being (Chuengsatiansup 2003).

The difficulty of reaching a trustworthy starting point for how the existential dimension should be understood in relation to health was a recurring item in the discussions in 1983 and 1998 (Nagase 2012; Tonil 2019). A fundamental obstacle in the attempts to establish the existential dimension in the medical societies and health organisations like WHO then was the lack of definitions that could be included in the prevailing scientific paradigm. When reading the protocol, it is clear that delegates were left to rely on their subjective judgment, depending on their own cultural background. At the meeting in 1983 e. g., the General Director had to consult the *Oxford English Dictionary* for a definition of spirit and spirituality (Tonil 2019). At the meeting in 1998, the delegates still tried to get a grip on the dimension by references to, for example, the “Spirit of St. Louis,” i. e., the aircraft Charles Lindbergh flew across the Atlantic (Nagase 2012). It is reasonable to assume that incorporating the existential dimension into the health definition was impossible then. WHO was not ready due to the lack of scientific knowledge and the lack of consensus among delegates who emphasized different origins for existential health: religious, spiritual and secular.

This was a time when Gro Harlem Brundtland was WHO's General Director (1998–2003); she had ambitions for precise measurement and research to gain evidence-based knowledge and technical excellence (Harton 2014). Brundtland's vision was that the organisation should be: "a focal point for the best research" (Harton 2014, 1620). At the time, the WHO research had just begun developing understanding, theories, and methods for the existential dimension of HQoL. Scientists in the WHOQOL-group, led by Dr Shekhar Saxena (later director of the WHOs Department of Mental Health and Substance Abuse), were in the process of including the existential dimension, called SRPB, in the concept of HQoL in manuals, surveys and empirical data (WHOQOL-SRPB Group 2006). In the appendix to the WHOQOL group position paper from 1995, there is a small footnote describing this existential dimension of the SRPB itéms, called facet, as followed:

> This facet examines the person's personal beliefs and how these affect his quality of life. This might be by helping the person cope with difficulties in their life, giving structure to their experience, ascribing meaning to spiritual and personal questions, and more generally providing the person with a sense of well-being. This facet addresses people with differing religious beliefs (e.g. Buddhists, Christians, Hindus, Muslims), as well as people with personal and spiritual beliefs that do not fit within a particular religious orientation. For many people religion, personal beliefs and spirituality are a source of comfort, well-being, security, meaning, sense of belonging, purpose and strength. However, some people feel that religion has a negative influence on their life. Questions are framed to allow this aspect of the facet to emerge. Examples:
>
> Muslims living in a Hindu area; a person with a terminal illness. (WHOQOL Group 1995)

Today, there are still strong forces among researchers who believe that WHO should include an existential dimension in its definition of health, despite the difficulties (Charlier et al. 2017). At the same time, questions are being raised as to whether WHO is ready for a true bio-psycho-social-spiritual model, even though it is deemed highly relevant in developing person-centred care (Saad, De Medeiros, and Mosini 2017).

Supportive environments in 'Health for All' strategies

In 1977, the WHO's General Assembly adopted objectives for 'Health for All by the Year 2000' (WHO 1991). Within the framework of the 'Health for all' strategy, a series of conferences followed that contributed to the development of health promotion work of relevance to the concept of existential public health. The existential dimension (called spiritual by WHO) received attention as a key dimension for supportive environments (WHO 1985:5,6; WHO 1991). The 1986 conference in Ottawa, Canada, was one of the starting points for the third public health revolution (Kickbusch and Payne 2003). The final document from the conference emphasised that

> Health promotion is the process of enabling people to increase control over and improve their health. To reach a state of complete physical, mental and social well-being, an individual or group must be able to identify and realise aspirations, satisfy needs, and change or cope with the environment. Health is, therefore, seen as a resource for everyday life, not the objective of living. (WHO 1986, 1)

Kickbusch (2007) highlights the central and urgent importance of the Ottawa conference's contribution to the public health view. She emphasises that the conference subtitle, "The Move Towards a New Public Health," was overlooked by many. A fundamental change from the WHO's original 1948 definition of health occurred then. Through the Ottawa conference, a view of health was established not as a goal but as a resource in daily life: "Health is created and lived by people within the settings of their everyday life; where they learn, work, play, and love" (WHO 1986, 3). According to Kickbusch, this perspectival shift constituted the third public health revolution (2007). She describes this revolution as

> The third public health revolution recognises health as a key dimension of quality of life. Health policies in the 21st century will need to be constructed from the key question posed by both the health promotion and population health movements. "What makes people healthy?" Health policies will need to address both the collective lifestyles of modern societies and the social environment of modern life and the quality of life of populations. (Kickbusch 2003, 386–387)

It is claimed, however, that several European countries lack the resources to carry out the third public health revolution. Professor Ulrich Laaser (2008) states that the development of public health work faces a challenge where:

> Public health is undergoing profound changes.
> *Goals:* from the reduction of disease and mortality to the increase of healthy life years and reduction of health inequalities.
>
> *Approach:* from a top-down prescriptive, administrative approach based on a knowledge transfer model to a participatory approach characterised by multi-component solutions addressing multiple causes at the socio-economic, environmental, and individual levels.

> *Actors:* professional experts and decision-makers are no longer the only relevant actors in dealing with population health, but are joined by a multi-disciplinary group including researchers, institutional decision-makers, professionals, civil society, and the private sector. (Laaser 2008, 470)

WHO believes that many different factors can affect health; "Political, economic, social, cultural, environmental, behavioural and biological factors can all favour health or be harmful to it" (WHO 1986, 1). The trend towards an increasingly complex view of health was in line with WHO's previous position. By emphasising health as a resource encompassing everyday life, where many factors – including cultural ones – can have a significant impact on health, the 1986 WHO conference opened up spiritual and existential dimensions of the concept of health, providing a more dynamic state of well-being that also included spiritual well-being alongside physical, social and mental well-being (Vang and Kristensson 2000).

Two international conferences followed that emphasised the 'Health for all' strategy: Adelaide, Australia, in 1988 and Sundsvall, Sweden, in 1991. The concept of "supportive environments," which was crucial in the reasoning of the third public health revolution, was concretised during the conference in Sundsvall. There, the final document states: "Thus action to create supportive environments has many dimensions: physical, social, spiritual, economic and political. Each of these dimensions is inextricably linked to the others in a dynamic interaction" (WHO 1991). The Sundsvall conference emphasised that people must become actively engaged to make their environment health-promoting and that the solution to our health issues goes beyond the traditional health systems and references to other contexts, with indigenous peoples often having a "unique spiritual and cultural relationship with the physical environment that can provide valuable lessons for the rest of the world" (WHO 1991, 2).

4.3 WE CAN DO IT! A manual for successful interventions

One of the results of the 1991 Sundsvall Conference was the handbook *We Can Do It!* Summarising 170 of the over 1 000 good public health initiatives presented during the conference and identifying common success factors. This handbook with a clear focus on the importance of creating supportive environments has subsequently been used as a manual for interventions.

While not diverging that much from other project guidelines, it does provide important insights into the specific public health field, such as detailing to a greater extent the meaning of the concept of supportive environments as well as highlighting the existential perspective. The authors believe that there is much to be gained by strategically working across borders, in order to, among other things, be able to clarify priorities, create new knowledge and clarify weaknesses in common structures.

Based on the examples presented, the handbook offers three models for strategic public health work, including the (Health Promotion Strategy Analysis Model – HELPSAM), a model that can be useful in developing existential counselling in institutions. The model consists of seven variables to take into account: 1 Developing new policies, 2 Laws and regulations, 3 Reorienting existing organisations, 4 Advocate 5 Collaborate and mediate 6 Enable 7 Mobilize / develop self- determining (Empowering) (Haglund 1996). These seven variables, in turn, relate to six areas where they are to be implemented: Approach, Effort, Goals, Arena, Tools and Expected Results (Haglund et al. 1993). Components that make up the environment are not just the visible structures and the services that exist. They also include spiritual, cultural, ideological, political, social and economic factors that constitute preconditions for health in the form of supportive environments (Haglund et al. 1993). Various aspects of supportive environments are explained, including certain general conditions being required for a supportive environment, such as psychosocial conditions that offer a sense of coherence, control and meaningfulness (Haglund et al. 1993). The existential dimensions are found both within the framework of the 'political environment' and partly in the description of the 'social environment'. A society's openness or closeness politically, whether that society is participatory or authoritarian, secular or religious, democratic or non-democratic – all are part of the political environment relevant for health and health promotion (Haglund et al. 1993).

Social support and care are clarified in three levels of support: the primary, the secondary and the tertiary. These levels are also called micro, mezzo and macro levels. The primary relates to family and close friends, the second to friends, relatives, and workmates and the third to society. The first level of family and close friends is of the utmost importance and must be strengthened when human power is weakened. The second and third levels also play a crucial role, not least in offering personal beliefs, cultural norms, and religious ideologies. This is described as follows:

> *Secondary* and *Tertiary Level Support* structures are established and developed depending upon the beliefs, cultural norms and political and religious ideologies that are prevalent in communities. Religious/moral values must be placed high in a community's life so that concern and commitment lead to the development of secondary support. (Haglund et al. 1993, 178)

WHO Measuring HQoL with an Existential Dimension

The World Health Organisation outlines the quality of life[5] based on the definition: "Quality of Life as individuals' perceptions of their position in life in the context of the culture and value systems in which they live and in relation to their goals, expectations, standards and concerns" (WHOQOL Group 2002a, 2). In line with this view, the existential dimension is inseparable from the other health dimensions. WHO's Evidence and Research Department of Mental Health and Substance Abuse developed a transcultural instrument, WHOQOL, to assess a person's health and quality of life during a period of the last two weeks. Early in the extensive development process of the instrument, the results revealed that the existential dimension had to be included in the assessment of HQoL: "(W)ere consistently suggested as important dimensions of quality of life [and thereby] Religion/ Spirituality/Personal beliefs' was included as a separate domain of Quality of Life (WHOQOL Group 1995, 1406). The WHOQOL instrument has 100 questions, including four SRPB questions, two about meaning in life and two about personal beliefs in difficult times (WHOQOL Group 1998).
WHO presented 2002 an additional module with 32 items to add to WHQOL for measuring the function of the existential dimension related to health and quality of life (WHOQOL Group 2002a). The advantage of the WHOQOL-SRPB is that this instrument was developed, and pilot tested in 18 countries around the world, which increases the credibility of the instrument's local applicability regardless of the cultural context. The SRPB dimension is based on eight main areas that are related to different clusters of four questionnaires. The main areas for measuring the SRPB dimension of HQoL are 1. Spiritual connection, 2. Meaning and purpose in life, 3. Experience of wonder, 4. Wholeness and integration, 5. Spiritual strength, 6. Harmony and inner peace, 7. Hope and optimism, and 8. Faith as a resource (WHOQOL Group 2002a).

The instructions for the WHOQOL-SRPB questionnaire outline questions concerning the existential perspective. Here it is stated that there are great differences in how to relate to these issues:

> These questions are designed to be applicable to people coming from many different cultures and holding a variety of spiritual, religious or personal beliefs. If you follow a particular religion, such as Judaism, Christianity, Islam or Buddhism, you will probably answer the following questions with your religious beliefs in mind. If you do not follow a particular religion, but still believe that something higher and more powerful exists beyond the phys-

5 When the WHOQOL group use the concept "quality of life" is it equal with the use of HQol in this text.

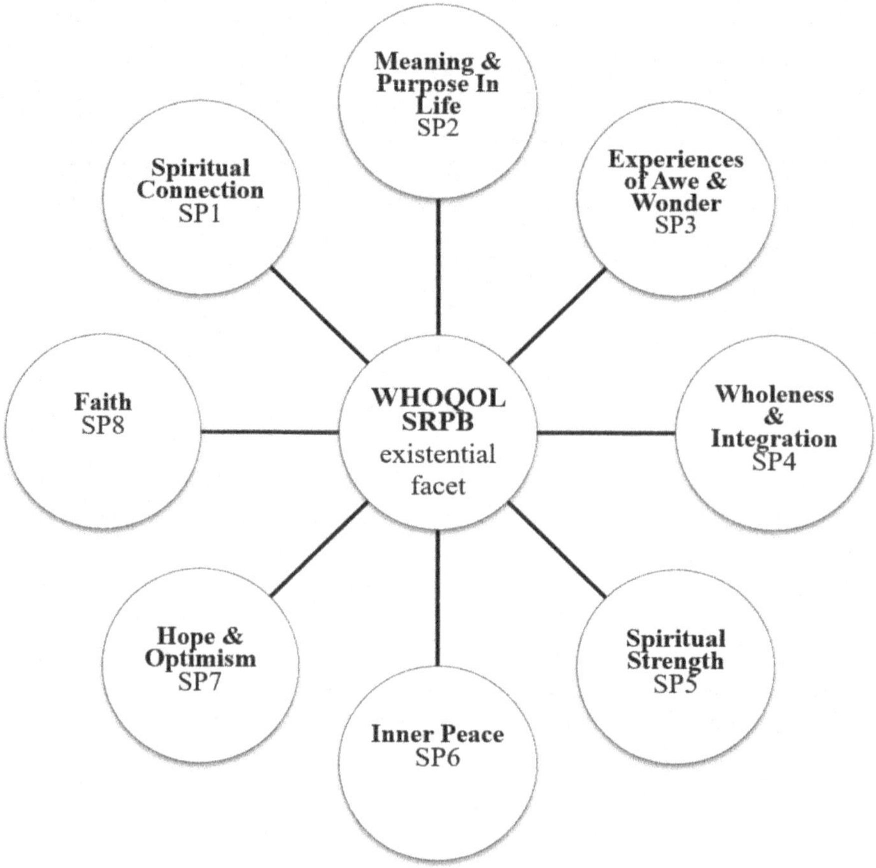

Fig. 1: The internal existential needs developed from the SRPB dimension (Melder 2012).

> ical and material world, you may answer the following questions from that perspective. For example, you might believe in a higher spiritual force or the healing power of Nature. Alternatively, you may have no belief in a higher, spiritual entity, but you may have strong personal beliefs or followings, such as beliefs in a scientific theory, a personal way of life, a particular philosophy or a moral and ethical code. While some of these questions will use words such as spirituality please answer them in terms of your own personal belief system, whether it be religious, spiritual or personal. (WHOQOL Group 2002b, 20)

The questions refer to the existential *function* rather than the *content* of existential beliefs, which allow it to be used to measure people with different religious and cultural backgrounds as well as people in a secular context. As such, the instrument is particularly relevant for multicultural and secular contexts, such as Sweden. In the global pilot study of 5,087 participants, a significant relation was found between the SRPB variable and self-rated health (WHOQOL-SRPB Group 2006). In one study, seven different instruments for assessing the quality of life were also reviewed and evaluated, but none of these instruments, except the WHOQOL-100 as the basis for WHOQOL-SRPB, was designed for intercultural use in contexts where existential health is included for self-rated health and quality of life (O'Connell and Skevington 2007). The WHOQOL-SRPB thereby represents a new criterion for investigating health (O'Connell and Skevington 2010).

WHOQOL is currently validated for 100 cultures and has also been used to measure the effect of changes over time, such as before and after interventions (Skevington and Epton 2018). Psychometric studies indicate that the SRPB dimensions can be divided into two different factors, one dealing with the religious/spiritual aspect, and one with the existential aspect which were found to be robustly associated with well-being independent of a person's religious, spiritual or personal beliefs or non-beliefs (Hammer, Wade and Cragun 2020). No Nordic country was included in the first pilot study, but translation, cultural adaptation and validation of the instrument are in process in both Sweden and Norway. (Melder et a. 2016: Berg Torskenæs & Kalfoss 2013). Survey translation work clarified the need for adaptation to the Swedish cultural setting. While the WHO is not the sole developer of surveys used to measure the existential dimension of HQoL, it is appropriate that it has developed an instrument in a variety of many different countries and cultures in order to adequately address secular and at the same time pluralistic cultural contexts.

A questionnaire that can measure HQoL, including the existential dimension in a context like Sweden, is needed. The WHOQL-SRPB questionnaire was considered most appropriate. A mixed method study was conducted to start a process of translation, cultural adaptation and validation of the WHOQOL-SRPB questionnaire and to evaluate interventions.

According to the WHOQOL group's instructions, forward and back translation, pre-testing, and pilot interviewing were carried out. The first version was completed by 170 individuals between the ages of 21 and 89 (m = 46.6), including 105 women, and comprised both healthy individuals and individuals with mental or somatic issues. The material is based on a convenience sample, so a final Swedish version required additional studies. It was discovered, however, that the SRPB items that used religious terminology needed adjustment. For example, 'spiritual being' needs to be replaced by 'spiritual dimension', 'belief' by 'your belief/idea', and 'higher and more powerful' explained as 'force/power dimension'. The pre-test results were useful in this process, especially qualitative data from individuals representing secular existential worldviews, including different philosophical and political traditions. The internal consistency reliability of the overall SRPB module was high (alpha = .97) as well as of the 8 aspects (alpha ranging .80–.97). Test-retest (n = 19) showed r = .83 (p\.01). There were strong correlations between all aspects, the overall SRPB module and the overall quality of life and general health perceptions. No difference was found between women and men in the overall SRPB module, but in the 'Connect' aspect, women scored higher (p = .02) whereas in 'Peac' men scored higher (p = .04) (Melder et al. 2016). The work with translation and cultural adaptation of the WHOQOL-SRPB survey for different subgroups of the Swedish context – for example, adolescents and the aged – is ongoing.

The results internationally and in the study above showed that the eight existential SRPB aspects in the WHOQOL-SRPB are central to existential health and HQoL. They could thereby be the existential foundation for a health intervention that in itself is non-religious but, depending on the participants, could be related to one or more religious, spiritual, philosophical, political or humanistic worldviews.

Existential health interventions in a secular context

Given that there is now an awareness that existential health matters and that concepts, policies and frameworks have been developed at a general level, we now need to apply this knowledge to designing specific models and methods for interventions that can be usefully implemented in a clinical setting. This section, therefore, outlines a possible approach.

New directions in research: towards interventions

While previous research on the existential health dimension has focused on discovering correlations that can be found between different existential aspects and illness, self-esteem and quality of life, etc., research today is becoming increasingly interested in interventions and promotions, in how existential health can be strengthened and in how this type of health promotion can and should be designed. In a context in which traditional arenas and strategies for existential mediation and religious values play decreasing roles in everyday life, new strategies need to be developed to support people in developing and maintaining a functional meaning-making system to gain existential health and thereby health in a broad sense. There has been development in both the creation of supportive environments and new existential interventions suitable for a secular context and for theorising about how existential health is created and maintained. The theory has been derived from the interpretation of the informants' descriptions in interviews and surveys about their perceived health and well-being (Melder 2011). The theory outlined in the model has been clinically tested for health promotion with respect to, for example, self-help groups and suicide prevention.

A new model for health determinants

The complexity of the social aspects that affect one's environment was addressed in a broad sense by Svanström and Haglund (Svanström 1979; Haglund and Svanström 1983), who developed a model for social health determinants (the SHD model). The model is based on the principle that health and ill-health are affected by different social levels related to the individual and his or her human limitations (Haglund and Isacsson 1982). The model is a rainbow-shaped semicircle with the individual and the primary micro level at the centre, followed by the mezzo, and the macro level, diagramming the individual's relationship to surrounding people and environments (Haglund and Svanström 1983). The model was then translated into English and became widely used.; today the model is well known. It is used, for example, in the Swedish Public Health Agency's Annual Report 2020 in a variant taken from a working report from the Institute for Future Studies 2007 (Pellmer, Wramner, and Wramner 2017; Public Health Agency of Sweden 2020; Dahlgren and Whitehead 2007).
The extensive research in recent decades about the existential dimensions significant for a variety of aspects on the micro, mezzo and macro levels support WHO's perspective on the 'Health for all' strategy. There are many studies on existential health and several on the social health determinants, such as the family that can convey that life is meaningful, a school that can instil hope, work that gives one a feeling of being part of a larger whole and leisure that can contribute to harmony and inner peace are all examples of interaction between social health determinants and existential aspects (Koening, King, and Carsson 2012). The existential dimension needs to be systematically included in theories and models of public health to get a better understanding so that efficient health intervention and political actions can be promoted. Inspired by the eight aspects of the SRPB dimension in WHOQOL the operationalisation of the concept was constructed (Melder 2012). It was noted earlier that prioritising defining the cognition, affections, and actions in spiritual, religious, or secular meaning-making systems of the existential dimension would have complicated the strategic and systemic approach. It is better to address existential health through designing models and interventions based on the functional aspect as a pragmatic method until a widely accepted definition can be found.

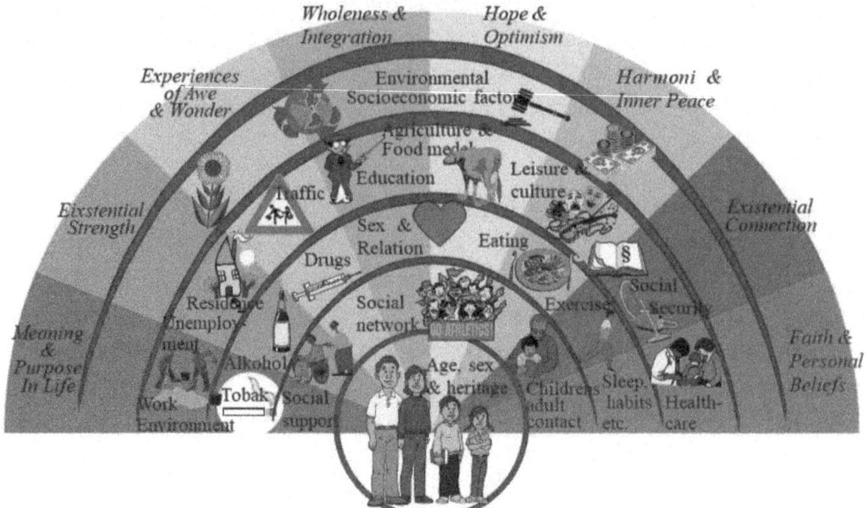

Fig. 2: Melder, C. (2019). **The SDH-SRPB Model:** Social determinants of health with the existential dimension.[a)] [a)] Based on Haglund, B. & Svanström, L. (1983). Samhällsmedicin – en introduktion. Illustration: Hammarström, B. & translation Melder, C.

The SDH-SRPB model was first published internationally in 2019, at the 9th conference for Nordic health promotion research (NHPRC) held in Roskilde, Denmark (Melder 2019). The intention behind the SDH-SRPB is to present a general model for the existential dimension exemplified by the eight SRPB aspects, which can be significant on different levels for different people and groups. There are other existential aspects that are relevant in the same way on the various levels for different people in different times and situations. This model can thereby aid new approaches and complement existing assessments and efforts. As such, the model suggests that the existential caregiver should be an agent for hope, maybe even an agent for meaning, harmony, and perhaps an existential connection among agents for other existential aspects that are missing in the context.

The existential health model

The psychological approach to this hypothetical model is inspired by Donald W. Winnicott a paediatrician and early psychoanalyst. He developed the foundation of the view of play held today as a necessary part of the child's healthy develop-

ment. He believed that play transformed into other activities as the individual grows up, such as those related to creativity, culture and religion (Winnicott 2005). Winnicott believed that these activities are essential for one's ability to reconcile his or her internal psychological world of dreams, personal needs, fantasies and wishes with the psychological experience of the external world with its reality, demands and facts. In between is what Winnicott called, the potential space, a 'play area' where the individual can interject the internal and external and develop systems to relate to the outside world and create meaning (Winnicott 1964). Good development of this potential space requires introjection between these external and internal spaces. The opposite is disintegration which, according to Winnicott, can lead to chaos and ill health (1988).
Melder's hypothesis-generating dissertation expanded Winnicott's theory into this model to describe the existential health dimension and an individual's meaning-making processes (2011). In brief, the process of creating and maintaining existential health is related to the possible unifying or splitting between two aspects. On the one hand, there are the images of the perceived external meaning-making structures in the form of cultural, political, philosophical, and religious conceptions, which are more or less reflected on or clear. There can also be everyday perceptions of what is right/wrong, good/bad, sick/healthy. On the other hand, there are also internal existential needs related to the need for wholeness, hope and harmony, and so on. etc. Where the external and the internal meet is the development of functional meaning-making systems possible. It is in this dimension that the existential health dimension develops. If the internal and external existential dimensions do not introject or an imbalance arises in the union, this affects the possibility of forming functional introjection processes between external meaning-making structures and the individual's existential internal existential needs. For example, if someone feels worthless, it does not matter how much he or she thinks that all people, regardless of gender, age and ethnic background, have the same value – thinking this will not constitute an existential health resource for this person. A person's cognition, emotion and action related to her existential dimension must be fairly consistent, to have good existential health. When the internal and external dimension affects or is affected by the other health dimensions (physical, mental, social, and existential), the process of reprocessing Introjection is crucial. This might happen when a person becomes sick, for example, is detained, enters the military, or enrols in higher education. It is easy to become vulnerable in those situations and existential counselling might be helpful.

A picture thus emerges of existential health based on a continuum between health and ill-health, largely due to how well internal existential needs are integrated with external meaning-making structures and other health dimensions.

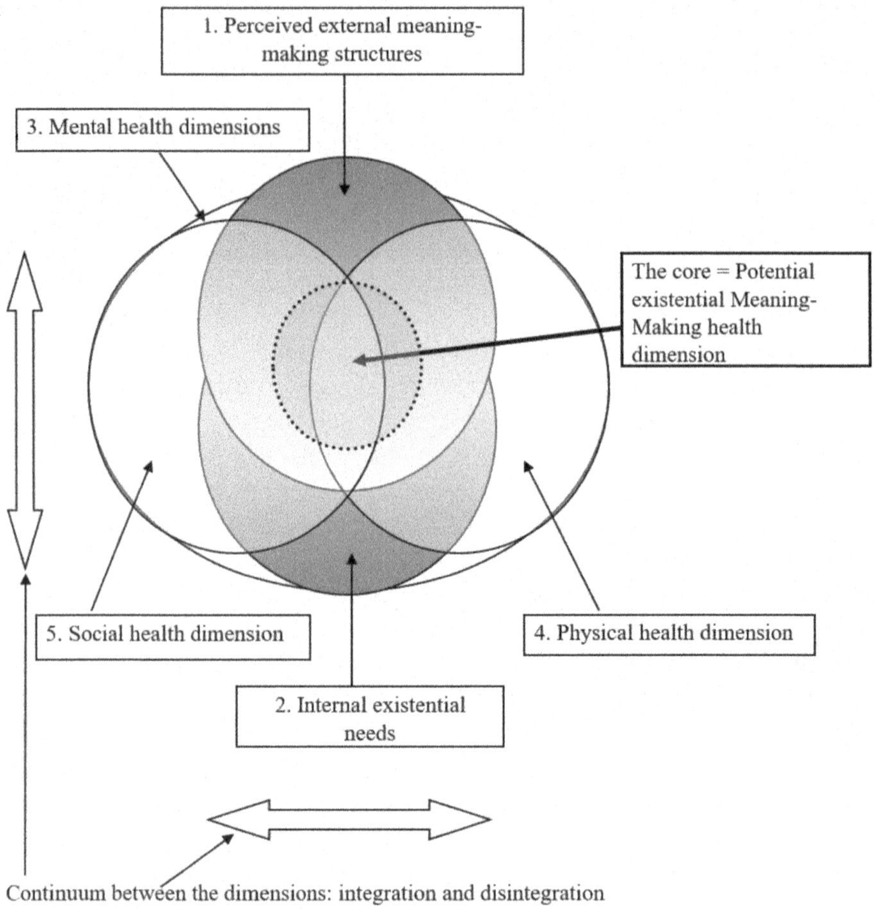

Fig. 3: The existential health model (Melder 2012, 253).

The different health dimensions have a mutual relationship, where the degree of interaction between the different dimensions affects how well the meaning-making processes work and vice versa. All health dimensions interact and can create opportunities for interaction as well as disintegration. In the innermost core of the health model lies the possibility of a potential existential dimension that is equivalent to Winnicott's potential space (2005). This potential dimension is crucial for the possibility of offering a functioning existential meaning-making structure in different situations to thereby promote existential health.

Structures for supporting functional existential health

There is a long tradition with positive results of working with different group interventions in institutional settings to facilitate the opportunities for creating a supportive environment (Ezhumalai et al. 2018). Studies show that group interventions have a high positive health outcome due to group social engagement and identification, and sustainability in the outcome is also more solid (Haslam et al. 2010; Zastrow 2009). The group intervention model was constructed, based on Melder's theory described above together with the eight existential aspects of WHOQOL-SRPB, to support the introjection of the perceived external meaning-making structures and the internal existential needs. In relation to existential interventions, it can be thus argued that a group that can share different thoughts and perspectives to support the group members in developing their own meaning-making structures in relation to their own existential needs is a useful resource.

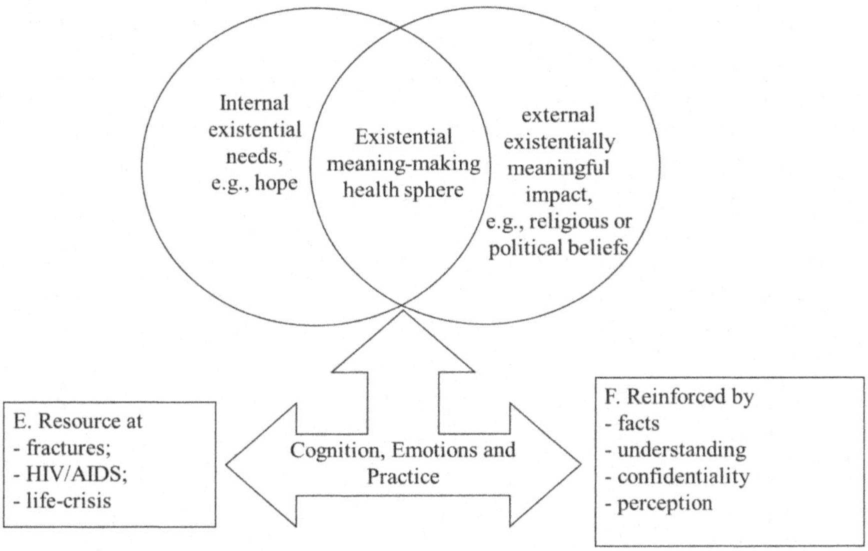

Fig. 4: Structure for existential health intervention (Melder 2011, 244).

The intervention needs a clear structure to be able to contain the introjection process, a structure that is the same in all cases. The more extensive the introjection process needs to be, the tighter the structure. To enable the process, the intervention needs input on different levels of knowledge. These are:

- *facts:* education about different external existentially meaningful structures.
- *understanding:* dialogue on the relation between existential meaning-making structures and the individual's inner existential needs.
- *confidentiality:* work with creativity and playfulness to introject inner existential needs and existential meaning-making structures.
- *perception:* various kinds of relaxation techniques lead to a deep form of knowledge in order to add confidentiality to the introjection in the existential potential dimension.

Designing two forms of existential health interventions

Using the model above, the existential health dimension has been strengthened in concrete ways, which thereby strengthens HQoL in a broad sense. By starting from the different aspects of the existential health dimension, operationalised in the eight SRPB aspects and the eight existential needs, the existential dimension has been included in a variety of supportive environments and counselling situations. The model has been further developed into two different interventions: a promotion and more extensive prevention to facilitate existential support.

An existential health tool was developed in 2013 to promote the existential dimension: *Dialogue Cards: Life Courage, Life Joy, Life Meaning*, in collaboration with Lena Bergquist at Västenskolan Västmanland. A couple of years later, the cards were developed further with the help of Anna-Karin Jeppsson and Thomas Sjöberg, based on their experience of working in psychiatry with the first version of these cards. Lena Bergquist has also developed the cards even more to include 'green cards' and pictures (Studieförbundet Vuxenskolan Västmanland). In the existential health promotion with the dialogue cards, knowledge levels have been summed up in *Thoughts*, *Feelings* and *Actions* in groups with 6 – 12 participants. Themes concerning the different existential aspects were discussed there once a week for 40 – 60 minutes over a period of eight weeks. The dialogue cards were used in a variety of groups such as self-help groups, secondary school students, employees in health care settings, different patient groups, and evening classes for the elderly.

Existential health promotion has spread organically, and a large body of experience of working with the dialogue cards has been generated. In local evaluations, participants and leaders are positive about the work with the dialogue cards. In the limited before and after studies done in the promotion groups with the WHOQOL-SRPB, positive changes have been reported, and the outcome varies among different groups (Melder 2014b). This in turn raises new questions, not least concerning an individual's ability to have a language for perceived external meaning-making structures and internal existential needs.

To prevent disorder and promote existential health, a more extensive intervention was also developed. This prevention has been tested on a small scale, in method development studies within the ordinary care process, with persons on long-term sick leave, and with persons with suicidal behaviours. In this small pilot testing of the prevention intervention, a schedule of three-hour meetings twice a week for eight weeks in groups of 5 to 12 participants was set up, covering one existential need a week. The WHOQOL-SRPB questionnaire was used for a 'before and after' study, and open-ended questions were added for qualitative evaluation.

In the intervention with people on long-term sick leave due to psychosocial ill health, the intervention took place in an activity centre where people are assigned activities like cooking and carpeting for the ones who are capable of such tasks and in general to meet people, so they break out of their isolation. In the intervention group, eight of the twelve participants answering the questionnaire before and after the intervention often had a hard time participating in any activities. The ten people in the control group answering the questionnaire at the same time as the intervention group and then again after eight weeks. Given this small number of participants, it is not possible to conduct a proper quantitative analyse. But it can be said that the intervention group increased their HQoL and the control groups HQoL decreased during the eight weeks. The suicide prevention intervention was a pilot group project conducted in a psychiatric hospital. The five participants, man, and women were between ca. 20 and ca. 50 years old; all of them had recently tried to commit suicide. On a group level, all health dimensions had increased. The group's satisfaction with their quality of life and the feeling that life was meaningful had increased from *Not at all* to *A little*. In the open-ended questions regarding what they did not like in the intervention, one reported that the relaxation activities were difficult. Other responses to that question were: "That it ended"; "Don't know, appreciate it so much, can't say anything bad"; "too few appointments" (Melder and Nyberg 2018). But most importantly, everyone was alive at the last check-up 15 months later.

These interventions were met with interest by both patients and practitioners. Even if the samples are small, there is a positive evolution in the participants' existential health and general HQoL, according to the WHOQOL-SRPB. And while these pilot studies are small-scale, their results are promising in that the participants generally emphasised the existential dimension as important for their HQoL and reported positive outcomes from the interventions. The quantitative improvement varies among the different groups, however. Given that the weekly topics were drawn from one of the existential themes identified above, with reference to the existential approach (i.e., function), rather than the content of existential beliefs, this makes such interventions applicable to both a secular context and a multireligious context. More systematic research on existential public health and the effect of these interventions is needed, however, to be able to generalise these tendencies.

The Covid-19 pandemic has increased awareness of the existential aspects of life. The SARS-CoV-2 virus and its consequences have demonstrated the importance of including the existential dimension in the perception of health. There are several consequences of this virus that we must now deal with in a way that is both efficient and sustainable, due to the expected increase in existential and mental ill-health. This increases the urgency to develop theories and models for including this dimension in the general concept of health and HQoL on the micro, mezzo and macro levels. That also includes having efficient ways to strategically and systematically make religious and non-religious people healthy in this dimension. The aim is to improve public health, and, for this task, a multiprofessional workforce is needed, including people trained in physical, mental, social, and existential healthcare working in close connection with researchers in this different field.

Conclusion

Existential challenges on micro- mezzo- and macro level has given us partly new experiences of life and death throughout society, such as not being present at the death of loved ones, the denial of physically present social support structures in dealing with grief, experiences of distance and digitalisation at traditional rites of passage that are designed to aid meaning-making structures surrounding death and life. This has been widely reported in the media and elsewhere as affecting widespread HQoL, including the existential dimension.

It has been argued that supporting environments (micro, mezzo and macro) are critical in a society's ability to meet HQoL at different levels. In non-secular societies, existential aspects of health can be met at different levels by religious support systems and structures. In a secular context, it is not obvious who has this responsibility, especially with respect to people without any religious affiliation. It becomes important to work in strategic and systematic ways to create supportive environments that can facilitate the creation of a functional meaning-making structure and thereby improve existential health. Secularity does not necessarily mean non-religiosity (and thereby the lack of religious support systems). Secular societies, such as modern Sweden, can be alternatively described as multicultural and multireligious. While some support systems can exist, existential health is not met systematically by existing public support structures/systems. The public support structures currently focus on psychosocial methods and techniques. By focusing on the existential aspects of HQoL, research thus argues that public support environments have the opportunity to operate from a different orientation than psychosocial support structures do.

Interventions based on theory and research show that including the existential dimension benefits HQoL. Thereby, systematically including theory development, research, and experiences from interventions within the field of existential health can lead to public support/care structures. New extended collaborations between interfaith and health communities and institutions can deal with the kind of existential issues that have developed into such societally widespread experiences where life is challenged on the micro-, mezzo-, and macro-level. Issues such as depression, isolation, poor mental health, lack of meaningfulness, etc., and their effects on HQoL in the time of crises could be systematically 'caught' in existentially oriented public care/support environments. This would reduce or manage the long-term negative effects of existential ill-health that affects HQoL in general. Not least of all and given that the eight existential aspects of the SRPB dimension can be found in many religious traditions throughout history, this model can also be used to systematise and improve research and practice within the field of interreligious existential care, as well as provide efficient and sustainable interfaith existential care in a variety of institutions.

References

Addiss, David, G. 2018. "Spiritual themes and challenges in global health." *Journal of Medical Humanities* 3/39: 337–348.

Association, American Psychiatric. 2013. *Diagnostic and Statistical Manual of Mental Disorders (DSM-5)*. Washington: American Psychiatric Publishing.

Bauereiß, Natalie, Stefanie Obermaier, Selçuk Ero Özünal, and Harald Baumeister. 2018. "Effects of existential interventions on spiritual, psychological, and physical well-being in adult patients with cancer: Systematic review and meta-analysis of randomised controlled trials." In *Psycho-oncology* 11/27: 2531–2545.

Berg Torskenæs, Kristina, and Mary H. Kalfoss. 2013. "Translation and Focus Group Testing of the WHOQOL Spirituality, Religiousness, and Personal Beliefs Module in Norway." In *Journal of Holistic Nursing* 31/1: 25–34.

Brodie, Ernest Frank, Jr. 2016. *The Leader as a Shepherd: A Case Study of Ecclesiastic, Business, and Education Leaders*. ProQuest Dissertations Publishing.

Brooks, Samantha K., Rebecca K. Webster, Louise E. Smith, Lisa Woodland, Simon Wessely, Neil Greenberg, and Gideon James Rubin. 2020. "The Psychological Impact of

Quarantine and how to Reduce it: Rapid Review of the Evidence." *The Lancet (British Edition)* 395/10227: 912–920.

Browning, Browning, and Wilfred Francis Robert. 2009. *A dictionary of the Bible.* Oxford: Oxford University Press.

Brülde, Bengt, and Fors Filip. 2013. "Är lyckan grön?" *Ekonomisk debatt* 41/2: 45–46.

Campbell, James D., Dong Phil Yoon, and Brick Johnstone. 2010. "Determining Relationships Between Physical Health and Spiritual Experience, Religious Practices, and Congregational Support in a Heterogeneous Medical Sample." *J Relig Health* 49: 3–17. https://doi.org/10.1007/s10943-008-9227-5

Carey, Lindsay B., Timothy J. Hodgson, Lillian Krikheli, Rachel Y. Soh, Annie-Rose Armour, Taranjeet K. Singh, and Cassandra G. Impiombato. 2016. "Moral Injury, Spiritual Care and the Role of Chaplains: An Exploratory Scoping Review of Literature and Resources." *Journal of Religion and Health* 55/4: 1218–1245.

Charlier, Philippe, Yves Coppens, Jean Malaurie, L. Brun, Marc Kepanga, Van Hoang-Opermann, J. A. Correa Calfin, George Nuku, M. Ushiga, X.E. Schor, and S. Deo. 2016. "A new definition of health? an open letter of autochthonous peoples and medical anthropologists to the WHO." *European Journal of Internal Medicine* 37/2016–2017: 33–37.

Chipman, Leigh N.B. 2001. "Mythic aspects of the process of Adam's creation in Judaism and Islam." *Studia Islamica.* 5–25.

Chuengsatiansup, Komatra. 2003. "Spirituality and health: An initial proposal to incorporate spiritual health in health impact assessment." *Environmental Impact Assessment Review* 23/1: 3–15. DOI: 10.1016/S0195–9255(02)00037–9.

Cook, Christopher C. H. 2011. "Recommendations for psychiatrists on spirituality and religion. Position Statement PS03/2011." *London: Royal College of Psychiatrists.* www.rcpsych.ac.uk.

la Cour, Peter, and Hvidt Niels Christian. 2010. "Research on meaning-making and health in secular society: Secular, spiritual and religious existential orientations." *Social Science & Medicine* 7/71: 1292–1299.

Dahlgren, Göran, and Margaret Whitehead. 2007. "Policies and strategies to promote social equity in health. Background document to WHO-Strategy paper for Europe." *Institute for Futures Studies* 14.

DeMarinis, Valerie. 2003. *Pastoral Care, Existential Health, and Existential Epidemiology. A Swedish postmodern case study.* Stockholm: Verbum.

DeMarinis, Valerie. 2006. "Existential Dysfunction -as a Public Mental Health Issue for Post-Modern Sweden: a cultural challenge and a challenge to culture." In: Bent Holm (ed.) *Tro på teatret -essays om Religion og Teater, Religion i det 21 århundrede.* Köpenhavn: Köpenhavns Universitet. 229–243.

DeMarinis, Valerie. 2008. "The Impact of Post-Modernization on Existential Health in Sweden: Psychology of Religion's Function in Existential Public Health Analysis." *Archive for the Psychology of Religion* 30: 57–74. DOI:10.1163/157361208X316962

Dew, Rachel Elizabeth, Stephanie S. Daniel, Tonya D. Armstrong, David B. Goldston, Mary Frances Triplett, and Harold G. Koenig. 2008. "Religion/Spirituality and Adolescent Psychiatric Symptoms: A Review." *Child Psychiatry and Human Development* 39/4: 381–398. DOI: 10.1007/s10578–007–0093–2

Dobbelaere, Karel. 2002. *Secularisation: An Analysis at Three Levels.* Brussels: Peter Lang.

Dotevall, Rolf. 2020. *Sveriges Lag: Innehåller Författningar Som Trätt i Kraft Per Den 1 Januari 2020: Huvudboken Är Uppdaterad Till Och Med 29 November 2019 Med SFS 2019:826 Som Sista Tillagda SFS*. Upplaga 8 ed. Lund: Studentlitteratur.

Ezhumalai, Sinu, D. Muralidhar, R. Dhanasekarapandian, and Bala Nikketha. 2018. "Group Interventions." *Indian Journal of Psychiatry* 60/8: 514–521. DOI: 10.4103/psychiatry.IndianJPsychiatry_42_18

Fisher, Roger S. 2016. "Women's Playthings: The Meaning of δούλευμα in Soph. Ant. 756, Eur. Ion 748, and Eur. Or. 221" *Philologus* 160/2: 197–216. https://doi-org.ezproxy.its.uu.se/10.1515/phil-2016-5011

Forsman, Anna K. 2014. "Främjande av psykisk hälsa och förebyggande av psykisk ohälsa." In: Susanne Rolfner Suvanto (ed.) *Äldres psykiska hälsa och ohälsa. Prevention, förhållningssätt och arbetsmetoder.* Stockholm: Gothia Fortbildning AB. 17–22.

Geels, Anton, and Owe Wikström. 2017. *Den religiösa människan: en introduktion till religionspsykologin.* Stockholm: Natur och Kultur.

Genisis. 2001. Bible, H. *Authorized King James Version.* London, and New York, nd.

Gerhardt-Strachan, Karina. 2022. "Exploring the place of spirituality in Canadian health promotion." *Health Promotion International* 37/1: 1–10. DOI: 10.1093/heapro/daab027.

Hagevi, Magnus. 2017. "Religious Change over the Generations in an Extremely Secular Society: The Case of Sweden." *Review of Religious Research* 59/4: 499–518.

Hagevi, Magnus. 2020. "Utan egen erfarenhet av kyrkor, om församlingens omvärld." In: Marie-Anne Ekedahl (ed.) *Livshjälp i en orolig tid. Själavård i forskning och beprövad erfarenhet.* Stockholm: Libris. 169–201.

Haglund, Bo J. A. 1996. "Stödjande miljöer för hälsa – ett strategiskt begrepp för det hälsofrämjande arbetet." *Socialmedicinsk tidskrift* 2/3: 91–99.

Haglund, Bo J. A., and Sven-Olof Isacsson. 1982. *Kommun diagnostik: en utgångspunkt för offensivt hälsoarbete: erfarenheter från tvärsnittsundersökningen hälsoprofil Skaraborg.* (HPS 77), Stockholm: Spri.

Haglund, Bo J. A., and Leif Svanström. 1983. *Samhällsmedicin – en introduktion.* Lund: Studentlitteratur.

Haglund, Bo J. A., Bosse Pettersson, David Finer and Per Tillgren. 1993. "We Can Do It! The Sundsvall handbook." *From the 3rd International Conference on Health Promotion Sundsvall, Sweden June.* Sweden: Repro Print AB, Solna.

Hammer, Joseph H., Nathaniel G. Wade, and Ryan T. Cragun. 2020; 2019. "Valid Assessment of Spiritual Quality of Life with the WHOQOL-SRPB BREF Across Religious, Spiritual, and Secular Persons: A Psychometric Study." *Psychology of Religion and Spirituality* 12/4: 440–450. DOI:10.1037/rel0000266

Hanrieder, Tine. 2017. "The public valuation of religion in global healthgovernance: spiritual health and the faith factor." *Contemporary Politics* 23/1: 81–99. http://dx.doi.org/10.1080/13569775.2016.1213076

Harrington, Anne. 2005. "Uneasy Alliances: The Faith Factor in Medicine; the Health Factor in Religion". In: *Science, Religion, and the Human Experience.* Oxford: Oxford University Press. DOI: 10.1093/0195175328.003.0015

Haslam, Catherine, S. Alexander Haslam, Jolanda Jetten, Adam Bevins, Sophie Ravenscroft, and James Tonks. 2010. "The Social Treatment: The Benefits of Group Interventions in Residential Care Settings." *Psychology and Aging* 25/1: 157–167. DOI: 10.1037/a0018256

Holmes, Emily A., Rory C. O'Connor, V. Hugh Perry, Irene Tracey, Simon Wessely, Louise Arseneault, Clive Ballard, et al. 2020. "Multidisciplinary Research Priorities for the COVID-19 Pandemic: A Call for Action for Mental Health Science." *The Lancet. Psychiatry* 7/6: 547–560.

Horton, Richard. 2014. "Offline: The Third Revolution in Global Health." *The Lancet (British Edition)* 383/9929: 1620–1620.

Hummer, R. A., R. G. Rogers, C. B. Nam, and C. G. Ellison. 1999. "Religious Involvement and U.S. Adult Mortality." *Demography* 36/2: 273–285.

Inglehart, Ronald. 2018. *Cultural evolution: People's motivations are changing, and reshaping the world.* Cambridge University Press.

Inglehart, Ronald. 2021; 2020. *What Is Replacing Religion? In Religion's Sudden Decline: What's Causing it, and what Comes Next?* New York, NY: Oxford University Press. DOI: 10.1093/oso/9780197547045.001.0001.

Inglehart, Ronald, and Christian Welzel. 2010. "Changing mass priorities: The link between modernisation and democracy." *Perspectives on Politics* 8/2: 551–567. DOI: 10.1017/S1537592710001258

Jager Meezenbroek, Eltica, Bert Garssen, Machteld Berg, Dirk Dierendonck, Aiaan Visser, and Wilmar Schaufeli. 2012; 2010. "Measuring Spirituality as a Universal Human Experience: A Review of Spirituality Questionnaires." *Journal of Religion and Health* 51/2: 336–354. DOI: 10.1007/s10943–010–9376–1

Jakob, Beate, and Birgit Weyel. 2020. *Spirituality, mental health, and social support: a community approach.* Berlin: De Gruyter.

Janlert, Urban. 2000. *Folkhälsovetenskapligt lexikon.* Stockholm: Natur och kultur i samarbete med Folkhälsoinstitutet.

Kickbusch, Ilona. 2003. "The Contribution of the World Health Organization to a New Public Health and Health Promotion." *American Journal of Public Health* 93/3: 383–388.

Kickbusch, Ilona. 2007. "The move towards a new public health." *Promotion & Education* 14/9. DOI: 10.1177/10253823070140020301x:

Kickbusch, Ilona, and Lea Payne. 2003. "Twenty-first century health promotion: The public health revolution meets the wellness revolution." *Health Promotion International* 18/4: 275–278. doi:10.1093/heapro/dag418

Koening, Harold G., King, Dana E., and Carsson Verna B. 2012. *Handbook of religion and health.* Oxford: Oxford University Press.

Kostenius, Catrine, and Cecilia Melder. 2019. "Existential health: A valuable dimension when promoting health throughout the life-course in Sweden." *WAIORA. Promoting Planetary Health and Sustainable Development for All. 23rd International Union for Health Promotion and Education (IUHPE) conference book.* http://urn.kb.se/resolve?urn=urn:nbn:se:ths:diva-352

Laaser, Ulrich. 2008. "Editorial: Global Health and Health Diplomacy." *Journal of Public Health Policy* 29: 467–473. DOI: 10.1057/jphp.2008.36

Larson, James, S. 1996. "The world health organisation's definition of health: Social versus spiritual Health." *Social Indicators Research* 2/38: 181–192.

Lewis-Fernández, Roberto, Neil Krishan Aggarwal, Ladson Hinton, Devon E. Hinton, Laurence J. Kirmayer, and American Psychiatric Association. 2016; 2015. *DSM-5 Handbook on the Cultural Formulation Interview.* First edition. Washington, DC: American Psychiatric Publishing, Inc.

Lynch, James J., Katz Mikael, and Sylven Schmidt. 1983. *Det brustna hjärtat: Medicinska konsekvenser av ensamhet och isolering*. Stockholm: Natur och kultur.

Lynch, James J. 1977. *The broken heart: The medical consequences of loneliness*. New York: Basic Books.

Lövheim, Mia, and Liv Ingeborg Lied. 2018. "Approaching Contested Religion." In: Knut Lundby (ed.) *Contesting religion. The Media Dynamics of Cultural Conflicts in Scandinavia*. Berlin: De Gruyter. 65–82.

Marliani, Rosleny, Zulmi Ramdani, and Jam'an Muhamad Hasan Imran. 2019. "Validation of Happiness Scale Convergence in Santri through Multi-Trait Multi-Method Analysis." *Psikohumaniora: Jurnal Penelitian Psikologi* 4/2: 143–156.

Medin, Jennie, and Kristina Alexanderson. 2001. *Begreppen hälsa och hälsofrämjande: En litteraturstudie*. Lund: Studentlitteratur.

Melder, Cecilia A. 2011. *Vilsenhetens epidemiologi – en religionspsykologisk studie i existentiell folkhälsa*. Uppsala universitet, Teologiska institutionen. Acta Universitatis Upsaliensis. http://urn.kb.se/resolve?urn=urn:nbn:se:uu:diva-134249

Melder, Cecilia A. 2012. "The epidemiology of lost meaning: A study in the psychology of religion and existential public health." *Scripta Instituti Donneriani Aboensis* 24: 237–258. DOI: 10.30674/scripta.67417

Melder, Cecilia A. 2014a. "Bättre och bättre dag för dag – Existentiell hälsa på äldre dar." In: Susanne Rolfner Suvanto (ed.) *Äldres psykiska hälsa och ohälsa: Prevention, förhållningssätt och arbetsmetoder*. Stockholm: Gothia Fortbildning. 36–63.

Melder, Cecilia A. 2014b. "Utvärderingsrapport: Existentiell hälsa – erfarenheter från ett metodutvecklingsprojekt inom Västmanlands läns Landsting. Landstinget i Västmanland, Kompetenscentrum för hälsa." *Samordningsförbundet Västerås*. http://www.samordningvastmanland.se/vasteras/insatser-i-samverkan/Existentiell_Halsa.shtml.

Melder, Cecilia A. 2019. "It's time to rewrite the model of social determinants of health." Oral presentation. *The 9th Nordic Health Promotion Research Conference (NHPRC) Book of Abstract* 24. Denmark, Roskilde.

Melder, Cecilia A. 2020. "Aktiv livshjälp. Andligvård i folkhälsans tjänst." In: Marie-Anne Ekedahl (ed.) *Livshjälp i en orolig tid. Själavård i forskning och beprövad erfarenhet*. Stockholm: Libris. 93–137.

Melder, Cecilia, Regina Santamäki Fischer, Björn Nygren, and Valerie DeMarinis. 2016. "Validating WHOQOL-SRPB in Sweden: Instrument adaption for measuring existential aspects of health-related quality of life [HRQL] in secular contexts." *Quality of Life Research* 25: 100.

Melder, Cecilia, Ida Jyrell, and Fredrik Söderqvist. 2016. "Measuring adolescents health-related quality of life [HRQL] in a secular context-introducing a Swedish WHOQOL-SRPB-adolescent instrument." *Quality of Life Research* 25: 88.

Melder, Cecilia, and Catrine Kostenius. 2013. "Existentiell hälsa, *Konferens material*." Sweden, Region Jönköping

Melder, Cecilia, and Catrine Kostenius. 2016. "Existential health – developing and evaluating." *Saúde e Sociedade*. São Paulo, v.25: 568–569.

Melder, Cecilia, and Ulla-Karin Nyberg. 2018. "Introducing an existential based suicide prevention, developed for secular contexts." *11th Nordic Conference in Psychology of*

Religion conference. Abstract book. Norway Biri. http://findresearcher.sdu.dk/portal/files/144158790/Abstract_Honne_konf_2018.pdf

Moehling, Krissy K., Mary P. Nowalk, Richard K. Zimmerman, Joyce T. Bromberger, Chyongchiou J. Lin, Samantha E. Ford, and Marnie Bertolet. 2021. "Spirituality, Quality of Life and Frailty in Community-Dwelling Adults ≥ 50 Years." *Psychology of Religion and Spirituality.* https://doi.org/10.1037/rel0000387

Moreira-Almeida, Alexander, Avdesh Sharma, Bernard Janse van Rensburg, Peter J. Verhagen, and Christopher C. H. Cook. 2016. "WPA Position Statement on Spirituality and Religion in Psychiatry." *World Psychiatry* 1/15: 87 – 88.

Nagase, Masako. 2012. "Does a Multi-Dimensional Concept of Health Include Spirituality. Discussionson WHO's 'Definition of Health' (1998)." *International Journal of Applied Sociology* 2/6: 71 – 77. DOI: 10.5923/j.ijas.20120206.03

van Norren, Dorine, and Christopher Beehner. 2021. "Sustainability leadership, UNESCO competencies for SDGs, and diverse leadership models." *International Journal of Development and Sustainability* 10/1: 24 – 49.

Northup, Lesley A. 1990. "The Challenge of the Chaplaincy." Tyson Granvill (ed.) *Military Chaplains' Review. The History and Traditions of Chaplaincy.* U.S. Dept. of Defense, US Army Chaplaincy Services Support Agency. 3 – 14.

O'Connell, Kathryn A., and Suzanne M. Skevington. 2007. "To measure or not to measure? Reviewing the assessment of spirituality and religion in health-related quality of life." *Chronic Illness* 3: 77 – 87. DOI: 10.1177/1742395307079195

O'Connell, Kathryn A., and Suzanne M. Skevington. 2010. "Spiritual, religious, and personal beliefs are important and distinctive to assessing quality of life in health: A comparison of theoretical models." *British Journal of Health Psychology* 15: 729 – 748. DOI: 10.1348/135910709X479799

Oden, Thomas C. 1992. "The historic pastoral care tradition: A resource for Christian psychologists." *Journal of Psychology and Theology* 2/20: 137 – 146.

Okkenhaug, Berit. 2004. *Själavård: en grundbok.* Örebro: Libris.

Oman, Doug, and Syme, S. Leonard. 2018. "Weighing the Evidence: What Is Revealed by 100 + Meta-Analyses and Systematic Reviews of Religion/Spirituality and Health?" In: Oman Doug (ed.) *Why Religion and Spirituality Matter for Public Health.* Springer International Publishing. 261 – 281. https://doi.org/10.1007/978-3-319-73966-3_15

Pellmer, Kristina, Håkan Wramner, and Bengt Wramner. 2017. *Grundläggande folkhälsovetenskap.* 4th edition. Stockholm: Liber AB.

Pettersson, Thorleif. 2006. "Religion in Contemporary Society: Eroded by Human Well-being, Supported by Cultural Diversity." In *Comparative Sociology.* 5/2,3: 231 – 257.

Pettersson, Thorleif. 2016. "Religion och samhällspraktik. En jämförande analys av det sekulariserade Sverige." *Socialvetenskaplig tidskrift* 16/3 – 4. DOI: 10.3384/SVT.2009.16.3 – 4.2497.

Public Health Agency of Sweden. 2020. *Folkhälsans utveckling – årsrapport.* http://www.folkhalsomyndigheten.se/publicerat-material/publikationsarkiv/f/ folkhalsans-utveckling-arsrapport-2020/.

Rapinchuk Kyle D. 2012. "The Servant Motif and Moses in Hebrews 3:1 – 6." *Society Milwaukee.* Wisconsin Evangelical Theological.

Saad, Marcelo, Roberta de Medeiros, and Amanda Cristina Mosini. 2017. “Are we Ready for a True Biopsychosocial-Spiritual Model? the Many Meanings of ‘Spiritual’.” *Medicines (Basel, Switzerland)* 4/4: 79. DOI: 10.3390/medicines4040079
Sakenfeld, Katharine Doob. 2006. *The New Interpreter's Dictionary of the Bible*. Nashville, Tenn: Abingdon.
SALVe. 2014. *Survey of adolescent life Vastmanland*. Västerås: Center for Clinical Research.
Sarkadi, Anna, Lisa Sahlin Torp, Anna Pérez-Aronsson, and Georgina Warner. 2021. “Children's Expressions of Worry during the COVID-19 Pandemic in Sweden.” *Journal of Pediatric Psychology* 46/8: 939–949.
Saxena, Shekhar, Kathryn O'Connell, and Lynn Underwood. 2002. “A Commentary: Cross-Cultural Quality-of-Life Assessment at the End of Life.” *The Gerontologist* 42/342: 81–85.
Schaff, Philip. 1883. “Nicene and Post-Nicene Christianity. From Constantine the Great to Gregory the Great A.D. 311–600 Vol III.” In: *History of the Christian Church, Volume III*.
Shattuck, Eric C., and Michael P. Muehlenbein. 2020. “Religiosity/Spirituality and Physiological Markers of Health.” *Journal of Religion and Health* 59: 1035–1054 https://doi.org/10.1007/s10943-018-0663-6
Shaw, Quentin. 2009. “On aphorisms.” In *British Journal of General Practice*. 59/569: 954–955. DOI: 10.3399/bjgp09X473312
Shiner, Larry. 1967. “The concept of secularisation in empirical research.” *Journal for the Scientific Study of Religion*. 6/2: 207–220. DOI: 10.2307/1384047
Skevington, Suzanne M., and Tracy Epton. 2018. “How will the sustainable development goals deliver changes in well-being? A systematic review and meta-analysis to investigate whether WHOQOL-BREF scores respond to change.” *BMJ Global Health* 3 (Suppl 1), e000609. doi:10.1136/bmjgh-2017–000609
Skevington, Suzanne M., Richard Emsley, Svenja Dehner, Ian Walker, and Stuart E. Reynolds. 2018; 2019. “Does Subjective Health Affect the Association between Biodiversity and Quality of Life? Insights from International Data.” *Applied Research in Quality of Life* 14/5: 1315–1331. DOI: 10.1007/s11482–018–9649–5
Solhi, Mahnaz, Esmaeil Fattahi, Mahnaz Pouresmaeil, Hadi Darvishigilan, Sedighe Rastaghi. 2019. “Letter to Editor: A Comprehensive Definition of Spiritual Health.” *Health, Spirituality and Medical Ethics* 6/3: 2–2.
Sorgenfrei, Simon, and David Thurfjell. 2021. “Inledning.” *Mångreligiositet och sekularitet i svenskt polisväsende, vård, skola och offentlig förvaltning*. En forskningsöversikt. Södertörns högskola. 5–6. http://urn.kb.se/resolve?urn=urn:nbn:se:sh:diva-44285
Svanström, Leif. 1979. “Arbetsmedicin.” In: Karl-Erik Fichtelius (ed.) *Allmänläkarboken*. Studentlitteratur: Lund. 279–297.
Svenska Akademien. 1926. *Ordbok över svenska språket* (8). Lund: Gleerups förlag.
Toniol, Rodrigo. 2019. “Minutes of the spirit. the WHO and instituting spirituality.” *Conference Proceedings, 18th IUAES World Congress: World (of) Encounters: The Past, Present and Future of Anthropological*. 5428–5453.
United Nations (UN). 1989. *General Assembly. Convention on the Rights of the Child. Annu Rev Popul Law* 16/95. 485–501. PMID: 12344587.
Vader, John-Paul. 2006. “Spiritual health: the next frontier.” *European Journal of Public Health* 16/5: 457. DOI: 10.1093/eurpub/ckl234

Vang, Johannes, and Margareta Kristenson. 2000. "The concept of self-rated health." In: Peter Nilsson, and Kristina Orth-Gomer (eds.) *Self-rated Health in a European Perspective. FRN-rapport* 2: 15 – 27. Stockholm: Forskningsrådsnämnden.
Weaver, Andrew J., Kenneth I. Pargament, Kevin J. Flannelly, and Oppenheimer Julia E. 2006. "Trends in the scientific study of religion, spirituality, and health: 1965 – 2000." *Journal of Religion and Health* 45/2: 208 – 214. DOI: 10.1007/s10943 – 006 – 9011 – 3
WHOQOL Group. 1995. "The World Health Organization quality of life assessment (WHOQOL): position paper from the World Health Organization." *Social Science & Medicine* 41/10: 1403 – 1409.
WHOQOL Group. 1998. "WHOQOL User manual." *Department of Mental Health and Substance Abuse.* Geneva: World Health Organization.
WHOQOL-SRPB Group. 2002. "Users Manual, Scoring and Coding for the WHOQOL SRPB Field-Test Instrument." *Department of Mental Health and Substance Dependence.* Geneva: World Health Organization.
WHOQOL-SRPB Group. 2006. "A cross-cultural study of spirituality, religion, and personal beliefs as components of quality of life." *Social Science & Medicine* 62: 1486 – 1497. DOI: 10.1016/j.socscimed.2005.08.001
Willander Erika, Hannah Bradby, Sandra Torres, and Pernilla Jonsson. 2019. "Conditions for Religious Pluralism in Swedish Hospital Chaplaincy: A Research Note." *Journal of Health Care Chaplaincy* 25/3: 99 – 109. DOI: 10.1080/08854726.2018.1548853
Winiger, Fabian and Simon Peng-Keller. 2021. "Religion and the World Health Organization: An Evolving Relationship." *BMJ Global Health* 6/4.
Winnicott, Donald W. 1964. *The Child, the Family, and the Outside World.* Repr. ed. Harmondsworth: Penguin.
Winnicott, Donald W. 1988. *Human Nature.* Taylor & Francis.
Winnicott, Donald W. 2005. *Playing and Reality.* New edition. London: Routledge.
World Health Organization (WHO). 1946. *Constitution* (Document 1). www.who.int/governance/eb/who_constitution_en.pdf
World Health Organization (WHO). 1985. "WHA37.13." In: *Handbook of Resolutions and Decisions of the World Health Assembly and the Executive Board.* Vol. II 1973 – 1984 (WHA37.13 The Thirty-seventh World Health Assembly).
World Health Organization (WHO). 1986. *Ottawa Charter for Health Promotion*, First International Conference on Health promotion, Ottawa, November 21, 1986. http://www.who.int/hpr/NPH/docs/ottawa_charter_hp.pdf
World Health Organization (WHO). 1991. *Sundsvall Statement on Supportive Environments for Health, Third International Conference on Health promotion*, Sundsvall, Sweden, June 9 – 15, 1991. http://www.who.int/healthpromotion/conferences/previous/sundsvall/en/print.html
World Health Organization (WHO). 1998. *Executive Board, 101:st session*, Geneva, January 19 – 27, 1998. www.who.int/iris/handle/10665/255825
World Health Organization (WHO). 2005. *The Bangkok charter for health promotion in a globalized world.*
World Value Survey Association. 2021. "The seventh wave of World Value Survey." Retrieved from https://www.worldvaluessurvey.org/
Zarei, Fatemeh. 2021. "Promoting Spiritual Health: Using Poetry as a Coping Strategy for Iranian Women Post-divorce." In: Hope Corbin, et al. *Arts and Health Promotion: Tools*

and Bridges for Practice, Research, and Social Transformation. SpringerLink. 41–52. https://doi-org.ezproxy.its.uu.se/10.1007/978-3-030-56417-9_3 021. 1–52.
Zastrow, Charles H. 2009. *Social Work with Groups: A Comprehensive Workbook.* 7th edition. Belmont: Cengage Learning.

Su Yon Pak and Gregory Snyder[1]

Uncomfortable wholeness: Buddhist chaplaincy education at a Protestant seminary

Abstract: How can theological education respond to the shape-shifting and expanding nature of chaplaincy? What is the tension between maintaining professional standards while allowing space for new forms of chaplaincy to emerge, especially in increasingly interreligious contexts? What pedagogical innovations need to be developed to support training of chaplains? This chapter highlights the Master of Divinity program with the focus on training of Buddhist chaplains at Union Theological Seminary (NYC), a historically liberal Protestant seminary. It articulates the Buddhism and Interreligious Engagement program, structure, and rationale in the context of Buddhist chaplaincy in the U.S. The authors explore interreligious pedagogical interventions that allow meaningful religious difference to endure while cultivating the possibility for connections to be realized across that difference.

Introduction: The many changing roles of chaplaincy

> In the fall of 2011, I took my class to downtown Manhattan, to Occupy Wall Street where people had been gathering to protest social and economic inequalities. Seeing the need to care for those encamped in Zuccotti Park, some of our students had begun to organize as "protest chaplains." They were not ordained, nor even fully trained. But they saw the need and felt compelled to fill that need. So, after a brief training with the Disaster Relief chaplains on trauma and interreligious spiritual care, they took turns providing "ministry of presence" for those who were occupying Wall Street. My students were learning theology in praxis, in real time.[2]

The above story illustrates the shape-shifting and expanding nature of chaplaincy and the need for us to pay close attention to it. So, we begin with some con-

1 While this is a co-written article, Gregory Snyder took the lead writing all the parts on Buddhist formation/self-inquiry and Su Yon Pak the parts that pertain to Christian formation, chaplaincy, and MDiv standards.

2 While this story is from Su Yon Pak's teaching experience, Joerg Rieger and Kwok Pui-lan have a fuller description of the role of chaplains in the Occupy Wall Street movement (2012, 68).

 https://doi.org/10.1515/9783110717365-010

textual observations. As chaplains become more diverse in terms of religion and world views, so too do the contexts where they work. There are chaplains at the airport, colleges and universities, fire and police departments, prisons, hospitals, hospice, nursing homes, social service agencies, family services, military installations, unions, businesses, seaports, racetracks, truck stops, movement spaces like Occupy Wall Street, Black Lives Matter, and Standing Rock, and online and on the mobile app, like Vennly (bevennly.com). In addition, the COVID-19 pandemic has brought chaplains to the frontlines of the battle in ways that demystified their roles and made them highly visible. In 2020 – 21, many news outlets covered stories about chaplains, their work, their commitments, and their life as the pandemic altered how people were cared for, died, processed grief and loss, and ritualized death. The chaplain's role, along with healthcare professionals, was at the center of the pandemic.[3]

The changing nature of chaplaincy is both a product of and the impetus for the changing religious landscape of the U.S. With the increasing number of Americans claiming "spiritual not religious" or "nones" or "dones" with organized, institutionalized religion (Pew Research Center 2015), chaplaincy is changing in response to the larger movements to reorganize religious life as we know it. More people are seeking spirituality outside of institutional faith communities, bringing religion into public and often secular spaces. However, within spaces that traditionally might have been regarded as secular, many are seeking deep spiritual heritage and training. The current embodiment of spiritual practice regularly defies the traditional categories of religious heritage.[4] Navigating this often-conflicted space, chaplains have become "priest(s) of the secular" (Sullivan 2014, 3) or "twenty-first century's indispensable ministers without portfolio" (Sullivan 2014, 3).

Currently, chaplaincy in the U.S. is developing in two seemingly opposing directions: First, in efforts to move toward professionalization, standardization, and certification, chaplaincy is becoming more regulated by the state via degree and certificate granting bodies. Secular institutions in which chaplains work are likewise highly regulated. Religious traditions engaging chaplaincy in the U.S. are increasing, complicating the formal process of training and certification. What does the increasing interreligious complexity of chaplaincy education

3 For a collection of news about chaplains, see Chaplaincy Innovation Lab, "Chaplaincy in the News." https://chaplaincyinnovation.org/chaplaincy-in-the-news.

4 The Chaplaincy Innovation Lab has taken up addressing chaplaincy as it is being transformed in recent years. Wendy Cadge and Michael Skaggs wrote a case statement for the Chaplaincy Innovation Lab with a helpful overview of the changing landscape of chaplaincy (2018).

mean when many of the assumptions in the professionalization, standardization, and certification process remain Protestant (Sullivan 2014, x)?

Second, chaplaincy is proliferating in new contexts previously unimagined, such as movements like Black Lives Matter or Standing Rock as mentioned above, where chaplains are organized on an ad hoc and temporary basis through organically and more loosely formed networks and social media. These movement spaces are also becoming deeply. Chaplains' varying training is democratizing chaplaincy. While all the competencies of a skillful trauma-informed chaplain are needed in these fast-changing and turbulent spaces, there is no certifying body that credentials such chaplains. That they are highly unregulated raises further questions about effective forms of education.

As regulators, how can we maintain the standards so critical to accountability while creating space for new forms of chaplaincy to emerge? As professional colleagues, how do we support the solid work of traditional chaplaincy and incubate experimentation, like chaplaincy through mobile apps? As educators, how do we create a pedagogy that allows so many meaningful religious differences to endure while cultivating the possibility for connections across those differences? In this emerging territory, how do we take seriously all these intersections and provide a formal education that lays a foundation for this work? Such questions inform Union Theological Seminary's Master of Divinity program that aims to train chaplains across religious traditions, in general, and Buddhist chaplains, in particular, with the interreligious perspectives, interpersonal, self-inquiry, spiritual care, justice commitments, and meaning-making competencies necessary to flourish in this quickly changing field. This chapter explores the opportunities and challenges of a Buddhist chaplaincy program in a historically liberal Protestant seminary.

The context of Buddhist chaplaincy in the U.S.

The Master of Divinity (M.Div.) in Buddhism and Interreligious Engagement (BIE) at Union was born of the relationship between these fundamental questions and the need to educate ordained Buddhist clergy and lay leaders for the complex American religious context. What does sangha (community of spiritual friendship) look like in America, and how do the various expressions of ordained Buddhist clergy relate to it? How do Buddhist clergy function effectively in a society whose religious language, rules of engagement, and polity are so fundamentally Christian that its assumptions are largely invisible? Should Buddhists concern themselves with U.S. credentialing bodies or abide by traditional Buddhist/Asian means for recognizing authority?

Various traditions with an array of sangha relationships have arrived in the U.S. with immigrant Buddhist communities since the early 1800s, blending in complex and contested ways. During the twentieth century, Vinaya-bound[5] monastics supported by the *dana*[6] of a wider lay community, married Zen priests with family temples, and Tibetan gurus in exile –for example– have all landed on U.S. shores tasked with either supporting immigrant heritage[7] communities or navigating the transmission of the Buddhadharma to Western converts. When supporting immigrant communities, ordained Buddhists often find themselves responsible not only for teaching the Buddhadharma but in the role of purveyors and custodians of the entirety of a transplanted culture. Moreover, they are doing so as their communities adapt to often hostile social, economic, and political realities in the U.S. It is likely that most of them were not trained in all the aspects required for the immense breadth of work required here, ranging from cultural support to social services to responding to hate crimes against community members within a foreign context.

While sangha–laity[8] relationships are complicated by new pressures within heritage communities, the Asian expressions of these roles and relationships are often misunderstood, confused, or rejected entirely in so-called convert communities. In convert communities, the complexities of the traditional Buddhist roles of lay and monastic are even more complicated. While the primary relationship between laity and monastics in Asian communities is usually one of devotion, Western, mostly white, lay Buddhists have often either devalued or exoticized devotional practices, rationalized the dharma outside of the cosmologies supportive of devotion, and insisted on taking up the meditative and text-based practices of monastics as lay practitioners (Glieg 2019). Traditional roles of monastics and laity are further blurred because many Japanese and Korean clergy (called priests in the U.S.), are trained monastically while marrying and

5 *Vinaya* refers to the code of conduct adhered to by those who have joined the formal Buddhist monastic community, or *sangha*, as *bhikku* and *bhikkhunī* (monks and nuns).

6 *Dana* refers to generosity, and here specifically, to the act of laity supporting the formal *sangha*.

7 Throughout this article, *heritage* is used to refer to Buddhist practitioners who were born into a Buddhist family of Asian countries where Buddhism is practiced. *Convert* refers to Buddhist practitioners who became Buddhist and are not of Asian heritage. While categories of heritage and convert are popular shorthand, the binary erases important groups like Asian-American practitioners who choose to become Buddhist when their family of origin is not, and European- or African-American practitioners born into families already practicing Buddhism.

8 *Sangha* here specifically refers to the orders of monks and nuns, which would be the traditional usage of the term.

inhabiting what early Buddhism would have regarded as a lay life.[9] These clergy care for temples and families rather than living in a monastic community under the authority of the full Vinaya. Even though the underlying assumptions and orientations are distinct, clergy arrangements of the priestly kind can potentially fit neatly into the Protestant expectations regarding clergy-congregation relationships. Further, many European-descended converts bring Protestant expectations to Buddhist temple leaders, expecting not only dharma talks and times for meditation, but family rites of passage, community engagement programs of social betterment that fit with Western expectations. While these aspects of religious life would be worked out in their traditional contexts, they are unclear in America. Consequently, any common path to understanding how ordained Buddhists are to relate to a lay community in the U.S. vanishes at the moment it is proposed.

Buddhism also spans the same aforementioned changing landscape of religion, both conditioning and conditioned by it. Buddhist practitioners include the deeply devout, insistently secular, multi-generational, newly converted, practice-oriented, study-oriented, ritual-oriented, individual, familial, upholders of the sangha jewel, bedroom-corner sitters, mantra reciters, mindfulness practitioners, the apolitical and the socially engaged. One may even find all of these practicing together in a single temple, seeking guidance from a single teacher. Each of them is in some way trying to understand human life and find relief from *dukkha*, often bringing personal as well as historic, societal *karma* into the work of transformation. Monastic training is often insufficient to address this complexity, especially considering that an increasing number of millennial Buddhist practitioners are requesting dharma teachers and clergy to bring the Buddhadharma to our collective karma born of a legacy of colonialism, genocide, slavery, white supremacy, and misogyny that remains unaddressed in many of our bodies and lives. Regardless of the depth of training and insight, the highly diverse complexities of American society mean Buddhist training communities often struggle to prepare those who will effectively act as clergy for the American context. Leav-

---

9 Here we are drawing a different ordained/lay distinction than is typical in Christianity. The distinction of monastic/lay is the original distinction within Buddhism where monastics take up the renunciant path and the laity are involved in everyday life. However, the rise of ordained non-monastics, predominantly in East Asia, creates a new distinction between priest and lay that is somewhat in tension with the original distinction, resulting in what in the Buddhist context would be lay priests. The meaning of lay then floats between a dialectical relationship with both priest and monastic, recognizing this more recent distinction while honoring the formative and dominant one.

ing this complexity unaddressed risks ignoring the diverse needs of the American Buddhist community.

While we need chaplains trained broadly enough that they are able to adapt to the varying needs of our sanghas, requests for Buddhist teachings and guidance also come to us from beyond the Buddhist communities. Certainly, what we consider to be traditional venues for chaplaincy work – hospitals, prisons, and schools – are increasingly calling on Buddhists to support these spaces. However, Buddhists are also being requested to serve in many burgeoning contexts that are shifting how we think of chaplaincy itself. This shows up in both secular ways (such as giving mindfulness training), as well as religious (teaching formal meditation to Black Lives Matters activists). While more traditional expressions suffer from limited credentialing bodies in the U.S., more secular manifestations often lack appropriate training or at least have no common clarity regarding satisfactory education (Cadge and Skaggs 2018). In both cases, the field of chaplaincy may be uniquely positioned to navigate this multifaceted, emergent terrain.

Add to this a nation that is becoming increasingly syncretic religiously. Many sanghas have a considerable number of multiple belongers (Rajkumar/Dayam 2016). At the Brooklyn Zen Center, where Greg is the senior priest, devoted Buddhist practitioners are also active in the religions of Hinduism, Catholicism, Protestantism, Islam, African ancestral and animist traditions, Paganism, Humanism, and more broadly held Rational Materialist views. Not only do Buddhist clergy need to be trained to lead a sangha in a multi-religious society, they also require the skills to lead a multi-religious sangha.

Master of divinity in Buddhism and interreligious engagement—program structure and rationale

The M.Div. is a professional degree most commonly required for ministers, chaplains, and religious leaders. At Union, the M.Div. program is the largest of all degree programs. Taken full-time, it is a three-year degree that requires 78 credit hours, including 40 to 44 credit requirement in Bible, Church History, Theology, Practical Theology, Interreligious Engagement, 6 credits of field education, and an option to complete a thesis or thesis project. Whereas the curriculum was composed of four classic fields in theological education—Bible, History, Theology, and Practical Theology— in 2013, the faculty adopted a fifth, namely the interreligious engagement field. Membership in this field is made up of faculty from other traditional fields to emphasize the multidisciplinary nature of this endeavor. This also ensures that the work of interreligious engagement occurs across the broader seminary curriculum. The focus and goal of the interreligious engagement field demonstrate the particular methodology embodied at Union:

- The focus of this field is engagement with non-Christian religious traditions potentially spanning a range of disciplines in the seminary curriculum: scripture, theology, worship, ethics, spirituality, etc. The focus of the field on substantive engagement of Christian professionals with different aspects of religious practice and thought of other traditions distinguishes this field from more purely academic approaches to comparative religion, religious pluralism and the like in non-seminary contexts.
- The goal of this field of study is to prepare religious and sociocultural leaders for a multireligious world. Equipping students to draw connections between interreligious dialogue, spirituality, social justice, and other practices is a distinctive feature of this field (as opposed to an exclusive focus on comparative theology). Drawing upon the diverse expertise of a large number of Union's faculty, the interreligious engagement field of study offers courses that focus on specific religious traditions and practices, comparative and dialogical topics, theology of religions and comparative theology.[10]

Creating this new multi-disciplinary field signaled the seminary's commitment to educating religious leaders, including chaplains, who will be ministering in increasingly multi-religious contexts. Strengthening interreligious knowledge became an essential and urgent commitment in ministerial formation. In addition, the fifth field, and subsequent creation of two new tracks to the M.Div., namely, Buddhism and Interreligious Engagement (BIE) and Islam and Interreligious Engagement (IIE), responded to the expanding religious identity of our students and faculty. To further support chaplaincy training, in 2020, Union created a new chaplaincy concentration that overlays the BIE course of study with chaplaincy training. This new concentration combines Union's historic strengths of the psychology and religion discipline and the newer Interreligious Engagement field.

The newly designed flexible M.Div. is a culmination of several years of faculty grappling with the increasing diversity of students, both in terms of vocation and religious identities. Union needed an M.Div. program what would satisfy the learning needs of traditional students seeking ordination in Christian denominations as well as unaffiliated, humanist, Buddhist, and Muslim students seeking to work in various contexts including hospital, hospice, higher education, mili-

10 Excerpted from the full proposal to faculty brought for discussion and vote on November 20, 2013.

tary, prison, and care facilities. Currently, Union offers four tracks in the M.Div. program:[11]

- **Ministerial leadership** prepares students for ordination or other credentialed ministry. Those interested in preparing for non-credentialed ministry, non-profit leadership, or vocations in contexts outside of or beyond a church will find alternative courses that will prepare them for their own calling.
- **Islam and interreligious engagement** prepares students for diverse leadership roles with and in Muslim communities. These roles include religious and spiritual leadership; chaplaincy at universities, hospitals, or prisons; professional counseling (with further clinical training); teaching; and careers in interreligious/interfaith cooperation, policy-making, social justice advocacy, journalism, non-profits, and government.
- **Buddhism and interreligious engagement** prepares students for diverse leadership roles with and in Buddhist communities as well as bringing Buddhist practices and principles to communities that may not identify as Buddhist. These roles include religious and spiritual leadership; chaplaincy at universities, hospitals, or prisons; professional counseling (with further clinical training); teaching; and careers in interreligious/interfaith cooperation, policy-making, social justice advocacy, journalism, non-profits, and government.
- **Anglican studies** prepares individuals for diverse leadership roles within the Episcopal Church, including ordination, chaplaincy, or other ecclesiastical ministries.

Both the Buddhism and Interreligious Engagement concentration and Islam and Interreligious Engagement concentration are embedded in and expanded from the traditional M.Div. curriculum with the four-fold (now five-fold) discipline/field structure of Christian theological education. The historical identity, ethos, curriculum, and culture of Union where Buddhist chaplain formation occurs is still Christian and, more specifically, Protestant. The creation of two additional tracks required two dynamic accommodations in the curriculum. First, Union's M.Div. program goals and outcomes, which are grounded in Christian theological education, needed to be reinterpreted to provide room and rationale for two new tracks. Similarly, both the Buddhism and Islam concentrations needed to work creatively within the curriculum map framed by the M.Div. program goals and outcomes that are based on the Association of Theological Schools (ATS) educa-

11 See M.Div. program guide for complete M.Div. learning goals and outcomes on Union's website https://myunion.utsnyc.edu/myunion/forms.

tional standards for M.Div. programs[12] offered by an accredited theological school. Union's M.Div. program goals give a fuller picture of the curricular frame. They address competency in four learning areas: *religious heritage, cultural context, personal and spiritual formation,* and *capacity for ministerial and public leadership. Religious heritage* includes scriptural, historical, and theological perspectives of Christian traditions as well as interreligious awareness and substantive interreligious engagements. Competencies in *cultural context* include social and cultural understandings necessary for contemporary theologies, the life of the church, and promotion of justice in the world. *Personal and spiritual formation* develops one's own spiritual life and practices as well as guides the spiritual formation of others. *Capacity for ministerial and public leadership* includes developing one's own ministerial identity, interpersonal intelligence, various arts of ministry, and contextually nuanced interpretation of religious traditions informed by interreligious engagement.[13]

The reason for developing an M.Div. BIE program within this broader context is to support those who wish to become Buddhist-literate chaplains, who are entering into leadership as dharma teachers or sangha leaders, or who are already ordained monastics relocating to the U.S. and wanting to be educated for our cultural context. The challenge was to construct a curriculum that balances structure and flexibility to address these varying needs.

The Buddhist core coursework needed to be broad enough to work across many traditions, cultures, and contexts without losing depth and within the limitations of a burgeoning program. In addition, skills-based courses and practicums historically rooted in a Protestant context had to adapt to Buddhist student needs while Buddhist professors must be in dialogue with instructors and facilitators to support this broadening. Finally, the program is Buddhism *and Interreligious Engagement*, meaning that IE skills must be articulated and reinforced throughout the coursework.

Only the specifics of the BIE program vary considerably from its Christian counterpart. Thus, the Bible requirement has expanded to include Sacred Texts (courses like "Zen Buddhist Texts" and "Reading Early Buddhist Texts");

12 For the complete list of M.Div. program standards, see Association for Theological Schools Commission on Accrediting Degree Standards. https://www.ats.edu/uploads/accrediting/documents/degree-program-standards.pdf. In June 2020, ATS revised the standards of accreditation which can be found here: https://www.ats.edu/uploads/accrediting/documents/standards-of-accreditation.pdf#pagemode=bookmarks.

13 For the complete M.Div. learning goals and outcomes, see https://utsnyc.edu/wp-content/uploads/MDiv-Program-Guide-2022-23.pdf, 3–5.

History now includes "Global Buddhist Histories," and Theology, "Buddhist Religious Thought."

Our BIE students study not only their own sacred texts but also those of other faiths, including Christianity, Islam, Hinduism, and Judaism along with indigenous spiritual practice and thought. In the first year, BIE students take an "Introduction to Christian Theology"; in learning how Christianity has critically engaged its tradition, they gain skills in which many Buddhists are not trained. "Introduction to the Bible" and "Zen Buddhist Texts" provide basic exegetical skills and hermeneutical lenses for engaging sacred texts. Buddhist Religious Thought introduces the grounding dharmic concepts of Buddhism. The first-semester requirement of "Religions in the City" gives all M.Div. students the opportunity to visit and practice with other faith traditions in New York City while being instructed in the foundational theories and methodologies of Interreligious Engagement.

In the first year, our "Introduction to Buddhist Meditation Practices" addresses spiritual formation. It introduces BIE students to a wide array of Buddhist meditation practices through primary, mostly early Pali texts. Each week they take up a different practice, until they have basic knowledge of the interrelationship of these practices and how they can be used in their work. Learning basic language and concepts through such practice-based engagement orients their future Buddhist studies appropriately. "Introduction to Pastoral and Spiritual Care" serves as a foundational course in how to work in a pastoral context, critical to chaplaincy and lay sangha service.

Finally, through "Socially Engaged Buddhism," a study of colonial and postcolonial Buddhist social movements in Asia and "Comparative Buddhist–Christian Liberation Theologies," which compares Christian liberation theology and Socially Engaged Buddhist movements, students explore community organizing and an array of justice issues through Buddhist frames. The first year is designed to provide the necessary foundations for the many possible needs and directions a Buddhist student might choose to take through their time at Union. Our current recommended program path for M.Div. BIE students follows:

> **FIRST YEAR**: The first year focuses on foundations in Buddhist thought and practice, Christian thought and practice, Interreligious Engagement and Spiritual/Pastoral Care, which collectively prepare BIE students for education pathways in the ensuing years. Specific capacities cultivated: meditation practices, self-inquiry, pastoral/spiritual care, IE methodologies and praxis, familiarity with texts and religious language across traditions, exegesis, hermeneutics, constructive theology, historical and social contextualization. The first semester provides the basic experiences and tools for a depth of learning within and across traditions.

First-year Fall Semester:

- Introduction to Buddhist Meditation Practices
- Religions in the City: Introduction to Interreligious Engagement
- Introduction to Pastoral & Spiritual Care
- Introduction to the Bible

First-year Spring Semester:

- Buddhist Religious Thought
- Foundations in Christian Theology
- Socially Engaged Buddhism
- Christianity in Historical Perspective

SECOND YEAR: With a focus on developing pastoral imagination and a capacity for theological reflection in field practice, the second year continues to deepen, broaden and integrate all of the capacities introduced in the first year. While there is a stronger focus on Buddhist texts and history in the second year, it is informed by IE frames developed in the first. Having basic skills in meditation and pastoral care in the first year are critical supports for the second.

Second-year Fall Semester:

- Buddhist Sacred Text Requirement, e.g. Zen Buddhist Texts, Reading Early Buddhist Texts: Ethics, Meditation, and Wisdom, etc.
- Buddhist Global Histories
- Field Education Seminar I
- Practical Theology or Additional IE Requirement

Second-year Spring Semester:

- Buddhist Concentration Requirement*
- Field Education Seminar II
- Practical Theology or Additional IE Requirement
- Buddhist Concentration Requirement or General Elective

A unit of Clinical Pastoral Education is highly recommended during the summer after the first or second year.

THIRD YEAR: In the third year, students focus on the integration and articulation of practical and academic aspects of their education as they formulate an engaged Buddhist vision of chaplaincy and leadership.

Third-year Fall Semester:

- Buddhist Concentration Requirement or General Elective (4 courses)

Third-year Spring Semester:

- Thesis
- Buddhist Concentration Requirement or General Elective (2 courses)

For students in the BIE-Chaplaincy concentration, they are required to complete courses in Psychology and Religion in addition to the BIE course requirements. The following are examples of Psychology and Religion courses:

- Introduction to Pastoral and Spiritual Care
- Pastoral Listening Practicum
- Chaplaincy
- Professional Ethics for Spiritual Care
- Trauma Informed Pastoral and Spiritual Care
- Death, Dying, and Bereavement
- Buddhism and Psychoanalysis: A Healing Partnership

The following are examples of Buddhist concentration electives:[14]

- Buddhist Psychology: Healing Intergenerational Trauma, Difficult Emotions, and Colonial Mentality
- Reading Early Buddhist Texts: Ethics, Meditation, and Wisdom
- Indo-Tibetan Buddhism
- Community Engaged Buddhism: Organizing for an Alternate Housing Future
- Buddhist-Christian Dialogue: Rereading of Parables and Stories in Buddhism and Christianity
- Comparative Buddhist-Christian Liberation Theologies
- Asian Theologies
- Double Belonging (focuses on Buddhist-Christian dialogue)
- Introduction to Self-Inquiry
- Integrative Path Personal & Social Healing: Buddhist Phenomenology
- Chaplaincy Through Theravada Lens
- Guided Readings in Buddhism

Throughout this program, Buddhist students are navigating the tensions of learning their own religious practice alongside those of others. Conflicting basic assumptions and analytical frames come into glaring relationship, highlighting areas where one's own unconscious assumptions require nuance and clarification to oneself, where foreign frames support, complicate, or confuse this clarification, where differences eventually resolve, and where the questions of one religion may simply not be the questions of another. While knowledge of other religions is cultivated, we suggest that wholeness of one's own faith is found through this process of interreligious learning. Wholeness as a process of deepening roots in a tradition is an alternative to purity of faith. While the process of becoming whole through engagement is uncomfortable, if not deeply painful and ungrounding, it is this path that cultivates the stable roots and flex-

14 Pali and Sanskrit courses are offered as summer intensives and also fulfill these requirements.

ibility in both the chaplain and religious tradition itself that is so desperately needed in our world. We tend to grasp our traditions as identities. In engaging other traditions, these identities are destabilized. In the best case, we open our grasp and connect to the other. Both of these processes are painful because they take us into the unknown. The typical egoic response to the unknown is resistance, and then we move through fear, grief, and loss before experiencing the joy of connection. One cannot truly commune with the other without first releasing and grieving one's grasped identities. Students come to realize that traditions and convictions are strengthened through this clarifying process of respectful interreligious engagement that often challenges our very core.

Successful implementation of the BIE program depends on this uncomfortable wholeness or "practical vulnerability" as our colleague John Thatamanil proposes, the posture of openness to the claims and aims of the other religious tradition(s) and a "commit[ment] to remain[...]in such intimate proximity" to those traditions (Thatamanil 2016, 356). It is an openness even to take on the practices of the other tradition "in order to see and to know as the other does" (Thatamanil 2016, 356). This "truth-seeking inquiry" respects the other persons and traditions toward mutual transformation (Thatamanil 2016, 358). It leads to interreligious wisdom.

Such interreligious wisdom is now essential for all chaplains. Educating for that interreligious wisdom is complex and contextual, and offers opportunities for creative pedagogical method. Thatamanil offers one such method for teaching Hindu-Christian Dialogue and courses on religious diversity. He frames his courses using "a medical model" of questions derived from Buddha's Four Noble Truths and invites students to put those questions to any text or thinker: "How does this text/thinker diagnose the human predicament? What is the etiology of that predicament? What is the prognosis? What is the therapy?" (Thatamanil 2016, 361). Bringing these questions to our own and others' traditions is an opportunity for sincere respect and deepened respect.

Educating toward wholeness: Interreligious engagement capacity-building for Chaplains

We turn now to discuss the interreligious engagement of capacities that transpire when offering Buddhist education within a historically Protestant seminary. First, we explore a Christian practice of theological reflection as one method to cultivating pastoral-moral imagination. Second, we explore the notion of self-inquiry, a central practice and capacity within the Buddhist tradition.

What resonance and dissonance do theological reflection and self-inquiry have when they are employed across religious traditions?

One of the fundamental goals of a seminary education is cultivating "pastoral imagination" in students, the multi-dimensional capacity that integrates the head, heart, and the spirit in response to the pastoral situation itself. To cultivate this imaginative capacity, we exercise four formative practices. First, one practices sustained engagement with sacred texts and practices of one's tradition(s). From this engagement, a pastor should be able to (re)interpret the sacred texts and traditions for this contemporary life and context. Second, one develops an understanding of human nature and a solid appreciation "of what makes human beings tick, of who people are and how they operate" (Dykstra 2008, 52). This practice also requires one to know oneself through a disciplined examination of one's conditioning as well as one's formation, discernment, spiritual practices, and theological reflections on those practices. Third, one hones skills for complex understanding of organizations and institutions—what they are, how they operate, both on a day-to-day level as well as on a longer-term strategic and structural level—to align the mission and values of the organization with organizational practices.[15] And the fourth practice offers a historical, contextual, and critical understanding of the world that the church/faith communities exist to serve. These four practices are woven together with a desire to know what it means to worship God and are context-specific.

Yet the term "pastoral" is limiting to our diverse student body for whom "pastoral" signifies "Christian" and "parish." Instead, what is needed alongside pastoral imagination is its prophetic partner—"moral imagination"— which requires clear-eyed analyses of power of systems, structures, and relationships and how they create injustices and inequalities, which values sacred dignity and agency of all people, and which fuels our fight against injustices. Moral imagination believes in the power of life over death, freedom over captivity. It is fueled by our courage to ask and enact, "what if?".[16]

While the imaginative capacity is in the function and the realm of the mind, moral imagination relies on bodily knowing, memories, and stories that live in

15 See the four-frames approach to organization and leadership by Lee Bolman and Terrence Deal. They advocate for identifying, understanding, and reframing four distinct frames (structural, human resource, political and symbolic) that operate in organizations and leaders. The skills of reframing these distinct frames give us a more comprehensive picture about a complex organization (2017).

16 Kelly Brown Douglas advocates for the prophetic religious tradition of the African American communities—moral memory, moral identity, moral participation, and moral imagination—as a way to break the racist structures, patterns, and practices in the society (2015).

our bodies and also the spaces in and through which our bodies move.[17] It is an integrative, embodied capacity for practical wisdom, *phronesis*. It is also the most difficult knowledge to learn and teach, especially in an interreligious space where our bodies move and present themselves very differently from each other.

While connecting the imaginative capacity to the full embodiment of wisdom aligns nicely with the Buddhist tradition, in the Dhammacakkapavattana Sutta, the Buddha was clear that there are three kinds of knowing: intellectual understanding, the process of deepening with that understanding into the body through practice, and then finally a deeply embodied knowing that is the foundation of one's actions in the world. Imagination, or what Buddhists would call *upaya* (skillful means) emerges from the full embodiment of the Buddhadharma. Buddhism brings to moral imagination 2600 years of practices whose primary aim is the embodiment of a clarified wisdom – moral, epistemological and ontological – compassion, and skillful means necessary to alleviate *dukkha*, or suffering for self and others. This process is the foundation for any skillful Buddhist chaplain whose ongoing practice would unfold *upaya* and the moral imagination.

However, a question for Buddhists is always one of societal context when it comes to *upaya*. The Buddha challenged caste bias regarding access to religious authority allowing all castes into the sangha and changing the cosmological genesis story with the Aggañña Sutta (Sujato 2018). Yet he did not openly challenge slavery as far as we can tell. Chinese Zen monastics both defied and supported the violence of imperial governments. Japanese monastics were divided across World War II aggression, some openly preaching in its favor. Sri Lanka gave birth to A.T. Ariyaratne and the Sarvodaya movement as well as monks effectively calling for genocide of the Tamil. A reluctant Buddha admitted that women were equal to men and gave them access to the monastic order. Yet, it is arguable that women have never received equal treatment or institutional support throughout the history of Buddhist practice. So when we speak of devotion to no harm and the liberation of all beings, do we also mean economic, political, racial, and gender violence? Are we also speaking about issues of justice? If so, how do we train Buddhist clergy to cultivate the moral imagination necessary to address these issues?

To this point, the tradition of cultivating pastoral and moral imagination, at least as it is understood and taught at Union, offers rich opportunities to Bud-

---

17 See Mai-Anh Le Tran (2017, 16–17) for a discussion on "testifying bodies" and "teaching bodies."

dhist students. The first point mentioned above includes the ability to "(re)interpret the sacred texts and traditions for this contemporary life and context" (Dykstra 2008, 52). The work of theology, as a necessary component of the context-specific spiritual practice of ministry, is one of the primary gifts that Union has to offer Buddhist clergy, especially where liberation, womanist and other theologies engaging a socially critical lens are concerned. While Buddhist students would likely translate theology into the framework of *upaya*, the engagement of social liberationist thought and movements for the purposes of ending *dukkha* is relatively recent to Buddhism, at least as gauged by surviving texts. Moreover, the consideration of the social positions of those giving and receiving the teachings as a frame for critiquing and considering skillful adaptations to varying contexts is critical to a Buddhadharma that does not inadvertently cause harm. Over time, Buddhism has always adapted to its context. But it is something else to train Buddhists how to do so consciously, thoughtfully, and effectively.

On the second point of ensuring a "disciplined examination of one's conditioning," while the training of Buddhist chaplains requires psychological nuance and skills likely missing in monastic training, Buddhism brings a great deal to the examination of conditioning. As the latter will be dealt with in the discussion of self-inquiry, we do not mention it here. However, it cannot be overstated how important training in transference/counter-transference and other Western psychological insights is for Buddhist chaplains and leaders who so often require support with egoic confusion and moral clarity.

Regarding the third point that pastoral imagination must include a "complex understanding of organizations and institutions," (Dysktra 2008, 52) those from traditions like Soto Zen who have worked their way up through the ranks and understand how monastic organizations function are the minority. Most incoming Buddhist students have few skills in administering institutions, nor are they aware of the tradition's positions on institutions.

Finally, one of the most important areas of exchange for BIE students at Union is the fourth aspect of pastoral imagination—that of developing "a historical, contextual and critical understanding of the world." This ties into the first point regarding the work of theology, but especially focuses on understanding the complexity of this moment and place in history so that we can respond skillfully. As an example, one cannot effectively teach the dharma without harm in the U.S. if one is not familiar with our history of racial violence. One cannot be an effective Buddhist chaplain without this knowledge. Any expression of the Buddhadharma must be both located and universal.

Moreover, karmic liberation requires the understanding of karmic conditions. Without a knowledge of the karmic effects of one's society and collective history, those effects will be internalized, unconsciously framing our expression of the Buddhadharma and thereby potentially causing unintentional harm when such views give rise to unconscious intentions and consequent actions. A Buddhist education that does not take into account histories of social violence reduces karma to a theory of individualized seeds and fruits that are divorced from the broader social reality that is the context from which a particular person's karma unfolds. The social, historical, and critical training emphasized in this aspect of pastoral imagination promotes a real-life reflection of *pratityasamutpada*,[18] allowing for *upaya* and *karuna* (compassionate action) to manifest in ways that meaningfully address the suffering of the world. For the Buddhist leader and chaplain in the U.S., this education must be central so that further harm is reduced.

A seminary education brings this wide array of knowledge to Buddhist students. That knowledge is spread across far too many courses to explicate here. To illuminate how this training might unfold for a BIE student, we turn to one aspect of training around pastoral imagination: theological reflection.

Theological reflection and moral imagination across traditions

How do we cultivate pastoral-moral imagination in students? Theological reflection is one practice that is at the heart of pastoral formation. In Su's work as a theological field educator, she witnesses the transformative capacity of reflecting and thinking theologically and of creatively bringing to bear the full resources of one's religious tradition(s) in shaping students' practice of spiritual care, their understanding of the other, and their cultivation of pastoral imagination. Theological reflection has a wide range of goals including personal and communal transformation, community building, accompaniment, and making sense of suffering (Foley 2014, 34:72). It is a life-long work that improves with practice. Whether it is called "reflective believing" (Foley 2015), "making faith sense" (Kinast 1999), "knowing-in-action" (Bounds 2008), or "pastoral cycle" (Holland and Henriot 1983), theological reflection is an exploration of individual and communal experiences in conversation with the wisdom of our religious traditions. It surfaces our beliefs, theology, perspectives, and actions as well as those of the

18 Often translated as dependent origination, *pratityasamutpada* in its simplest form is the Buddhist teaching that all *dharmas* – here best translated as phenomena – arise in causal relationship with all other dharmas. No dharma is ever ultimately independent.

traditions. Another way of thinking about it is to ask the questions: Where is God in this situation? Where is God present? Absent? What is God calling us to do? This action-reflection-action method confirms and challenges, orients and disorients for the sake of expanding our understanding both of our experiences and of our tradition. The result is a new understanding and meaning for our lives.

This process critically engages the whole self in context, employing traditions/disciplines of inquiry. While there are many different ways to do theological reflection, Patricia O'Connell Killen and John De Beer's method is particularly effective: a) one narrates an experience; b) in contemplation and engaging feelings that arise, one lets the heart of the matter emerge; c) one explores and reflects on the heart of the matter with traditions and disciplines of inquiry; d) one allows new insights to emerge; e) one structures action that arises out of this reflection (Killen and De Beer 1994).

Because theological reflection begins with experience, contemplation on that experience necessarily involves embodied knowledge. Feelings, emotions, bodily sensations, and images assist in exploring the heart of the matter. Theological reflection then engages our intellect as we put critical theological frameworks as well as our traditions in conversation with the heart of the matter. This rigorous exchange can create a disorienting, liminal space, yet one from which new insights emerge from which we return to practice (Cameron, Reader, Slater, and Rowland 2012). And when theological reflection is done together across religious traditions, the assumptive world framed by this Christian method may collide with others' world views and cosmologies and challenge or affirm them.

Edward Foley has taken up the task of exploring theological reflection across religious traditions by moving away from tradition/religion-specific terminologies. He calls this "reflective believing" by which he means, "a meaning-making practice, exercised in light of one's individual or shared wisdom-heritage, that honors the experiences and stories of its participants" (Foley 2015, 92). Engaging the head, the heart, and the hands, Foley asserts that reflective believing is an "invitation to intimacy as spiritual community" (Foley 2015, 42).

In Su's field education seminar class, she introduces this method of theological reflection as an essential tool of engagement for ongoing pastoral reflection and formation. When she teaches this method to Buddhist students in her class, she is acutely aware that even though she has broadened this process for non-Christians, it still bears the imprint of Christian practice. At the same time, this practice is at the heart of building capacity for practical wisdom for chaplaincy and any ministry vocation. This circular movement of practice, reflection, and return to practice is a life-long reflective art form which becomes a habitus (Pak 2020).

How might a Buddhist student utilize theological reflection for their own pastoral formation? Ian Case, a Buddhist student in the M.Div. BIE program was a field education intern at the Manhattan Detention Complex, a New York City jail that detains people awaiting trial. For one of his verbatims, Ian wrote a theological reflection on an encounter with the detainee in jail. We wanted to understand more fully, how he experienced doing theological reflection as a Buddhist. We asked Ian to write a second-order reflection on theological reflection process for this chapter.

Some reflections on Buddhist theological reflection

Ian Case (M.Div. '20 Buddhism and Interreligious Engagement Concentration)

As an American convert Buddhist, there is already a certain kind of "translation" or "cultural rearticulation" that necessarily functions as an aspect of my spiritual path. While I wasn't brought up in a specific faith tradition or in an especially religious household, I was certainly raised in an overall Christian cultural context. Taking up a Buddhist practice meant learning a different vocabulary, embodying new ritual forms, and relating to others within a new ethical framework—and approaching all of this from a position and a mind/body that had been enculturated by Christian assumptions (not to mention the other dimensions of my social conditioning). For the most part—especially during the first few years of my practice—this rearticulation happened implicitly and automatically.

That being said, the reality of studying Buddhism at a largely Protestant seminary did not come as that much of a shock to the system. I was already used to navigating across this difference. The main effect of being at Union has been to make me more sensitive and deliberate about the process. I was lucky to be able to take a course on Buddhist-Christian liberation theology during my first semester, and this class served as a primer for doing this kind of interreligious rearticulation in an academic setting. It also became very clear that "translation" is not always possible or preferred. Traditions also need to be understood and appreciated on their own terms. My rearticulation became more nuanced, more careful.

Another effect of studying at Union was that I began to think about Buddhism "theologically," as an integrated system of philosophical/psychological/ethical teachings and practices that is always dynamically situated in history and social contexts. I understood Buddhist soteriology not as salvation but as liberation from suffering (which may be variously defined depending on context).

When I was first introduced to the practice of theological reflection, I understood "theology" within this Buddhist context and I saw the reflection as a process of meaning-making within that frame. My first attempts at the practice—during my first year—were a bit intellectual and forced. I felt as if I was searching my own archives of the Buddhist tradition for a teaching that would fit the situation. And then I would try to extract some insight from the teaching to apply to the situation in question.

Once I started doing these reflections in the context of chaplaincy, however, the process became much more organic and natural. As I reflected on the pastoral situation, I would make an effort to completely let go of all of my preconceived ideas of how the situation *should* develop or what I *should* do. At the same time, I would bring my awareness to my body and allow sensations and energies to arise. In this sense, this part of the process was very much about not knowing and renunciation—giving up any notion of control and just being open to what emerges in the moment.

Eventually, something *does* emerge. Sometimes I will see the situation with more clarity, or I'll see some aspect of my own conditioning that is functioning in the situation (and which I missed before). These feel like gifts that arise from the reflective process and the beginning of a kind of meaning-making. As more of the heart of the matter is revealed in this process then a conversation with my tradition (and with my own experience of practice) can start to happen. Again, this is not necessarily willful. Connections and resonances become evident. In the best case, there is a resonance not just with the teaching but also with my embodied understanding of the teaching. As the conversation develops, this will often generate deeper insights into the situation and the overall pastoral plan. Sometimes a response is clarified.

This stage of the process can be understood as confessional in a certain sense. In the Zen tradition, I understand confession to have two aspects: first I must acknowledge the action in question (see it clearly) and then I must take responsibility for it. As I let the situation or interaction speak to me, I begin to see emerging themes (and my own karmic tendencies) more clearly. I may see where the suffering is. Once this happens, I can begin to take responsibility for my part or I might see areas where agency is possible for those I am serving. I can also take responsibility for whatever aspect of the teaching is illuminated in the process; I can own that as one possible interpretation of the living encounter.

The process of theological reflection is iterative and ongoing, supporting more skillful responses from a position of humility and not knowing.

Here, Ian clearly articulates many of the themes so far expressed in this paper as he respectfully engages traditional chaplaincy training around pastoral-moral imagination and theological reflection from his own Buddhist positionality. In fact, his insight about theological reflection that leads to the Buddhist notion of confession is a powerful enhancement of the reflective process that could have only come about through interreligious encounter.

Practicing self-inquiry across traditions

What of the skills and capacities that Buddhism brings to a seminary and chaplaincy training program? For starters, it brings a long history of systematic inquiry into the nature of self and being; the threefold training of *sila* (ethical discipline), *samadhi* (mental discipline) and *prajna* (embodied, phenomenological realization) provide a path for taking full responsibility for who we are in the world. *Ethical discipline* is not only aimed at transforming behavior from unwholesome to wholesome, but morality as a practice is itself a mirror to the self-clinging mind, meaning that *sila* is a support for the mind's unbinding, greater stability, deeper realization, and final liberation. In turn, the gathering and stabilizing of mental factors in *samadhi* cultivate a fertile garden for moral clarity and dharmic insight. To lie, steal, or otherwise act in unwholesome ways destabilizes the mind, causing us to falter on our path to freedom. Third and finally, the deepening realization of *pratityasamutpada* delivers the mind from its obsession with, and grasping of conventional and ultimate truths, and points human life right back to relational morality and the immediacy of our interconnected life. To do this transformative work with integrity requires each of us to do as the thirteenth-century Zen Buddhist monk, Eihei Dogen, instructed and "learn the backward step that turns your light inwardly to illuminate the self" (Waddell and Abe 2002). For the sake of shorthand, we will refer to Dogen's "backward step" as self-inquiry.

While there is certainly a strong encouragement of moral commitment at Union, of theological reflection and voice, of critical engagement with the text, analysis of power, interreligious engagement, and social justice work on all fronts, from a Buddhist perspective Union lacked the cultivation of self-inquiry that matures the self-knowledge and capacities necessary to engage the painful, demanding, spiritually transformative work of constructive theology and social change. In some cases, it seemed clear this was a barrier to deepening theological and moral commitments as well as cultivating key capacities for chaplaincy. Many non-Buddhist students have felt comfortable taking Buddhist courses to develop these capacities. Many have very skillfully integrated them into their own spiritual formation. Usually at least one third of participants in the course, "Introduction to Buddhist Meditation Practices" are non-Buddhist. However, courses in Buddhist practice do not necessarily support non-Buddhist students in developing self-inquiry language and skills within their own tradition.

After much discussion with colleagues about this matter, this perceived need led Greg to create the course, "The Practice of Self-Inquiry," which draws from multiple religious traditions as well as European and African phenomenology, existentialism, and post-structuralism for guidance on how to think about self-inquiry within one's own tradition. Beginning with Husserl, we worked our way through Butler, Dostoyevsky, Ellison, Foucault, Plato, the Buddha, Descartes, Fanon, de Beauvoir, hooks, Ignatius, Al-Ghazzali, Sankaracarya, Suzuki, Dogen, and others, exploring the various potential objects of inquiry, methods of suspension of investment in those objects, the reliability of the observer/narrator, normative versus liberative teleologies, rational, imaginative and phenomenological methodologies, skepticism, theories of body, decolonization, gendered experience, and examples of Hindu, Muslim, Buddhist and Christian inquiry models. Then we asked students to address the following issues in the formation of a personal methodology of self-inquiry:

- *What is the self:* How does the student understand the self ontologically? Where is it experienced and what is the nature of what is being located?
- *A theory of body is a theory of perception:* Taking the suggestion from Merleau-Ponty, how does the student understand and experience the body as it relates to the self and experience of a world (Merleau-Ponty 2002)?
- *Suspension:* Informed by writings of Eihei Dogen, Edmund Husserl, and others, student's look at what it is to cultivate a stable witness for their experience as a phenomenological foundation for the process of self-inquiry (Husserl 2012).
- *Teleology:* What is the purpose of the inquiry? Is it soteriological, aimed at pure knowledge, moral betterment, etc.? How does the aim affect the means by which it is obtained?
- *Confession and renunciation as process of inquiry:* All self-inquiry requires a form of confession and renunciation to maintain a reliable inquiry. This is especially the case when morality is centered. For the student, is confession and renunciation normalizing, cultivating, liberatory, or otherwise?
- *Scene of address:* Who is being addressed in the inquiry? Is it to yourself? God? An imagined moral other? A communal other? Ancestors? The Earth? Non-human sentient beings?
- *Epistemological method:* Is the inquiry phenomenological with regard to direct observations? Is it rational with regard to metaphysical conclusions? Is it imaginative, or does it claim some other method? How do you discern and articulate the difference as you shift from one to another? —
- *Reliability of Inquirer:* How does one discern and account for reliability of the inquirer, whether it be a manifestation of resistance, deception, forgetfulness, ignorance, the mere fact of our conditioned nature, or, as Butler suggests, when the subject is not the authority of their own account due to lack of memory in early life (Butler 2009)?
- *Responding to Resistance:* What are the methods and practices the student will use to address resistance to more difficult threads of inquiry?
- *Social Critique:* If the "I" is a function of norms and conditions, then self-inquiry includes engaging social conditioning and therefore becomes a form of social critique. How is this navigated with clarity? Where does moral responsibility lie when the self is a site of social reproduction?
- *Exposure/*being (intimate and anonymous) *vs. narrated self* (published & substitutable). The former, which is basic experiential presence, cannot be narrated even though it structures all narrated accounts of self.

These areas of thought were treated methodologically, not simply theoretically. Students were asked to uncover how they understood *suspension* of mundane mental processes within their practices, critically engaging Husserl (2015) as only one example to frame the problem. Were students engaging in rational, imaginative, phenomenological, another, or multiple methods of inquiry? How did they deal with resistance to process? What is the teleological trajectory that guides the process – salvation, clarity, liberation, moral normativity? What was their method for confessing errors (however they define them) and renouncing them in order to reconnect with the path? What or who is the "scene of address" as Butler (2009) describes it? In other words, who are they unconsciously addressing in their inquiry? How do they ensure the reliability of their self-inquiry process? These, among many other questions, resulted in one of the most exciting, productive, and rewarding classes Greg has ever facilitated. He was privileged to watch a very religiously diverse group of students work diligently together to create personal methodologies of self-inquiry that seemed very much to clarify and deepen their spiritual paths. We asked two students in the class to write a reflection about the process of self-inquiry for this chapter. Hear what students said about the process:

Reflection on interreligious engagement and spiritual formation: A Christian student's perspective

Kristine Chong (M.Div. '19, Ethics concentration)

Given my family's history of migration (triggered by U.S. militarism and neocolonialism in the Korean peninsula) and embeddedness in the Christian church (my father is an ordained pastor), my seminary journey can be characterized as a constant negotiation of my Christian tradition/identity with the multiplicities of my historical-racial schema. Having begun the work of examining and integrating my ancestral and historical spiritual roots in other courses and engagements at Union, taking Professor Snyder's course on "The Practice of Self- Inquiry" during my last semester of the M.Div. program at Union was a pivotal experience. I consider the course to be a capstone of my seminary education, as it offered a site of assessment, articulation, and affirmation of my formation as a Korean American diasporic womxn of Christian upbringing training to be a chaplain in an interreligious and postmodern context.

Engaging in the self-inquiry process enabled me to systematically assess my own practices and assumptions as a Christian-raised, multiply-formed practitioner. As the class introduced self-inquiry practices from various religious traditions as well as non-religious phenomenological thinkers, the focus on metapraxis as the locus of engagement was generative for students to articulate our understanding and the aim of our self-inquiry. Learning the methods of self-inquiry gave vocabulary to my existing practice – such as suspension, subjectivity of self, bodily presence, discernment, confession, and scene(s) of address – and the assumptions, worldviews, and habits that both underlie and orient self-inquiry practices. Since self-inquiry is a crucial component to how I as a chaplain ground and prepare myself when engaging with people, having diverse frameworks and sources to understand my practices (such as that of the Examen), prepares me to be a more self-aware and spacious spiritual caregiver.

Moreover, articulating my self-inquiry process facilitated new insights about my formation, discernment, and theological reflections as a developing chaplain. Examining my self-inquiry practices reflected my spiritual development at an institution like Union, a historically Protestant seminary oriented towards interreligious theological education. My practices encompass Christian ones, such as the Examen[19] (as taught by Professor Roger Haight, S.J.), centering prayer[20] (as introduced by my peers) – as well as other traditions, including mindfulness meditations (as facilitated by Professor Tara Chung) and rituals that incorporate indigenous Korean traditions such as *Tonghak* ("Eastern Learning")[21] and shamanism. Dialoguing with multiple sources and traditions has helped me to trace lineages and identify new linkages between my existing self-inquiry practices and my ongoing formation as a chaplain who will interact with people of diverse and multiple religious identities. As I cultivate a deeper connection and sense of my multitudinous identity and history, I have a richer reservoir of resources to utilize for spiritual care.

A key realization I had through the self-inquiry class was how significant the Zen Buddhist practice of living by vow is for my self-inquiry process and chaplaincy work. Living so that "life is itself a vow," a practice that is endless, helps me to dismantle a capitalist and neoliberal worldview prominent in Christian theologies that focus on a linear, progressive trajectory and teleology (Okumura, 2012, 30). In fact, my struggles of feeling like chaplaincy is "not productive or effective enough" are grounded in an output-oriented economy. Thus, living by vow – which for me is comprised of *imago dei* (the view that every person/being is created in the image of God/mystery) and *jeong* (a Korean concept of right-relation that encompasses compassion, affection, solidarity, and vulnerability) – enacts a relational, ethical, and care-oriented metapraxis that undergirds my chaplaincy ethos. I would not have come to this realization and integration without a co-learning interreligious space, nor without a Buddhist instructor and colleagues.

Amidst the various values of interreligious engagement, challenges also existed in the self-inquiry class. The sets of "conditioning moral norms" entangled in the "prevailing ma-

---

19 The Examen is an ancient Christian practice of daily prayerful reflection and discernment of God's presence, as conceived and taught by Ignatius of Loyola (who founded the Society of Jesus order, or the Jesuits) in the sixteenth century.

20 Centering prayer is a form of contemplative prayer and meditation that developed from mystical traditions within western Christianity, such as the Desert Mothers and Fathers and the fourteenth-century treatise, *The Cloud of Unknowing*. Centering prayer focuses on interior silence and letting go of words, images, and emotions, with the exception of using a sacred word to symbolize one's intention of inward receptiveness to divine presence and action (Thompson, 2014, 47–48).

21 *Tonghak* was an indigenous political, social, economic, and religious movement in Korea in the late 1800s. An amalgamation of various religious and philosophical ideologies – including shamanism, Neo-Confucianism, Buddhism, Taoism, and western learning (Christianity) – *Tonghak* preached a message of equality for all people and a heaven on earth. The movement led to the Tonghak Rebellion of 1894, a massive peasant uprising against a corrupt and exploitative government during a time of growing Japanese and western interventions and economic polarizations between wealthy farmers and peasants.

trix of ethical norms and conflicting moral frameworks" that we read in Judith Butler's work were very real in the classroom; they showed up across various standpoints regarding race, gender, sexuality, and citizenship (Butler, 7). Particularly resonant for me was the intersection of race and religion, as reflected by the majority white representation of non-Christian (typically Buddhist) students in the room. This composition raised questions of how to be together and acknowledge differences across multiple markers, without overlaying or misattributing differences solely to one category. The notion of *uncomfortable wholeness* manifested in manifold ways: the discomfort of being together among differences; the discomfort of acknowledging who were absent in the room; the discomfort of disrupting the concept of what "wholeness" means or looks like; the discomfort of the dangers and realities of appropriating other traditions. These discomforts point to the hard work that is required for interreligious engagement, and the need for new sets of norms, intentions, and practices that account for diversity, division, and kinship.

And yet, amidst the challenges, the self-inquiry process ultimately affirmed my formation as a Christian chaplain. The power and value of presence – of showing up – is the core of my chaplaincy work, and this was embodied in the class. Self-inquiry is about presence for one's present being in the world. It offers a space of rest, awareness, care, and healing for deeper self-knowledge and toward "moments of unconditioned love and spacious awareness" (King 2018, 126). Such a state is what frees, motivates, and sustains my self-inquiry practice and my work of spiritual accompaniment with people who are in transition, crisis, or trauma.

Uncomfortable wholeness

Reamogetje Ngoepe (M.Div. '19 Psychology and Religion Concentration)

The self-inquiry class helped me realize that prayer, and specifically praying in tongues, is to what I turn to suspend, to inquire about myself. I find myself praying in tongues, under my breath or somewhere on bended knees when I'm in distress, seeking clarity, questioning, wrestling. This knowing has had a profound impact for me, enabling me to understand the pivotal role of prayer in my personal knowing; I now pray more frequently, more intentionally.

In reflecting on our self-inquiry processes, we were encouraged to reflect across an array of variables to understand the different ways in which our processes are impacted. Starting off with the aim of our self-inquiry processes – mine being to foster relationship through intimacy and accountability with God, myself and others. Societal conditionings also play a pivotal role in inquiry, and for me, race embodied culturally through language was the most impactful; navigating and negotiating feelings of inferiority, traumatization, [and] imposed and appropriated language. So it is necessarily at this social location [that] my self-inquiry process meets me. Further pressing on me was what it means to speak in another language (tongues) that subverts and disrupts when my own language and culture has been colonized.

To interrogate my process further, I will reflect on the following variables: my scene of address, accountability, reliability, confession, and body.

To draw from Judith Butler in *An Account of Oneself*, my scene of address takes two forms: the person being addressed as well as the location of address. My scene of address is God, and the location within which it takes place is wherever I am praying. Throughout this process there is a narration from God, the person exposed to that narration, and a new narration of self I beget from this encounter. It is in this process of narration from God as well as my own thoughts (and those of others if communal prayer) that various forms of reflection and revelation take place. This reflection could be expressed through a poem, fleshing out an idea, receiving an affirming word for someone.

Butler distinguishes between exposure and narrated self – helping us connect more authentically with that which is true about ourselves vs. merely taking in what is said about it. Butler says in terms of language, "the very terms by which we give an account, by which we make ourselves intelligible to ourselves and to others, are not of our making" (Butler, 21). In naming this, she challenges us to find our true voice in a sea of clutter. Resmaa Manekam expands on this to relay how it's even more critical to engage with our narrations of self in relation to trauma that has been passed down; in how we lose the location of trauma, thereby losing ourselves and finding false comfort in telling and believing stories about us that are not (no longer) true about us.

In reflecting on my reliability as an inquirer and what I'm most resistant to, it is letting go of the narrations about generational racial trauma that provide a false sense of comfort vs. a truly healing narrative. I feel like I would be giving up and losing a big part of myself if I lost the narrative that has lost its location.

I reflect on my confession process as one that should enable me to sufficiently explore vulnerable parts of me. I borrow Foucault's notion of gnostic self as a hermeneutic of self – a notion of self that is more curious, open and seeking. A sense of self that is more likely to recover a sense of self after trauma and internalized inferiority. Phillis Sheppard, a black psychoanalyst, mentions how culture is a medium within which our sense of self grows, [and that] if this is compromised it can result in a "compromised developmental trajectory and a failure to develop a healthy and firm sense of self, with an ambivalence, or hostility towards one's own culture, gender, race and sexuality" (Sheppard 2011, 120). For healing to occur within this reality, it would be helpful to have a self able "to discover the truth inside oneself, to decipher the real nature and the authentic origin of soul…." (Foucault 2016, 2–16, 55).

My confession process is also intertwined with the people to whom I am accountable. It is my hope that it also illuminates those things that get in the way, the things that cause me to resist and cloud my reliability as an inquirer. The people who I confess to are God, my analyst, and close friends, community. I have recently started praying with a group of black women on campus and it has been one of the most enriching experiences I have had in Seminary. As we share what's heavy on our hearts, our prayer items, praying for each other, I feel the spirit moving and my sense of knowing and connectedness deepening.

My theory of body remains an area of growth and interrogation for me. I perceive body as experience, having a history. I also perceive the body as having knowledge to navigate its historical conditioning, to know how to move to survive.

Otto Rank, an Austrian psychoanalyst, suggests that the oldest form of speech is akin to prayer, and of speaking in tongues that it is "an actual creation through words of the soul" (Rank 1989, 267). Telia Anderson asserts that "if black women's howling or moaning is a prediscursive linguistic disruption, awaiting entry into proper language, speaking in tongues is one of the most powerful forms of post discursive speech… to disrupt the continuity of known speech and to travel beyond the boundaries that restrict black women's agency" (Anderson 2001, 124). This emergence of subversive and disruptive language evokes healing, and therefore, a new kind of knowing.

While it certainly has its limitations in terms of inclusivity and scope, we consider this course a very practical example of how Buddhist competencies can become both core and transformative within the current seminary context. This was not an easy class. Class meetings were uncomfortable, at times contentious, but overall surprisingly and profoundly healing for many participants as they understood their traditions more deeply and engaged them through emergent methodologies. They were able to come forward in the confusing, profound, and sometimes terrifying complexity of a process that unfolds who we are right in front of us. Students engaged inquiry both personally and collectively with great courage and grace. It was an honor to be a part of this process with them.

Conclusion

In closing, we return to an earlier question: How to create a pedagogy that allows meaningful religious difference to endure while cultivating the possibility for connections to be realized across that difference? The above methods of formation provide guidance here. Both theological reflection and self-inquiry are processes not only of formation but of pedagogy. They are normative as structures, but not overly determinant in terms of content and tradition. Any interreligious pedagogy must allow for deep engagement in the particularity of one's tradition while being vulnerable to the same depth and particularity of the other's traditions. It requires a normative structure that holds differences and allows for multiple religious convictions and expressions to flourish. However broadly conceived and applied it is, we realize that no normative structure can be fully divorced from a tradition. Recognizing this, those engaging interreligiously must enter this formational space with the "practical vulnerability" mentioned above. Counterintuitively, it is precisely the normative structure that allows for the creativity of interreligious wisdom to emerge in its religious specificity.

While the above frame of self-inquiry could be argued to be Buddhist, or dharmic, the space held by the normative structure is open enough to allow for practitioners of other traditions to both recognize themselves and find voice within this structure. Similarly, the frame of theological reflection is primarily Christian, but broad enough for practitioners in other traditions to fully engage the particularities of their own traditions for meaning-making.

Navigating the initial foreignness of these formational processes, one endures the discomfort of a stranger until one's integrity and wisdom emerge. This pedagogical method requires the faculty to engage "practical vulnerability." In fact, this co-authored paper arises out of our interreligious relationship where we live out this vulnerability. This has given birth to an incredibly creative friendship that models this process for our students. Such relationships are the beating heart of interreligious engagement, the reason Buddhism is able to flourish in a historically Protestant seminary and the path leading to a religious life that values wholeness borne of respectful relationship over harmful, exclusionary notions of purity.

References:

Anderson, Telia U. 2001. *African American Performance and Theatre History.* New York, NY: Oxford University Press.

Bolman, Lee, and Terrance Deal. 2017. *Reframing Organization: Artistry, Choice and Leadership.* 6th edition. Hoboken, NJ: John Wiley and Sons.

Bounds, Elizabeth. 2008. "Theological Reflection in Contextual Education: An Elusive Practice." In: Theodore Brelsford, and P. Alice Rogers (eds.) *Contextualizing Theological Education.* Cleveland, OH: The Pilgrim Press.

Butler, Judith. 2009. *Giving an Account of Oneself.* New York, NY: Fordham University Press.

Cadge, Wendy, and Michael Skaggs. 2018. "Chaplaincy? Spiritual Care? Innovation? A Case Statement." *Working Paper, Department of Sociology, Brandeis University.* http://chaplaincyinnovation.org/wp-content/uploads/2018/12/Cadge-Skaggs-2018.pdf

Cameron, Helen, John Reader, Victoria Slater, and Christopher Rowland. 2012. *Theological Reflection for Human Flourishing: Pastoral Practice and Public Theology.* London: SCM Press.

Chaplaincy Innovation Lab: www.chaplaincyinnovation.org.

Douglas, Kelly Brown. 2015. *Stand Your Ground: Black Bodies and the Justice of God.* Maryknoll, NY: Orbis Press.

Dykstra, Craig. 2008. "Pastoral and Ecclesial Imagination." In: Dorothy C. Bass, and Craig Dykstra (eds.) *For Life Abundant: Practical Theology, Theological Education, and Christian Ministry.* Grand Rapids, MI: Eerdmans Publishing Co.

Foley, Edward. 2014. "Reflective Believing: Reimagining Theological Reflection in an Age of Diversity." *Reflective Practice: Formation and Supervision in Ministry* 34: 60–75.

Foley, Edward. 2015. *Theological Reflection across Religious Traditions: The Turn to Reflective Believing.* New York, NY: Rowman & Littlefield Publishers.

Foucault, Michel. 2016. *About the Beginning of the Hermeneutics of the Self.* Chicago, IL: University of Chicago Press.

Glieg, Anne. 2019. *American Dharma.* New Haven, CT: Yale University Press.

Holland, Joe and Peter Henriot, 1983. *Social Analysis: Linking Faith and Justice.* Maryknoll, Orbis Press.

Husserl, Edmund. 2012. *Ideas: General Introduction to Pure Phenomenology.* New York, NY: Routledge.

Killen, Patricia O'Connell, and John De Beer. 1994. *The Art of Theological Reflection.* New York, NY: Crossroad.

Kinast, Robert. 1999. *Making Faith-Sense: Theological Reflection in Everyday Life.* Collegeville, MN: The Liturgical Press.

King, Ruth. 2018. *Mindful of Race: Transforming Racism from the Inside Out.* Boulder, CO: Sounds True.

Merleau-Ponty, Maurice. 1958. *Phenomenology of Perception.* New York, NY: Routledge.

Okumura, Shohaku. 2012. *Living by Vow: A Practical Introduction to Eight Essential Zen Chants and Texts.* Somerville, MA: Wisdom Publications.

Pak, Su Yon. 2020. "Cultivating Moral Imagination in Theological Field Education." In: Kwok Pui-Lan (ed.) *Asian and Asian American Women in Theology and Religion.* Cham, Switzerland: Palgrave Macmillan.

Pak, Su Yon. 2022. "Through a Multi-frame Lens: Surviving, Thriving, and Leading Organizations." In: Wendy Cadge, and Shelly Rambo (eds.) Chaplaincy and Spiritual Care in the Twenty-First Century: An Introduction. Chapel Hill: The University of North Carolina Press.

Pew Research Center. 2015. "America's Changing Religious Landscape." https://www.pewforum.org/2015/05/12/americas-changing-religious-landscape/

Rajkumar, Peniel Jesudason Rufus, and Joseph Prabhakar Dayam (eds.). 2016. *Many Yet One? Multiple Religious Belonging.* Geneva, Switzerland: World Council of Churches.

Rank, Otto 1989. *Art and Artist: Creative Urge and Personality Development.* New York, NY: W.W. Norton and Company.

Rieger, Joerg, and Kwok Pui-lan. 2012. *Occupy Religion: Theology of the Multitudes.* New York, NY: Rowman and Littlefield Publishers.

Sheppard, Isabella P. 2011. *Self, Culture, and Others in Womanist Practical Theology.* New York, NY: Palgrave Macmillan.

Sujato, Bhikkhu, 2018. "Aggaññasutta." https://suttacentral.net/dn27/en/sujato

Sullivan, Winnifred Fallers. 2014. *Ministry of Presence: Chaplaincy, Spiritual Care, and the Law.* Chicago: University of Chicago Press.

Thatamanil, John. 2016. "Transreligious Theology as the Quest for Interreligious Wisdom." *Open Theology* 2: 354–362.

Thompson, Marjorie J. 2014. *Soul Feast: An Invitation to the Christian Spiritual Life.* Louisville, KY: Westminster John Knox Press.

Tran, Mai-Anh Le. 2017. *Reset the Heart: Unlearning Violence, Relearning Hope.* Nashville, TN: Abingdon Press.

Waddell, Norman, and Masao Abe. 2002. *The Heart of Dogen's Shobogenzo.* Albany, NY: SUNY Press.

List of Contributors

Naveed Baig

Naveed Baig is currently a PhD fellow at the Faculty of Theology, University of Oslo. He has served several years as a hospital chaplain at Rigshospitalet in Copenhagen, and has published on Islamic spiritual care, Islamic theology and Christian-Muslim dialogue in Denmark and beyond. Baig is presently conducting empirical research on Muslim patients' hospitalization with COVID-19 and how they perceive their sickness and tribulations. He teaches Islamic spiritual care at the University of Oslo.

Beret Bråten

Beret Bråten holds a master in sociology and a PhD in political science from the University of Oslo. She is associate professor at the Centre for Gender Research at the University of Oslo and researcher at Fafo – a social science research foundation. She did a postdoctoral project at the Health Services Research Unit (HØKH), Akershus University Hospital, Norway on palliative care in a multicultural society. Hospital chaplaincy services were part of the postdoctoral project. Bråtens research is focused on diversity, inclusion/exclusion and gender equality.

Pieter Coppens

Pieter Coppens is Assistant Professor at the Faculty of Religion and Theology, Vrije Universiteit Amsterdam. He lectures in the Islam-track of the Spiritual Care Master. His research focuses on the history of Qur'an interpretation and the history of Sufism. His current research project is on the origins, growth and dissemination of Salafi Qur'an interpretation since the 19th century.

Anne Hege Grung

Anne Hege Grung is Professor in Interreligious Studies at the Faculty of Theology, University of Oslo.

She holds a PhD in interreligious studies. In 2019 she was pivotal in establishing the master program "Leadership, ethics and counselling" at the University of Oslo, which provides training in chaplaincy and spiritual and existential care for a religiously diverse student group. She was the chair of the European Society for Intercultural Theology and Interreligious Studies (ESITIS) 2017–2022 and is presently member of the Steering Committee for the unit Interfaith and Interreligious Studies in the American Academy of Religion.

Nazila Isgandarova

Nazila Isgandarova is Assistant Professor at Emmanuel College of Victoria University in the University of Toronto. She has a Ph.D. from the University of Toronto, a Doctor of Ministry degree in pastoral counselling, marriage and family studies from Wilfred Laurier University, and a Master of Social Work from the University of Windsor. She is a Registered Psychotherapist at the College for Registered Psychotherapists of Ontario and a Registered Social Worker at the Ontario Social Workers and Social Service Workers. Isgandarova is the recipient of the prestigious Forum for Theological Exploration research award for her study on domestic violence against Muslim women, the Canadian Association for Spiritual Care Senior Research Award and the Society for Pastoral Counselling Research Award. Her book, titled *Muslim*

 https://doi.org/10.1515/9783110717365-011

Women, Domestic Violence, and Psychotherapy: Theological and Clinical Issues, was published by Routledge in 2018 and *Islamic Spiritual Care; Theory and Practice(s)* by Pandora Press in 2019.

Bikram Lalbahadoersing
Bikram Lalbahadoersing studied Psychology, Philosophy, and Sanskrit at the University of Groningen. For over 15 years he was chief editor of the radio programs of the Dutch national broadcasting organisation. Since 2010 he is head of Hindu chaplaincy at the Department of Justice.

Stef Lauwers
Stef Lauwers obtained a Ma in Religion and a Special Degree in Social and Cultural Antropology at Leuven, postmasters in Chaplaincy at Tilburg and Mindfulness at Nijmegen. He is also a qualified supervisor. He worked as a chaplain in healthcare and as a Buddhist chaplain in several Dutch prisons. For five years, untill August 2019, he was coordinator and lecturer of the postmaster program Buddhist Spiritual Care at Vrije Universiteit Amsterdam.

Anke I. Liefbroer
Anke I. Liefbroer is Associate Professor in Psychology of Religion and Spiritual Care at Tilburg School of Catholic Theology, Tilburg University. She obtained her PhD on 'Interfaith Spiritual Care' at the Faculty of Religion and Theology of the Vrije Universiteit Amsterdam. Before starting her PhD research, Anke I. Liefbroer obtained a MSc in Clinical Psychology at the University of Groningen and a MA in Religious Studies at the University of Amsterdam. She currently conducts research in spiritual care in palliative care.

Cecilia Melder
Cecilia Melder is Assistant Professor in Psychology of Religion at University College Stockholm. Her research focuses on Existential Public Health. She has a T.D. in Psychology of Religion at Uppsala University, Sweden. Her dissertation title is "Vilsenhetens epidemiologi -en religionspsykologisk studie i existentiell folkhälsa" ["The epidemiology of lost meaning – A study in Psychology of Religion and Existential Public Health in a Swedish context"]. Melder has specialist knowledge of existential health intervention and has created a method for intervention to support existential health and Health-related Quality of Life in general. She is now studying this intervention in different clinical settings. Melder is also a priest in the Church of Sweden since 1992.

Su Yon Pak
Su Yon Pak is Vice President for Academic Affairs and Dean, Union Theological Seminary in the City of New York. Dr. Su Yon Pak holds an Ed.D from the joint program of Teachers College Columbia University and Union Theological Seminary. She has revitalized the curricular and co-curricular work of field education. She was pivotal in creating the new chaplaincy concentration at Union and is the senior advisor to the Chaplaincy Innovation Lab. Her latest publication is a co-authored and co-edited volume, *Sister in Mourning: Daughters Reflection on Care, Loss, and Meaning* (Cascade, 2021). Her research interests include: aging and spirituality, Asian/Asian American women and leadership, integrative education pedagogies, interreligious chaplaincy education, and poetry as theological reflection.

Carola Roloff

Carola Roloff is Permanent Visiting Professor for Buddhism at the Academy of World Religions, University of Hamburg.

She holds a Ph.D. in Philosophy focusing on Tibetan and Buddhist Studies. From 2013 to 2018, she was part of the European Research project "Religion and Dialogue in Modern Societies." Since 2020, she has taught Buddhist Care Practices at the University of Oslo. Current focal points include Dialogic theology and practice, intra-Buddhist dialogue, and impulses and processes of recognition of Buddhist minorities in Europe.

Jussra Schröer

Jussra Schröer is Research Fellow at the Centre for Islamic Theology at the University of Tübingen in Germany. She studied at Jordan University in Amman and at the Catholic University of Applied Sciences in Cologne and has a PhD in the sociology of religion from the University of Cologne.

Since 2020, she has directed the master's programme "Islamic Practical Theology for Spiritual Care and Social Work". Her research fields include the significance of practice research and professionalism for Islamic Practical Theology for Chaplaincy and Social Work in Germany. Other research issues include gender and religion (the role of Muslim women theologians in the development of mosque communities in Germany).

Kosen Gregory Snyder

Kosen Gregory Snyder is Senior Director and Assistant Professor of Buddhist Studies at Union Theological Seminary in the City of New York.

He is an ordained priest and dharma-transmitted teacher in the Soto Zen Buddhist tradition. In 2016, Snyder was the founding director of the Master of Divinity program in Buddhism and Interreligious Engagement at Union Theological Seminary where he later founded the Thích Nhất Hạnh Program for Engaged Buddhism. He co-founded and is currently the senior resident priest at the Brooklyn Zen Center in Brooklyn, NY, as well as Ancestral Heart Zen Temple, a residential training center in Millerton, NY.

Gé Speelman

Gé Speelman was until 2021 Assistant Professor at the Protestant Theological University in Amsterdam, now retired. She taught religious studies and intercultural theology at the PThU, and her research is mainly in the field of Christian-Muslim encounters. Speelman has published on interreligious hermeneutics, dialogue of women and religiously mixed marriages. She is presently in the board of the European Society for Intercultural Theology and Interreligious Studies (ESITIS).

Index

 https://doi.org/10.1515/9783110717365-012